TPH

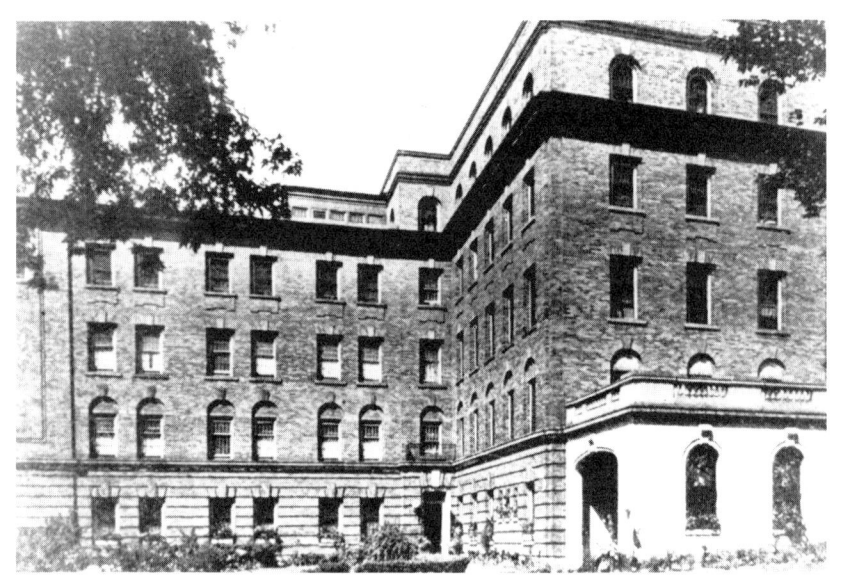

Toronto Psychiatric Hospital
QSMHC ARCHIVES ON THE HISTORY OF PSYCHIATRY

To support the publication of this volume, funds have been contributed in memory of Mary V. Jackson, MD, and Susan Strathy Wilson, Dip.O.T.

TPH

History and Memories of the Toronto Psychiatric Hospital, 1925-1966

Edited by
Edward Shorter
Hannah Chair in the History of Medicine
Faculty of Medicine
University of Toronto

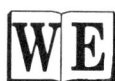

Wall & Emerson, Inc.
Toronto, Ontario • Dayton, Ohio

Copyright © 1996 by Edward Shorter

All rights reserved. No part of this publication may be reproduced or transmitted in any form or by any means, electronic or mechanical, including photography, recording, or any information storage and retrieval system, without permission in writing from the publisher.

Orders for this book and requests for permission to make copies of any part of this work should be sent to: Wall & Emerson, Inc., Six O'Connor Drive, Toronto, Ontario M4K 2K1 Canada. Phone: (416) 467-8685; Fax: (416) 696-2460; E-mail: wall@tor.hookup.net.

Canadian Cataloguing in Publication Data

Main entry under title:

TPH : history and memories of the Toronto Psychiatric Hospital, 1925-1966

Includes bibliographis references and index.
ISBN 0-921332-45-9

1. Toronto Psychiatric Hospital - History.
I. Shorter, Edward.

RC448.063T67 1996   362.2'1'0971354109   C96-930134-0

Printed in Canada.

1 2 3 4 5 6   04 03 02 01 00 99 98 97+96 95

Table of Contents

List of Photographs vii

Preface viii
    Edward Shorter

1. The Recent Revolution in the History of
   Psychiatry 1
       Edward Shorter

2. Origins of the Toronto Psychiatric Hospital .. 19
       Cyril Greenland

3. C. B. Farrar: A Life 59
       Edward Shorter

4. The Life of the Toronto Psychiatric Hospital . 97
       Roger Baskett

5. Farrar and the American Journal of
   Psychiatry 155
       Peter Faux

6. Recollections of a Patient at TPH: Snakepit . 171
       Peter Keefe

7. Experiences of a Student Intern at TPH 183
       W. Clifford M. Scott

8. Memories of a Nurse 187
       Claire A. (MacKid) Muller

9. Nursing 193
       Margaret L. Gorrie

10. Psychology 218
    Hugh McLeod and Andrew Boyd

11. Social Work 239
    Mora Skelton

12. Occupational Therapy 259
    Judith Friedland

13. The Outpatient Department 271
    Donald Coates

14. The Children's Service 292
    Edward J. Rosen

15. The Mental Retardation Clinic 296
    Mora Skelton

16. The Forensic Clinic 304
    R.E. Turner and Erika Steffer

17. Farewell to TPH 316
    Charles Roberts

Index 321

List of Photographs

Toronto Psychiatric Hospital .... Cover and ii

C.B. Farrar's childhood home 60

Clarence B. Farrar as a boy 61

Farrar at Kraepelin's clinic in Heidelberg 64

Keys to the wards of the Heidelberg psychiatric clinic 65

Members of Kraepelin's clinic in Heidelberg 66

In Nissl's laboratory at Heidelberg 67

Farrar at Trenton State Hospital 73

Farrar as a family man 77

Farrar on a Toronto street 81

C.B. Farrar and Duncan Graham 121

Aldwyn B. Stokes 123

John Dewan 128

Mary Victoria Jackson 283

Canadian psychiatrists with Judy LaMarsh 289

Kenneth G. Gray 305

Charles A. Roberts 317

Preface

Edward Shorter

Little is known of the history of psychiatry in the first half of the twentieth century. While we are well informed about such distant matters as the origins of the asylum in the nineteenth century or the early days of Freud's psychoanalysis, more recent periods are largely a blank. How widely applied were the new physical therapies of the 1930s, such as lobotomy and electroshock? When did psychiatry begin to reach out to the other mental-health professions? How was psychiatry itself transformed by such societal forces as the increasing emphasis upon individual rights? Such larger questions have not been satisfactorily addressed because we simply do not know enough about individual doctors and patients acting in concrete settings. A few pages of textbook information are no substitute for precious knowledge about what real people were actually doing and experiencing.

The Toronto Psychiatric Hospital, known as TPH, was a mirror of these larger trends. It came into existence at a time when psychiatry was scarcely differentiated from neurology, when society's interest in psychiatry revolved around the criminally insane, the retarded, and the removal of acutely ill patients from the streets. TPH closed its doors at a time when the the adjective "psychiatric" had been extended to a much wider range of personal malaise than in 1925, when new biological doctrines were moving the discipline of psychiatry much closer to medicine, and when concerns about patients' welfare and rights had achieved equal weight with society's desire for order. TPH, located at 2 Surrey Place in the city's downtown, was founded in 1925 and closed in 1966 with the establishment of the Clarke Institute of Psychiatry. TPH's first director was Clarence B. Farrar, a psychiatrist trained at Johns Hopkins University and a well-known psychiatric editor. Farrar was succeeded in 1947 by the distinguished English clinician Aldwyn Stokes. John Dewan was director from 1960 to 1964. TPH's last director, Charles Roberts, closed the hospital two years later. These men are all interesting and even riveting figures. Yet the emphasis of the book is not on them and their works. It is rather on what the hospital did, its life, and on the conflicts that swirled about it.

In Canada, the first half of the twentieth century saw a tug-of-war between European and American influences. Was the nation's scientific culture primarily an offshoot of Britain and the continent, or of America? This tug-of-war also surged back and forth in the corridors of TPH, a hospital founded by people who had been profoundly influenced by German examples, yet whose first director was an American. While the giants of English and continental psychiatry towered over TPH before the Second World War, in the postwar years it was clearly the great American scientific train that pulled TPH and the rest of Canadian psychiatry.

The present volume attempts to analyze these developments rather than to memorialize them. TPH shared much that was positive and forward-looking (and some that was awful and misguided) of the psychiatric doctrines of its day. Its medical staff tried to give care of a high scientific standard, while at the same time coping with meddling bureaucrats, penuriously distributed funds, and a chronic inadequacy of space and beds. Moreover, the doctors' perceptions of what they were about often differed sharply from those of their patients.

There are also many non-psychiatric stories in this book. Psychiatrists at TPH worked alongside—first as bosses, then as colleagues—many other health-care professionals. Thus the occupational therapists, psychologists, social workers, nurses, and other specialists also have their chapters, and the stories they tell are full of insight into professional worlds of which outsiders have little inkling. In giving readers an inside view of a psychiatric hospital from these many viewpoints, the present volume breaks new ground. The typical can be astonishing.

But even though TPH is a typical story, it is a story that matters. TPH is important in the history of Canadian psychiatry because it trained several key generations of psychiatrists who would carry to other centers the science they had learned at TPH. It is important in the history of Canadian psychiatric *care* because it pioneered the participation of the other health-care professions.

The archives of TPH have largely disappeared. Although the records of individual patients have been preserved, the administrative correspondence on which the history of such a hospital would normally be based has vanished. In telling the story of TPH we therefore have chosen a two-pronged strategy: a group of historians, working with published sources and manuscript materials in other archives, recount the main lines of the narrative. A number of individuals who themselves experienced life at TPH also give their accounts, bringing something of the history of their various disciplines together with their own recollections. Hence, it is a volume of history and memories.

This volume would never have seen the light of day without the persistence and insight of Cyril Greenland, who as part-time Director of Social Work at TPH from 1960 to 1966, recognized the importance of the story. Researching the story would not have been possible without the generous financial support of the Clarke Institute of Psychiatry and its president and psychiatrist-in-chief, Paul Garfinkel. We also gratefully acknowledge grants from the Laidlaw and the Jackman foundations. Joan Farrar, the widow of Clarence B. Farrar (TPH's first director), kindly granted access to her husband's private papers. Jack Griffin and Michael Bliss were generous enough with their time to comment on various chapters. Indispensable in finding materials were Shannon Davy and Lisa Thompson. The administrator of the History of Medicine Program, Andrea Clark, has been a font of energy and goodwill in typing manuscripts and coordinating phone calls. Susan Bélanger compiled the index. I should like to acknowledge the editorial skill and sensitivity to language of Erika Steffer, who, functioning as a kind of subeditor, set about reducing the cacophony of many voices while according individual contributors their own distinctive styles.

Finally, the publication of this book would not have been possible at all without a publication subsidy generously contributed by friends of the history of psychiatry.

1

The Recent Revolution in the History of Psychiatry

Edward Shorter[*]

The quickening of interest in the history of psychiatry in the last two decades has been truly extraordinary. Consider how the pace has leapt in the last few years. In 1990, a major new journal, *History of Psychiatry*, was established, published by the Royal College of Psychiatry in England. Several other major journals, such as *Social History of Medicine* and *Psychological Medicine*, regularly have contributions on the history of psychiatry, and there has been a virtual outpouring of books on psychiatry's past, ranging across institutions, famous physicians, and the history of various psychiatric diseases. Berrios and Tischler write, "scholarship on the history and philosophy of psychiatry...has reached new heights. This not only shows in the number of publications but also in their quality which compares well with that achieved in other fields of psychiatric research."[1]

As for non-psychiatrists, an index of the new popularity of the history of psychiatry is its detachment from the traditional history of medicine. On university campuses the history of psychiatry is being incorporated into undergraduate teaching, not in faculties of medicine, but in courses on the social history of medicine in faculties of arts and sciences. For undergraduates it is not so important to integrate changes in psychiatry within medicine as a whole, but rather within society as a whole. The history of psychiatry for many humanists and social scientists is not so much part of the history of medicine as it is a way of charting the social and emotional misadventures the modern population has endured at the

---
[*]Edward Shorter received his Ph.D. in History from Harvard in 1968. Since 1967, he has taught history at the University of Toronto, where he is now Hannah Chair in the History of Medicine. Among his more recent books are, *From Paralysis to Fatigue: A History of Psychosomatic Illness in the Modern Era*, published by the Free Press in 1992, and *A Century of Radiology in Toronto*, published by Wall & Emerson in 1995.

hands of the professions and of the state. (This, I must say, is not my own view, but it fairly characterizes the history of psychiatry at most arts faculties.)

What accounts for this remarkable surge of interest? Is it part and parcel of a rising trend of interest in the history of medicine in general? Not really, for interest in the history of other medical specialties, such as surgery or dermatology, has not accelerated.

Is it the result of the public's growing interest in mental health, the result perhaps of an increased tendency to accept mental illness as on par with all other medical illnesses? Not at all. The stigmatization of psychiatric illness on the part of the general public is only somewhat less than a hundred years ago. Witness the efforts of patients with the "disease-of-the-month syndrome" (and here I mean such diagnoses as Chronic Fatigue Syndrome and Multiple Chemical Sensitivities) to give themselves organic-sounding diagnoses and resolutely to avoid anything that smacks of psychiatric illness.[2]

This resurgence in psychiatric history is more complicated, involving the interaction between changes within psychiatry itself and changes in the wider world. In order to understand this burgeoning interest in the history of psychiatry we must deal both with psychiatrists themselves and the world they inhabit.

Think for a moment about how psychiatry itself has changed. For anyone trained in psychiatry in the 1950s or 1960s, the current psychiatric landscape offers a vision as different as the dark side of the moon is from the light. A number of what were considered in the 1950s and 1960s to be age-old verities have now crumbled.

In the 1950s, one of the great verities was the relative uselessness of medication in major psychiatric illness. It is true that before 1952, no drugs were effective in the treatment of schizophrenia, and nothing except opium offered relief in the treatment of major depression. The sedatives and hypnotics then on the market palliated the symptoms in some of the psychoneuroses, and therewith the list of effective medications was at an end. The introduction of chlorpromazine in 1952 began an epoch as new and momentous for psychiatry as the epoch in medicine commencing in 1935 with the first sulfa drugs.

For years after the arrival of chlorpromazine, mainline psychiatry (still heavily under the influence of the psychoanalyst) struggled against the neuroleptics. Tales are legion of the lack of interest encountered by pharmaceutical company Smith Kline and French (as it was then called) in the mid-1950s when it introduced chlorpromazine among leaders of the psychiatric profession in the United States. Only much later did the demonstrated efficacy of the new neuroleptics, anti-depressants, and mood stabilizers sweep away resistance and "biological psychiatry" began a new era.

Another of the great verities of the 1950s and 1960s was the uselessness (indeed the abusive nature) of electroconvulsive therapy (ECT). It was in the 1960s that ECT went into what seemed a terminal decline, vilified by both academic critics and by the anti-psychiatry movement of those years.[3] ECT then experienced a comeback in the 1980s and is now the therapy of choice for major depression.

A third eternal verity from the 1950s and 1960s was the election of psychoanalysis as the therapy of choice among the psychotherapies. So complete was the identification among psychiatry, psychoanalysis, and psychotherapy that the general public today still believes a psychiatrist is a psychoanalyst. I hope this observation will not be construed as a value judgment on my part, but I think it is fair to say that in the 1970s and 1980s psychoanalysis has, rightly or wrongly, been dethroned from its kingship of the psychotherapies, turning into *uno inter pares,* one among equals. To note this encapsulization and marginalization of psychoanalysis from mainline psychiatry is not to comment on its intellectual validity. Yet, the fact remains that psychiatry in the last twenty years has evolved along biological lines. This evolution has anachronized the methods of someone like Frieda Fromm-Reichmann, the noted German analyst of the Chestnut Lodge Clinic, who attempted to alleviate schizophrenia through psychoanalysis.[4]

Thus, the psychiatry of the 1990s is a vastly different enterprise from that of the 1960s. It is a psychiatry firmly ensconced in the saddle of the neurosciences, much closer to the mainstream of medicine than ever before. It is, as well, a psychiatry with a higher self-image, confident in its ability to alleviate psychotic illness with medications whose mechanisms are becoming known.

In the history of psychiatry as well, the 1960s contained certain supposedly eternal verities. One verity was seeing the history of psychiatry in the context of the class struggle. Applying the Marxism of the "new left" (then so much in vogue), many historians tried to fit the history of psychiatry into the larger combat of bourgeoisie and proletariat, the class struggle. (The very words now bring a smile to the lips.) In this fight to the finish, psychiatrists were seen as being on the side of the bourgeoisie, and the object of the history of psychiatry was to unmask and discredit the discipline as a tool in class warfare. Klaus Dörner, author of *Madmen and the Bourgeoisie* (first published in German in 1969), rumbles the doctors' plot against the proletariat already in the eighteenth century.[5] This dogmatic view of psychiatry as an agency in the class struggle would be overturned and left behind in the 1970s and 1980s as many new historiographical currents swept aside the angry young men and women with their set agendas.

A second familiar verity to historians of psychiatry in the 1950s and 1960s was the history of psychiatry basically as a history of psychoanalysis. The story's ending, for these historians, was the triumph of Freud's doctrines in the university clinics of the 1940s and 1950s. This was true teleological history, history progressing inevitably to a fitting end-place. And older histories of psychiatry possess this strong odour of teleology, as the supposedly misguided doctrines of Theodor Meynert and his ilk gave way unstoppably to the wisdom of Freud. For Berlin-trained analyst Gregory Zilboorg, who practiced in New York and wrote the *History of Medical Psychology*, a standard older text, the story is over once we reach Freud, "the Second Psychiatric Revolution," as Zilboorg calls it.[6] Ilza Veith, whose history of hysteria was once a standard work, could scarcely wait in her tale until the dawn of psychoanalysis. She became impatient with Freud's precursors and berated them for not seeing the light.[7] Pouring the history of psychiatry into the history of psychoanalysis imposed a singularly limiting straitjacket, one even more confining than the class struggle. Marxist writers, at least, attempted to draw interesting links between medical ideas and larger social structures, whereas the prism of psychoanalysis focused all light upon the interior: upon the internal evolution of psychoanalytic ideas. Reuben Fine's *History of Psychoanalysis* is a perfect illustration;[8] not one word is said about the position of women in Vienna at the turn of the century.

A third eternal verity in the history of psychiatry in the 1960s insisted that the state used psychiatry as an agency of social control: psychiatrists were not just pawns of the bourgeoisie, in other words, but also of the state-builders. This approach did possess a Marxist flavour, but it was principally from the pen of Michel Foucault, whose book *Madness and Civilization* (published in French in 1961) imputed to psychiatry this sinister cultural and political cast. Psychiatrists, hand in hand with the state, emerged in Foucault's work not so much as agents of class oppression as of cultural oppression. Foucault's psychiatrists took innocuous variations in behavior along the band of normal and redefined them as pathological, locking up those whose lifestyles challenged the mores of middle-class civility. Foucault, in particular, called attention to the "great confinement," a bestial lockup of the poor and undesirable, culminating in the work of William Tuke in England and Philippe Pinel in France. In this great lockup, said Foucault, modern psychiatry experienced its birth pangs.[9]

The most articulate proponent of the historical view of psychiatry as unfair confinement has been the University of California sociologist Andrew Scull, who, to his credit, has become a subtler and more elegant thinker as he has continued to research over the years. Scull's *Museums of Madness*, a history of nineteenth-century asylums in England, published in 1979, created something of a sensation among scholars. Scull portrayed the evil English asylum reaching out its tentacles to draw in patients who were not really ill at all, but either poor, dangerous, or deviant.[10] Of course, these were seeds that fell upon the fertile ground of angry young historians of the 1960s and 1970s, but, by the early 1990s, Scull had distanced himself from Foucault. And, with the range and depth of his knowledge, Scull has, in fact, established himself as one of the leading Anglo-American historians of psychiatry.[11]

The point is that this thesis of a "grand confinement" had an enormous impact upon the history of psychiatry. Twenty years ago it was really not on, not *bon ton*, to see psychiatry's past as anything else than yet another chapter in the history of oppression. Since then, Foucault has come under withering fire, and the tyranny of this fantastical thesis of the "great confinement" has been broken.[12] Therewith, the last of the three great verities of the sixties has lost its hold.

The parallel between the evolution of psychiatry itself and the history of psychiatry is an interesting one. After the 1960s, not only did psychiatry itself become freed of an explanatory paradigm that seemed more like philosophy than science, the history of psychiatry as well became liberated from various intellectual straitjackets that had stifled the life from the subject.

Are these twin acts of liberation related? Do they help us account for the recent burgeoning of the history of psychiatry? In part I think, yes. The new therapeutic self-confidence of psychiatry has deepened the curiosity of many psychiatrists themselves about the history of their field. It has given them a more positive appreciation of the intrinsic dignity of psychiatry, an understanding that psychiatry is a healing art with a mission to relieve suffering rather than a branch of the local police force. I would argue that reinforcing this awareness of the profession's essential dignity requires some historical understanding of one's roots. The history of psychiatry allows practitioners to embrace praiseworthy sources of continuity and to cut off dead branches that have failed to flourish. Thus, if we ask what causes the burgeoning interest in the history of psychiatry among psychiatrists themselves, it is the therapeutic confidence accompanying the new biological psychiatry. This self-confidence has provoked a re-examination of what has proven vital or superfluous in the discipline's evolution.

But what about humanists and social scientists? These are writers who little appreciate (and are indeed often suspicious of) the new therapeutic benefits the discipline has to offer. Why the quickening of interest among them? Here we must look to causes outside the evolution of psychiatry itself. One of the great intellectual agendas of modern times has been linking changes in "mentalities" (how cultures work and how individuals subjectively assess their fates) to "structural" changes. By structural, I mean the basic structures of society such as how people make their living, whether they live in cities or the countryside, and how easily they can communicate. If, for example, people turn to fascistic doctrines (as they did in the 1920s), that would be an example of change in mentalities. The social historian's first impulse in explaining fascism would be to look at changing social structures, to see what was happening to the lower middle class, to traditional life in the village, and so forth.

Until recently, Marxist models offered the most promising means of explaining changes in the superstructure of thought and action in terms of changes in the underlying substructure of society. Then, in the 1970s and 1980s, these Marxist models started to become discredited among intellectuals, shortly before their actual collapse in Eastern Europe. A whole generation of social historians who treasured the agenda of understanding changes in mentalities in terms of changes in structures, was cast more or less adrift. They began to search for other kinds of evidence, other explanations.

One can imagine that 30 years ago someone like Roy Porter (to name a brilliant English social historian of medicine of today) would have ended up writing about "the making of the English working class" (the title of the classic study on that subject in 1964 by Edward Thompson, a distinguished and now deceased English social historian).[13] One can also imagine that Thompson himself, had he been born 30 years later, might have ended up writing about the subjective experience of mental illness in eighteenth-century England (Porter's current subject). So I think that discrediting Marxism freed up intellectual energies to search elsewhere for data and for arguments.

If Marxism and the class struggle have ceased to serve, where do we search now for arguments and explanations? The agenda remains the same: understanding the intimate lives of people in the past in terms of the world they inhabited. However, historians today are no longer interested in whether people joined labour unions or how they felt about the class struggle; now researchers want to know how people felt about their bodies, their body images, their perceptions of illness and wellness, their attitudes towards disorders of the mind-body relationship and disorders of the mind, and whether women encountered these themes differently than men.

This new agenda seeks out in first line the enormous and largely untapped medical literature of the past. Social historians of medicine are not principally interested in the classic agenda of medical history: the study of great doctors and their triumphs, in combination with, it must be said, a rather plodding kind of institutional history that described the evolution of this health-benefits plan or that dermatology clinic. The classical history of medicine had little sense of outside forces impinging upon the autonomous "internal" development of science and medical organization.

The new agenda is quite different. A major item on it is identifying the causes of the growing "medicalization" of society, of people's growing psychological dependency upon medical care in situations where they previously had sought non-medical kinds of relief or coped autonomously without intervention. (One considers the work of Claudia Huerkamp on the rise of doctors in the nineteenth century or of Reinhard Spree on the growing dependency of the German population upon health care systems.[14]) Other historians have become fascinated by individuals' subjective appreciation of their bodies or the objective social representation of the body. Historians with these concerns attempt, for example, to link changing patterns of anorexia nervosa to changing modes of bodily image.[15] Still other researchers are interested in the relationship between social prejudice and medicine. Medicine has a long history of providing apparent "scientific" confirmation of ideological prejudice, bolstering, for example, nineteenth-century medical notions about women and Jews as being somehow biologically inferior.[16]

Such examples of apparently scientific ideas serving to perpetuate prejudice and discrimination have been present in psychiatry over the years. This is seen notably in women's encounter with psychiatry in the last century, for example in admissions to asylums for such problematic indications as "hysteria," or in gynecological surgery for mental illnesses attributed to the "reflex action" of the uterus and ovaries.[17] Elaine Showalter has argued that nineteenth-century hysteria represented merely a form of "proto-feminism" among women, a first forecasting of implicit revolt that would later become manifest in the political realm.[18]

It would be fair to say that none of these scholars has been primarily concerned with the classic agenda of the history of medicine, the "internalist" chronicling of the evolution of therapies and institutions (important though these matters are in laying a basis in fact for later speculation). Most of the new social historians of medicine are "externalists," trying to plumb medical sources for evidence that will confirm or deny the validity of larger theories that the historians themselves wish to investigate (e.g., feminism, how the growth of the professions changes society, or how change in family life produces change in bodily image and in sensitivity to bodily sensations). To answer these questions, historians must consult medical sources and understand something of medicine, biology, and disease as well.

Here, the history of psychiatry comes into its own, as opposed to the history of dermatology or of nephrology. Unlike other kinds of illnesses, psychiatric illness is directly influenced, or shaped, by the surrounding culture. Although certain characteristics of major psychiatric diseases remain the same across a wide variety of cultures and periods, other psychiatric symptoms and syndromes are heavily culture-specific, or gender-specific, or class-specific. One thinks, for example, of anorexia nervosa as being culture-specific, of classic "conversion" hysteria as gender-specific on the female side, and of sociopathy as gender-specific on the male side. The valetudinarian woman of the nineteenth century, abed for years or decades, was both gender- and class-specific. Most organic diseases, such as nephritis, polio, and pneumonia, possess none of these specificities.

But culture shapes psychiatrists, as well as their patients. Psychiatric theories are subject to the influence of fashion in a way that theories about pathological anatomy are not. Once the mechanism of pneumonia or nephritis became clear, these maladies ceased to be buffeted by trendy speculations about etiology. Not so in psychiatry, where the mechanisms of very few illnesses (outside of the organic brain syndromes) are clear. Psychiatric theories about causation may fluctuate wildly, the "schizophrenogenic mother" being in fashion one year, build-ups of aluminum in the brain the next year. Therefore, the interaction between psychiatric theory and society becomes a fascinating object of study. Did nineteenth-century psychiatrists such as Paul Julius Möbius incriminate women for "physiological weak-mindedness" as a result of bad science or as a result of male prejudice against the female gender?[19] One can see that post-Marxist historians with this new interest in medical data would turn electively to psychiatry rather than to dermatology.

In this explosion of interest in the history of psychiatry, among psychiatrists and historians alike, certain subjects have achieved pride of place. It is worth briefly reviewing these exciting new themes: (1) the history of psychiatric illness as such, (2) the internal evolution of psychiatry, and (3) the relationship between psychiatry and society.

Major interest has been shown in the evolution of psychotic and psychoneurotic illness. Several of the major mental illnesses have now found their historians. Stanley Jackson has written of the history of depression and of psychiatric views of it.[20] Markus Schär has situated the occurrence of manic-depressive illness in three centuries of Swiss life.[21] Fuller Torrey has speculated about the "modernity" of schizophrenia.[22] And, in a series of important articles, German Berrios, co-editor of the new journal *History of Psychiatry*, has attempted to come to grips with theoretical issues in delimiting given psychiatric diseases and syndromes.[23]

A capital issue in disease biography is the increase in the number of admissions to mental hospitals in the nineteenth century. This increase has given rise to debate between sociologist Andrew Scull and psychiatrist Edward Hare. Scull argues that mental hospitals reached out to successively less ill groups in the population (the poor, the criminal, and the deviant) in order to increase admissions and hence the power of the profession. Hare and others have attributed this growth in asylum populations to real increases in the incidence of schizophrenia, alcoholism, and neurosyphilis.[24] The outcome of this debate will determine one of the central questions in the history of psychiatry: was the rise of the discipline a response to a genuine growth in demand, or did an increased supply of influence-hungry psychiatrists generate more demand for their services, via their power to pathologize and confine?

As for the psychoneuroses, disease biographies have been legion. Some studies have shot off useful flares for clinicians today. For example, Harold Merskey has thrown cold water on the whole notion of "multiple personality disorder." Merskey went back to famous individual cases in the literature and identified most of them as artifacts of medical suggestion.[25] I myself have cautioned against treating such trendy diagnoses as "twentieth century disease" or "Chronic Fatigue Syndrome" as distinct diseases, but rather as partial aspects of the larger phenomenon of somatization.[26]

A second principal area of inquiry has been the internal evolution of psychiatry itself, the profession's organization and its elective historical venue of activity: the asylum. Gerald Grob has described psychiatry's rising distinctiveness as a discipline in the United States[27] and a three-volume work edited by William F. Bynum, Roy Porter, and Michael Shepherd provides coverage for Great Britain.[28] An overview of the history of psychiatry in Canada remains unwritten.

In tracing the history of the asylum the new social history of psychiatry has been most energetic. Far from the self-congratulatory chronicles of yesteryear, scholars writing histories of institutions today tend to be critical of care (often too critical, the authors having little sense of the real challenges in the management of psychotic illness). Historians now study the patients as well as the doctors, paying close attention to social background and diagnosis. This body of literature is enormous. I cannot pretend even to list all of the significant contributions. In terms of chronicling the private asylum in England, William Parry-Jones' pathbreaking monograph *The Trade in Lunacy* might be mentioned.[29] For Canada, we have Cheryl Krasnick Warsh's history of the Homewood Retreat in Guelph, Ontario, at the turn of the century.[30] In the history of the public asylum, Nancy Tomes' study of the Pennsylvania Hospital in Philadelphia is a model.[31] Anne Digby has given us a splendid study of the York Retreat[32] and S.E.D. Shortt has written a study of the asylum in London, Ontario, during the nineteenth century.[33]

If, on the plus side, these studies are hallmarked by their archival relentlessness and attentiveness to context, on the minus side they are marred by their relative lack of interest in psychopathology and in psychiatric diagnosis. Much of this literature fails to get beneath vague allusions to "lunacy," "madness," and "insanity." The causes of a disease such as neurosyphilis are vastly different from those of alcoholic psychosis; the presentations of mania and of de Clérambault's syndrome (also called erotomania) are quite distinct. Although the natural histories of these disorders diverge markedly, historians have lumped all of them pell-mell into the large pot of "lunacy." If progress is to be made in resolving the Scull-Hare debate, future historians of mental hospitals will have to pay much closer attention to the question: what did these patients actually have?

Finally, among new currents in writing the profession's internal history, it must not be forgotten that somebody actually has to tell the story. Somebody has to assemble the facts and say this happened after that, and on these dates, before lofty cultural interpretations of any kind may be attempted. One thinks of such important, basic building blocks in the history of Canadian psychiatry as John D. ("Jack") Griffin's history of the Canadian Mental Health Association or Harvey Simmons' work on mental health policy in Ontario.[34] Werner Janzarik's misleadingly titled book "Psychopathology as Basic Medical Science" conceals the fact that Janzarik and collaborators have assembled the complex story of the rise to dominance after 1900 of the Heidelberg school, a group of psychiatrists including Emil Kraepelin, who felt that the phenomenology of psychiatric illness, meaning its individual symptoms, had to be assessed before much headway could be made in figuring out causation.[35] Thus, in running after the new social history of psychiatry, one must not forget this tradition of careful scholarship on which all further speculation must be based.

The third area to have burgeoned in the 1980s and 1990s concerns relations among psychiatry, psychiatric symptoms, and the rest of society. How do medical and societal forces change the presentation of mental illness? How do social pressures change psychiatry? Here, the "English school," led by William Bynum and Roy Porter, has performed pioneering work. Porter's own book *Mind-Forg'd Manacles* (published in 1987) attends to the subjective experience of psychosis, neurosis, and dementia (all of which Porter denominates as "madness"). He examines how popular culture dealt with these aberrations, then watches the asylum and the discipline of psychiatry emerge from these folkloric roots.[36] Another powerful effort from the new social historians of psychiatry is Michael Macdonald's work *Mystical Bedlam* (published in 1981). Macdonald studies the psychiatric symptoms of the patients of a quackish seventeenth-century English figure named Sir Richard Napier, and asks to what aspects of English society might these patients have owed their symptoms.[37]

A whole gaggle of historians has waded into the history of the psychoneuroses, and rightly so, given that what constitutes "neurosis" is often in the eye of the beholder rather than being rigorously defined objective pathology. Both feminists and mainline historians have plunged into the turbulent broth of hysteria as a historical diagnosis. Carroll Smith-Rosenberg was perhaps the first of the professional historians to argue that hysteria was basically a cultural artifact imposed upon powerless women by powerful doctors, a baleful side-effect of an asymmetrical doctor-patient relationship.[38] Other historians have suggested that hysteria (strictly defined as physical conversion symptoms) has not gone away at all; despite enormous changes in the situation of women since the nineteenth century, it has merely changed forms. The tendency of women to somatize, or express psychic stress in the form of physical symptoms, is as great as ever, merely that the predominant symptoms have changed from fits and paralysis to pain and fatigue. Thus, the oppression of women in and of itself would not, in this view, constitute the immediate cause of hysteria.[39]

There have been other voices in the hysteria debate too. Mark Micale, for example, believes that English physicians avoided the diagnosis of "male hysteria" because "hysterical" behavior in men was simply not to be contemplated within the ironclad English definitions of sex roles.[40]

Barbara Sicherman and F.G. Gosling have both attempted to describe the social roles played by the diagnosis "neurasthenia." Sicherman calls neurasthenia a respectable rationale for "diagnosing and treating many types of stress."[41] Yet the hysteria and neurasthenia of many authors turn out to be a heterogeneous grab bag of symptoms and syndromes with little internal consistency. Writing a social history of such poorly differentiated entities would be like writing a social history of dust.

More sophisticated about psychopathology are the psychiatrists who have tried to link such diagnoses as neurasthenia to trends in nineteenth-century society. British psychiatrist Simon Wessely has likened such trendy diagnoses as "myalgic encephalomyelitis" (also called M.E.) and "chronic fatigue syndrome" to neurasthenia in the nineteenth century. Such terms, then and now, were produced by the patients' own striving for organicity, their need for some affirmation that they were not psychically affected, because mental illness carried such a stigma.[42] Psychiatrists Susan Abbey and Paul Garfinkel have seen nineteenth-century neurasthenia "as a manifestation of women's distress and their lack of satisfaction with life. The rise of neurasthenia," they write, "occurred in the context of significant changes in the role of women in the new industrial society..."[43]

One can scarcely imagine a more challenging subject than writing the history of the psychoneuroses, for here individual subjectivity is tangled together with surrounding social circumstance. Disentangling these issues requires great talent, and historians and psychiatrists bring different but complementary skills and sensitivities to bear upon this task. The optimum solution would be to have historically trained psychiatrists, and vice versa, an A-team of scholars such as Henri Ellenberger.[44] Yet, in North America, few have acquired this kind of dual training.

One final example will bring us back to our starting point. It was partly owing to the grip of psychoanalysis in the 1950s and 1960s that both psychiatry and the history of psychiatry failed to keep pace with their sister sciences. Precisely in the history of psychoanalysis, the last two decades have breathed new life, replacing inward-looking internalist perspectives with outward-reaching externalist ones. The same shift has happened to psychoanalysis as a discipline. It is one of the great ironies that, just as psychoanalysis has fallen out of favour among psychiatrists, it has never been more popular among humanists and social scientists. The outpouring of literature on Freud and his collaborators and on the history of the international psychoanalytic movement has been extraordinary. It is not for me to review this enormous corpus here. Suffice it to remark that, in step with the new critical spirit that has infused the history of psychiatry generally, a more inquiring attitude has replaced the hagiography that once characterized psychoanalytic scholarship. Paul Roazen's *Freud and His Followers* (first published in 1971) represented the opening salvo, to be followed by such heavyweights as Frank Sulloway, author of *Freud: Biologist of the Mind*.[45] The 1980s and 1990s have seen literature on the history of psychoanalysis whose tone is respectful but iconoclastic form a major channel of its own, parallel to, but independent of, the new social history of psychiatry.

One might build a bridge here, skipping from historiographical considerations to the man who was professor of psychiatry at the University of Toronto from 1925 to 1947, Clarence B. Farrar. There is a link between Farrar's life and these great historical currents in psychiatry, but first one might say a bit about Farrar, who died in 1970 at the extraordinary age of 95 at his home on Oriole Road in Toronto. He was an American, born in New York City, who came up to Toronto during the First World War as a consultant to the Canadian Army on shellshock. Farrar had, without doubt, an interest in the psychological side of psychiatry; in shellshock, of course, there was no brain lesion. Shellshock, a post-traumatic stress disorder, was psychogenic.

An interesting point about Farrar, however, is that soon after receiving his MD from Johns Hopkins University in 1900, he went to Germany to study with the founder of modern psychiatric diagnosis, Emil Kraepelin. Kraepelin was then professor of psychiatry at Heidelberg. The approach of the whole Heidelberg school went back to the need for careful description before one could launch grand generalizations about a phenomenon, and became known for its efforts to describe and understand individual symptoms. It was Kraepelin who put an end to the late nineteenth-century tendency to reduce psychiatric illness to brain disease. At the same time, Kraepelin and such co-workers as Franz Nissl were extremely interested in brain histopathology, for the brain, after all, is the substrate of the mind. When Farrar returned from Heidelberg in 1904, he had received thorough training in Kraepelin's psychological approach (influenced by Kraepelin's study with psychologist Wilhelm Wundt at Leipzig). Farrar also returned mindful of the emphasis upon neurohistology and neuropathology of the whole Heidelberg school. (Remember that Alois Alzheimer was also part of that school.)

Through Farrar's long career in North America ran some of the fundamental themes both in psychiatry and the history of psychiatry. Farrar was, for example, no great friend of psychoanalysis, preferring the more cautious wait-and-see approach that the Kraepelinians had adopted to the issue of causation. Farrar was extremely interested in exact description of mental illness and in the statistical approach to knowledge, and many of his statistical tabulations from the Toronto Psychiatric Hospital still survive. In short, Farrar represented much that was splendid, because it was so intensely scientific, about early twentieth-century psychiatry.

After Farrar's retirement in 1947, control of the commanding heights of psychiatry in Toronto passed to other hands, and a new phase commenced under Aldwyn Stokes. Farrar's views started to seem antiquated. But Farrar belonged to a grand tradition that situated psychiatric illness somewhere on a spectrum that began with neurobiology. The Kraepelinian school was not highly reductionistic; it did not reduce all mind disease to brain disease, but it did implicate biological and genetic factors, as well as drawing in stress and traumatic early development. Under Farrar, various physical therapies were attempted at TPH, in line with a biological model of psychiatric illness. Yet, in line with this eclectic view of causation, psychologists and social workers, for the first time in the history of psychiatry in Toronto, also had roles to play at TPH. Farrar's interest in psychogenesis was evidenced by his two-year tenure in the early 1920s as chief physician of the Homewood Sanitarium at Guelph, a private clinic for psychoneurosis.

Historians of psychiatry have largely forgotten about the intellectual richness of the Kraepelinian school. In standard histories, the years 1900 to 1940 are often impatiently brushed away as a reactionary period somehow still resistant to Freud's insights, the psychiatrists of the day incorrectly dismissed as fanatical pursuers of brain biology. It is in C.B. Farrar's personal history and in the history of the Toronto Psychiatric Hospital that one gains a sense of the richness of this school of psychiatry. Similarly, in the history of psychiatry, the reductionism of the 1960s caused the real scientific achievements of the period 1900 to 1940 to be overlooked. Under the influence of Foucauldians and Marxists, psychiatry became reduced to part of the capitalist state's apparatus of repression, and the devotion of many historians to the psychoanalytical model distracted their attention entirely from such figures as Kraepelin. It is striking that we still have no biography (major or minor) of Emil Kraepelin.

Later in this volume a brief biography is attempted of C.B. Farrar. The German scientific model which he attempted to import to Canada took root for 30 years at TPH and became the basis of the modern history of psychiatry in English Canada.

ENDNOTES

For monographs published prior to 1945, the publishers are not indicated.

[1] G. E. Berrios and G. Tischler, "History, Philosophy and Economics of Psychiatry," *Current Opinion in Psychiatry* 2: 641-43 (1989), quote p. 641.

[2] See Edward Shorter, *From Paralysis to Fatigue: A History of Psychosomatic Illness in the Modern Era* (New York: Free Press, 1992), ch. 12.

[3] See W. Vaughn McCall, "Physical Treatments in Psychiatry: Current and Historical Use in the Southern United States," *Southern Medical Journal*, 82 (3): 345-51 (March 1989). Elliot S. Valenstein, *Great and Desperate Cures: The Rise and Decline of Psychosurgery and Other Radical Treatments for Mental Illness* (New York: Basic Books, 1986).

[4] Ann-Louise S. Silver, *Psychoanalysis and Psychosis* (Madison: International Universities Press, 1989).

[5] Klaus Dörner, *Madmen and the Bourgeoisie*, Eng. trans. (Oxford: Blackwell, 1981).

[6] Gregory Zilboorg, *A History of Medical Psychology* (New York, 1941).

[7] Ilza Veith, *Hysteria: The History of a Disease* (Chicago: University of Chicago Press, 1965).

[8] Reuben Fine, *A History of Psychoanalysis* (New York: Columbia University Press, 1979).

[9] Michel Foucault, *Madness and Civilization: A History of Insanity in the Age of Reason*, Eng. trans. (New York: Random House, 1965).

[10] Andrew T. Scull, *Museums of Madness: The Social Organization of Insanity in Nineteenth-Century England* (London: Allen Lane, 1979).

[11] See, for example, Andrew Scull, "Psychiatry and its Historians," *History of Psychiatry* 2: 239-50 (1991).

[12] For views pro and contra Foucault see the essays in Arthur Still and Irving Volody, eds., *Rewriting the History of Madness* (London: Routledge, 1991).

[13] Edward P. Thompson, *The Making of the English Working Class* (London: Gollancz, 1964).

[14] Claudia Huerkamp, *Der Aufstieg der Ärzte im 19. Jahrhundert* (Göttingen: Vandenhoeck & Ruprecht, 1985); Reinhard Spree, *Health and Social Class in Imperial Germany*, Eng. trans. (Oxford: Berg, 1988).

[15] For example, Joan Jacobs Brumberg, *Fasting Girls: The Emergence of Anorexia Nervosa as a Modern Disease* (Cambridge: Harvard University Press, 1988); Walter Vandereycken, Ron Van Deth, Rolf Meermann, *Hungerkünstler, Fastenwunder, Magersucht: eine Kulturgeschichte der Ess-Störungen* (Zülpich: Biermann, 1990).

[16] See, for example, Sander L Gilman, *Difference and Pathology: Stereotypes of Sexuality, Race, and Madness* (Ithaca: Cornell University Press, 1985); Gilman, *Jewish Self-Hatred: Anti-Semitism and the Hidden Language of the Jews* (Baltimore: Johns Hopkins, 1986).

[17] See, for example, Wendy Mitchinson, *The Nature of Their Bodies: Women and Their Doctors in Victorian Canada* (Toronto: University of Toronto Press, 1991).

[18] Elaine Showalter, *The Female Malady: Women, Madness, and English Culture, 1830-1980* (New York: Pantheon, 1985).

[19] Paul Julius Möbius, *Über den physiologischen Schwachsinn des Weibes* (Halle, 1900).

[20] Stanley W. Jackson, *Melancholia and Depression: From Hippocratic Times to Modern Times* (New Haven: Yale University Press, 1986).

[21] Markus Schär, *Seelennöte der Untertanen: Selbstmord, Melancholie und Religion im alten Zürich, 1500-1800* (Zurich: Chronos, 1985).

[22] E. Fuller Torrey, *Schizophrenia and Civilization* (New York: Jason Aronson, 1980).

[23] German E. Berrios, "Descriptive Psychopathology: Conceptual and Historical Aspects," *Psychological Medicine*, 14 (2): 303-13 (May 1984); "'Depressive Pseudodementia' or 'Melancholic Dementia': a 19th Century View," *Journal of Neurology, Neurosurgery and Psychiatry*, 48 (5): 393-400 (May 1985); "The Psychopathology of Affectivity: Conceptual and Historical Aspects," *Psychological Medicine*, 15 (4): 745-58 (November 1985); "Melancholia and Depression During the 19th Century: A Conceptual History," *British Journal of Psychiatry*, 153: 298-304 (1988); "Historical Aspects of Psychoses: 19th Century Issues," *British Medical Bulletin*, 43 (3): 484-98 (July 1987).

[24] In response to Scull's *Museums of Madness*, see Edward Hare's "Was Insanity on the Increase?" *British Journal of Psychiatry*, 142: 439-55 (May 1983); for Scull's counter-rejoinder to Hare, see Scull, "Was Insanity Increasing?" in Scull, ed., *Social Order/Mental Disorder: Anglo-American Psychiatry in Historical Perspective* (Berkeley: University of California Press, 1989), pp. 239-49. For Hare's work on other components of the great increase in asylum populations, see his seminal articles,

"The Origin and Spread of Dementia Paralytica," *British Journal of Psychiatry*, 105: 594-626 (July 1959); "Schizophrenia as a Recent Disease," ibid., 153: 521-31 (1988).

[25] Harold Merskey, "The Manufacture of Personalities: The Production of Multiple Personality Disorder," *British Journal of Psychiatry* 160:327-340 (1992).

[26] Shorter, *From Paralysis to Fatigue*.

[27] Gerald N. Grob, *Mental Institutions in America: Social Policy to 1875* (New York: Free Press, 1973); *Mental Illness and American Society, 1875-1940* (Princeton: Princeton University Press, 1983).

[28] W.F. Bynum, Roy Porter, and Michael Shepherd, eds., *The Anatomy of Madness: Essays in the History of Psychiatry*, 3 vols. (London: Routledge, 1985-1988).

[29] William L. Parry-Jones, *The Trade in Lunacy: A Study of Private Madhouses in England in the Eighteenth and Nineteenth Centuries* (London: Routledge, 1972).

[30] Cheryl Krasnick Warsh, *Moments of Unreason: The Practice of Canadian Psychiatry and the Homewood Retreat, 1883-1923* (Montreal: McGill-Queen's University Press, 1989).

[31] Nancy Tomes, *A Generous Confidence: Thomas Story Kirkbride and the Art of Asylum-Keeping, 1840-1883* (Cambridge: Cambridge University Press, 1984).

[32] Anne Digby, *Madness, Morality and Medicine: A Study of the York Retreat, 1796-1914* (Cambridge: Cambridge University Press, 1985).

[33] S.E.D. Shortt, *Victorian Lunacy: Richard M. Bucke and the Practice of Late Nineteenth-Century Psychiatry* (Cambridge: Cambridge University Press, 1986).

[34] John D. Griffin, *In Search of Sanity: A Chronicle of the Canadian Mental Health Association, 1918-1988* (London, Ontario: Third Eye, 1989); Harvey G. Simmons, *Unbalanced: Mental Health Policy in Ontario, 1930-1989* (Toronto: Wall & Emerson, 1990).

[35] Werner Janzarik, ed., *Psychopathologie als Grundlagenwissenschaft* (Stuttgart: Enke, 1979).

[36] Roy Porter, *Mind-Forg'd Manacles: A History of Madness in England from the Restoration to the Regency* (Cambridge: Harvard University Press, 1987).

[37] Michael Macdonald, *Mystical Bedlam: Madness, Anxiety, and Healing in Seventeenth-Century England* (Cambridge: Cambridge University Press, 1981).

[38] Carroll Smith-Rosenberg, "The Hysterical Woman: Sex Roles and Role Conflict in 19th-Century America," *Social Research*, 39: 652-78 (Winter 1972).

[39] Shorter, *From Paralysis to Fatigue*.

[40] Mark S. Micale, "Hysteria Male/Hysteria Female: Reflections on Comparative Gender Construction in Nineteenth-Century France and Britain," in Marina Benjamin, ed., *Science and Sensibility: Gender and Scientific Enquiry, 1780-1945* (London: Basil Blackwell, 1991), pp. 200-39.

[41] Barbara Sicherman, "The Uses of Diagnosis: Doctors, Patients, and Neurasthenia," *Journal of the History of Medicine and Allied Sciences*, 32 (1): 33-54 (January 1977), quote p. 53; F.G. Gosling, *Before Freud: Neurasthenia and the American Medical Community, 1870-1910* (Urbana: University of Illinois Press, 1987).

[42] Simon Wessely, "Old Wine in New Bottles: Neurasthenia and 'ME'," *Psychological Medicine*, 20 (1): 35-53 (February 1990).

[43] Susan E. Abbey and Paul E. Garfinkel, "Neurasthenia and the Chronic Fatigue Syndrome: The Role of Culture in the Making of a Diagnosis," *American Journal of Psychiatry*, 148 (12): 1638-46 (December 1991), quote p. 1643.

[44] See Henri Ellenberger's magisterial work, *The Discovery of the Unconscious: The History and Evolution of Dynamic Psychiatry* (New York: Basic Books, 1970).

[45] Paul Roazen, *Freud and His Followers*, reprint (New York: New York University Press, 1984); Frank J. Sulloway, *Freud: Biologist of the Mind: Beyond the Psychoanalytic Legend* (New York: Basic Books, 1979).

2

Origins of the Toronto Psychiatric Hospital

Cyril Greenland[*]

> There can be no question though, that where the insane are concerned the public are not only indifferent, but terror stricken and very often heartless.[1]

Having been involved in the Ontario Asylum service since the age of seventeen, C.K. Clarke was acutely aware of what he called "the malign influence of politics over psychiatry."[2] Nevertheless, he never hesitated to use his political connections and considerable know-how to improve the life of patients and to advance the profession of psychiatry in Canada. His dream was to establish a world-class psychiatric centre, closely associated with a university, where acute mental illness could be treated under ideal conditions and where teaching and scientific research had the highest priority. This dream became a reality in December 1925 with the opening of the Toronto Psychiatric Hospital. C.K. Clarke, who died on January 20, 1924, did not live to enjoy the results of his labour. Today, the Clarke Institute of Psychiatry, which succeeded the TPH in May 1966, stands as an enduring memorial to this pioneer psychiatrist.

The following account of the prolonged and often frustrating attempts to build the Toronto Psychiatric Hospital is designed to do more than chronicle the determination of a small group of stalwarts lead by "C.K." as he was affectionately known. This chapter traces the tortuous path which the pioneers followed, with varying degrees of wisdom and fortitude, in order to establish psychiatry as a respected branch of medicine in Canada.

[*] Cyril Greenland, M.Sc., University of Wales; Ph.D., University of Birmingham, 1984, was part-time director of social work at TPH from 1960-66. He is professor emeritus of social work at McMaster University and co-founder (with Dr. J.D.M. Griffin) of the Archives on the History of Psychiatry and Museum of Mental Health Services (Toronto).

The Break-down of the Asylums

Massive overcrowding was responsible for the virtual breakdown of the asylums in the postwar years. This is why the building of the TPH assumed strategic importance as the linchpin of the new mental health system in Ontario. Taking the years 1914 and 1923 as examples, one can see that, over this period, the demand for mental hospital beds usually exceeded the supply.

Excluding the "Idiot Asylum" at Orillia, in 1914 there were nine mental hospitals in Ontario.[3] They had a bed capacity of 5,682 and an occupancy of 5,912. The Toronto mental hospital, with a bed capacity of 852, housed 991 patients. By 1923, including the newly commissioned hospital at Whitby, Ontario had a bed capacity of 7,821.[4] In the same year there were 8,002 patients in residence. Perhaps for the first time in its long history Toronto had 43 more beds than patients. This was due to the temporary relief afforded by the opening of the Whitby hospital.

Overcrowding had been endemic in Ontario's mental hospitals from the earliest days. When the Provincial Lunatic Asylum, the first purposely built asylum in Upper Canada, was opened in 1850 in Toronto, the expectation was that the mentally ill would be admitted, treated, and promptly returned to their former useful and productive lives. Instead, John Scott, the first medical superintendent, found himself in charge of an already overcrowded institution built to house 250 patients. Before the end of the first year, over 300 mostly pauper patients were accommodated. Scott reported that of the 308 patients under treatment in this period, "40 recovered, 13 were relieved or improved, 2 eloped, 20 died, and 233 remained."[5] A large proportion of the remaining patients were "in a state of dementia and, for the most part, harmless; there is no hope of their ever being restored." Scott felt that these chronic patients could be cared for elsewhere on a much cheaper basis.

A second chronic problem was political interference which resulted, for example, in Scott's resignation in 1853.[6] In addition to deciding who was to be hired and fired, the asylum's board of directors took upon themselves responsibility for awarding contracts for provisions. The result was an undisciplined staff and poor quality food for the patients. During the next hundred years, the Ontario asylums were managed under various political authorities, but opportunities for patronage were rarely absent.

Joseph Workman, medical superintendent of the Toronto Asylum from 1853 to 1875, frequently complained about overcrowding and political interference. At this point, C.K. Clarke arrived on the scene. Clarke, Workman's pupil, had become the assistant superintendent at the Rockwood Asylum, Kingston, in 1882.

Sickened by asylum politics, Clarke decided to resign from the government service. Then, on the morning of August 13, 1885, while he and William Metcalf, medical superintendent, were making their ward rounds, a patient, Patrick Maloney, stabbed Metcalf in the abdomen, inflicting fatal wounds. Following Metcalf's death, Clarke reluctantly withdrew his resignation and was appointed medical superintendent at Kingston. He accepted this appointment, he said, "in order to protect several hundred defenceless creatures from a political hireling who might be pitchforked into the position."

Clarke continued, "I love psychiatry, but hate politics: I felt that much could be accomplished if the politicians could be fought off with any degree of success."[7]

Clarke's exasperation was shared by some of his senior colleagues. The experience of T.J.W. Burgess (1849-1926), medical superintendent of the Verdun Protestant Hospital (now the Douglas Hospital, Montreal), was typical. In June 1907 he wrote:

> the appointment of outside practitioners to superintendentships for political purposes is a flagrant injustice to the patients, to the taxpayers, and to deserving juniors, of who[m] there are many in the service. No man should be given charge of an institution for the insane unless he has had special training in psychiatry and has shown a penchant for the work. I speak freely on this subject, gentlemen, because I myself have gone through the mill. Sixteen of the best years of my life were spent in the asylum service of Ontario, and when time and time again I saw myself passed over in favour of some outside man, though senior for promotion, I thought it was time to quit which I did. This was of course under the regime of the late government. Whether the present one would have treated me any better I cannot say, but I think it extremely doubtful.[8]

Considering that Clarke's father, Lieutenant Colonel Charles Clarke, was a "True Grit" member of the Legislative Assembly (1871–1894), Speaker of the Assembly (1880–1885), and Clerk of the Assembly (1901–1907), his antipathy to politics and politicians was, perhaps, inevitable. At the same time, because of his political connections, Clarke could afford to undertake major reforms which would have been quite impossible for anyone else. For example, in his 1893 annual report Clarke wrote: "during the summer we have been busy, under the direction of the Public Works Department, erecting a new hospital building where acute disease can be properly treated and quiet for convalescent patients secured."[9] In the same report, he made an eloquent plea to abandon the term "asylum."

> It is a difficult matter to get the non-professional and sometimes professional men to realize that an insane person is one suffering from a bodily disease just as much as a patient with typhoid fever. We have hospitals for patients suffering from fever, etc., why not hospitals for persons suffering from insanity?[10]

FROM ASYLUM TO HOSPITAL FOR THE INSANE

Although the notion of treating acute mental illness in hospitals instead of asylums was not entirely new in the 1890s, the move from asylum to hospital took many years and a great deal of effort. The first step was the opening in 1894 of the Beech Grove Infirmary in Kingston. Designed by C.K. Clarke, this was the first hospital unit in Ontario to serve acute cases as well as convalescent patients. It had 30 beds. A unique feature of this facility was that patients quarried and dressed the stone used in the building. Some 200 patients were involved in the building of Beech Grove, which took about two years to complete.

The mood of the times was reflected in Clarke's comments.

> Public opinion must back us up in our endeavours to advance the treatment and care of the insane, and while it is only fair that a rigid scrutiny of all expenditures should be made in the hope of checking extravagance, still the desire to have cheaply managed institutions should not for one moment endanger the welfare and chance of recovery of any person committed to our care.[11]

After a long period of gestation, Clarke's recommendation that the ominous word "asylum" be replaced by "hospital" was finally adopted by the government in 1907.[12] S.A. Armstrong, assistant provincial secretary, confirmed this policy at the formal opening of the Reception Hospital, Brockville, on August 16, 1916.

> ... This hospital, which is being opened today, is a splendid example of the policy of the Department with respect to the hospitalization of the Public Institutions of this Province. Public

opinion seems to be that a patient sent to a Hospital for the Insane is sent in reality to a House of Detention and not to a Hospital for treatment. We have been endeavouring in the years past to correct this impression in order that no stigma may attach to a patient admitted to an institution. To this end, the Government no longer uses the term "Asylums" but our public institutions are known today as "Hospitals for the Insane," "Hospitals for the Feeble-Minded," and "Hospitals for Epileptics," as the case may be. In addition to this, legislation has been passed which enables a patient to enter a Hospital for the Insane as a voluntary patient.[13]

Political interference in asylum management concerned Clarke, who dreaded the patronage appointments that accompanied changes of government administrations. This scenario recurred when the Liberals were defeated in 1905. True to form, the new Conservative government under J.P. Whitney lost no time in rewarding its supporters. The "political hireling" dreaded by C.K. Clarke was Edward Ryan, a surgeon, former mayor of Kingston, president of the local Conservative Association, and defeated candidate in the previous election. The sum of this experience was, it seems, sufficient to merit Ryan's appointment as medical superintendent of Rockwood Hospital. To facilitate this move, C.K. Clarke was transferred to the Toronto hospital where he succeeded Daniel Clark who, upon reaching the age of 70, conveniently resigned in September 1905.

A much more significant political appointment was that of William Hanna, KC, MPP (1862-1919). A staunch Conservative lawyer and MLA for West Lambton since 1902, Hanna was appointed provincial secretary and registrar general in February 1905. Through his inspectors, the provincial secretary was in those days required to monitor every aspect of the operation of the ten provincial asylums, which housed 6,280 patients, as well as the prisons and charitable institutions. Hanna's influence within the Whitney government was, of course, substantial.

Having established himself in Toronto, C.K. lost no time in making personal contact with Hanna. This arrangement was unusual, if not highly irregular. In those days, the medical superintendents were expected to communicate with the provincial secretary through his staff of inspectors who, in turn, reported to the assistant provincial secretary. However, as the most senior medical superintendent in the service and as associate editor of the *American Journal of Insanity* since 1904, Clarke obviously had exceptional authority. His status was enhanced in 1908 by his appointment as full professor of psychiatry and dean of medicine at the University of Toronto.

The Psychiatric Clinic

The high esteem in which Clarke was held is best illustrated by his informal correspondence with the provincial secretary. Writing privately to W.J. Hanna, from the Toronto Asylum on February 26, 1907, Clarke said:

> the enclosed will give you the most cogent "reasons why" for a Psychiatric Clinic, looking at the matter from a medical standpoint. Perhaps I have not arranged them in the best manner possible, but they were simply jotted down as they appealed to me.
>
> There are no doubt many other arguments to be brought forward, from your point of view, and it goes without saying that you will do more than justice to the subject, when you take it up.[14]

The sixteen-page memorandum that accompanied Clarke's letter reads like a modern briefing paper prepared for a cabinet minister. It contains very little "medical" information which would be unfamiliar to a well-read person. Clarke's arguments for establishing a psychiatric clinic in Toronto are mostly of an economic, political, and humanitarian nature. Clarke stressed the economic side:

> To build a complete new institution, for acute and chronic cases, near the city, means an enormous expenditure of money for a site alone, and the cumbersome elaboration of buildings to provide accommodation for acute and chronic cases, an arrangement which is not considered ideal...from the modern standpoint;...[15]

The solution, he argued, is to provide separate facilities for chronic patients using the cottage system (planned for Whitby) and to build a new psychiatric hospital modeled on Emil Kraepelin's clinic at Munich. "This is a new departure that marks a new era in Hospital history, not only in Canada but in America." Clarke estimated that the cost of the site at $75,000 and $100,000, and the construction costs (excluding the nurses' residence) at $300,000. Finally, said Clarke, "until more details have been acquired from their experiences in Germany, it will not be possible to approximate this closely."[16]

As Clarke confidently noted of this venture in 1907:

Ontario has an opportunity to score a veritable triumph if she will wisely accept the opening. With the reorganization of the University, the building of the Provincial Hospital, and the accepted policy that Toronto Asylum has outlived its usefulness, come the chance to do something that will, at last, lift psychiatry to its proper position, as one of the most practical and important branches of medical science. This would mean the establishment of a Psychiatric Clinic upon a site near the new Hospital. The building would be a self-contained establishment, under Government control, would embrace every modern requirement for the scientific treatment of acute cases of insanity—laboratories and lecture rooms and provisions for the prosecution of research work in pathology, physiology and psychology.

The educational side of the Clinic would be of just as great importance as the curative, and the general practitioner and student would have abundant opportunity to acquire some insight into the nature of mental diseases. The Clinic would have an intimate relationship with the Provincial University and Provincial Hospital and should also have a Dispensary Department.[17]

The article concludes with a promise of international recognition which the writer (who else but C.K. Clarke?) mistakenly assumed the government would find irresistible.

If Toronto University is to become as great a Mecca (and why not even a greater?) as Johns Hopkins, the Psychiatric Clinic is an absolute necessity, and there is no reason why we should not lead the way in America....[18]

THE WILLOUGHBY COMMISSION

Convinced by Clarke's petition, Hanna wasted no time in securing the support of the premier and cabinet colleagues. In April, 1907, the government allocated $100,000 towards the construction of the new facility which, it was estimated, would cost $400,000.[19] The next step involved appointing a commission to visit Europe in order to study the methods used in caring for the insane. On July 2, 1907, Hanna sent Clarke a government cheque for $2,000, covering the travel expenses of Clarke and Ryan, and wished them bon voyage.

Anticipating his trip to Europe, on May 29, 1907, Clarke wrote to his friend C.B. Farrar of the Sheppard and Enoch Pratt Hospital in Baltimore,

Maryland, requesting introductions to leading psychiatrists in Germany.[20]

The commission, including C.K. Clarke and Edward Ryan, was chaired by W.A. Willoughby, MPP, minister without portfolio. Since Ryan was the new medical superintendent at Kingston and an unabashed political appointee, his membership on the commission is understandable. Also, it must be said that, contrary to Clarke's dour predictions, Ryan was a relatively successful superintendent. He was also the founding president (1920-24) of the Ontario Neuropsychiatric Association. Except that he was Hanna's friend and political confrere, Willoughby's appointment to chair the commission is puzzling. Although he was qualified in medicine (Victoria College, 1867) and served as a Surgeon Lieutenant Colonel, Willoughby, a Conservative politician, devoted most of his time to local and provincial politics. He lacked experience or interest in asylums, and there is no evidence that he made any contribution to the commission except as a cipher. A similar thought must have occurred to the unnamed correspondent in the *Dominion Medical Monthly* of September 1907, who wrote:

> Just why the Hon. Dr. Willoughby has been selected to take part in this manoeuvre is not quite clear to the psychiatrists in Ontario, as he was never announced to be a specialist in this department of medicine, having so far been but a general practitioner in a small lake port town and a politician. However, the government is to be congratulated that it did not send three politicians.[21]

Clarke's personal letters to Hanna from Berlin confirm Willoughby's incompetence. For example, he said that "poor old" Willoughby was exhausted and confused by the ordeal. In a subsequent letter, Clarke added: "the poor old Doctor is quite a source of anxiety to me, as he is not well and requires no end of care..." In retrospect, it seems that Willoughby was seriously ill. He died in April 1908, aged 64, before the printer's ink on the commission's report was properly dry.

In the course of its work, the commissioners visited some of the most important university centres in Britain and in Europe. Their visits included hospitals and asylums in Germany, Zurich, and Paris; Berlin (Dalldorf, Buch), Munich (Eglfing), Tübingen, and Giessen; London and Derby in England; Edinburgh; and Dublin, Clonmel, and Waterford in Ireland.[22] As might have been anticipated, Clarke discovered his personal Mecca at Kraepelin's "Klinik" in Munich. In this respect, the commission's report is little more than an elaboration of the memorandum which Clarke prepared for Hanna in February 1907.

The commission's report concluded with four concise recommendations:

> *First:* The enlargement of the present staffs of physicians and nurses;
> *Second:* The isolation of the tuberculous;
> *Third:* The proper care and treatment of insane criminals;
> *Fourth:* The Psychiatric Hospital being the ideal institution for the treatment of all acute forms of insanity, we should recommend the establishment, as necessity arises, of such hospitals at University centres.[23]

CLARKE, JONES, AND KRAEPELIN

Did C.K. Clarke and Ernest Jones, who became famous as Sigmund Freud's first biographer, meet while visiting Kraepelin's Clinic in Munich in the summer of 1907? We know that Clarke, Ryan, and Willoughby were in Europe in July and August of 1907. Also, according to one scholar, Jones studied with Kraepelin in Munich for three months between 1907 and 1908.[24] Richard Paskauskas claims that Jones went to Munich to prepare himself for a possible career in Toronto. This is confirmed in a letter from Jones to Freud, dated May 13, 1908:

> I am working all day at the psychiatry Klinic. It will be very important for me in Canada for they think the world of Kraepelin and a government commission visited Europe recently and was most enthusiastic over his Klinic. They are going to build one on its model in Toronto and send their assistants over to Kraepelin to be trained. I therefore hope to get some position over there, which of course will be important for me both as regards standing and material.[25]

If they didn't meet in Munich, and there is no evidence of any correspondence before 1908, how did Jones know that C.K. Clarke desperately needed someone with his particular brand of training, skills, interests, and missionary zeal? The most likely explanation is that Kraepelin recommended Jones to Clarke. This is confirmed, more or less, in a letter dated October 23, 1908, from Clarke to Hanna:

> Dr. Ernest Jones has called upon me, after a warm note of introduction from Dr. Osler. He is also recommended by Dr. Mott, the celebrated English pathologist, who is head of the

pathological department at Claybury Asylum and is one of the best known living authorities on nervous and mental troubles. Other eminent English and German authorities have also recommended Dr. Ernest Jones to me. This young man is already recognized in literature as one of the most eminent authorities on functional nervous troubles, and has had exceptional opportunity for work in the greater laboratories of Europe, such as those at Munich Psychiatric Clinic, under Kraepelin and Alzheimer, also with Jung and Freud at Vienna.[26]

Within a week or so of meeting C.K. Clarke in Toronto, Jones was offered and accepted four appointments: pathologist (replacing J.G. FitzGerald) and clinical assistant at the Toronto Asylum; sessional demonstrator in applied physiology at the Faculty of Medicine; demonstrator in psychiatry; and unpaid assistant in the Department of Psychiatry, Toronto General Hospital. In an optimistic mood, Jones wrote to Freud (26 September 1908) "Clarke...has promised me a university appointment and also one in the new psychiatry clinic, which will be open in two years and of which he will be head."[27]

Having undertaken additional training in neuropathology with Kraepelin, Jones was well versed in Kraepelinian psychiatry as well as in neurology. Since Clarke was more experienced as an administrator than as a clinician, Jones, whose credentials were impeccable, was a perfect assistant and ally in providing a scientific basis for the practice of psychiatry. This goal was achieved, more or less, when Clarke, as dean of medicine and professor of psychiatry, adopted the English version[28] of Kraepelin's famous textbook for use in the Department of Psychiatry. Then, with the support of his friend, Clarke introduced Kraepelin's classification of mental diseases in 1909 into the Ontario Hospitals for the Insane. Thus, the modern scientific approach to psychiatry, developed in Germany by world-famous Kraepelin, served as the keel of Clarke's revolutionary plan to establish a psychiatric clinic in Toronto.

A NEW DEPARTMENT OF PSYCHIATRY

A brief description of Clarke's (proposed) new Department of Psychiatry was published in the *University of Toronto Monthly* in 1907–8. The "modern" methods outlined by Clarke follow the all too familiar medical model.

> Ordinarily, such an [insane] patient, when admitted to an institution, is at once put to bed and kept there for sometime, perhaps

a week or more, until his condition, physical and mental, is enquired into. His complete examination may take many hours; the psychological analysis alone occupying much time. His history from childhood up to date of admission is enquired into, and no sphere that is likely to afford information is left untouched. A careful analysis of blood and other body fluids, including even the cerebro-spinal fluid when necessary is made, and when all of the information that can be had is gathered together, the whole case is critically discussed at a conference of the staff, and the line of treatment mapped out. The amount of detail required would surprise one not conversant with the exaction of modern medicine. To do all this requires a large staff; a far larger staff than is generally found in asylums.[29]

Clarke's vision of modern psychiatry, circa 1908, was predicated on the ability to discover, by means of exact clinical tests, discreet causes of mental illness due to conditions such as neurosyphilis, toxicity, cerebral organicity, infections, and dementia praecox, etc. This was the challenge of modern psychiatry pioneered by Kraepelin in Europe and by Clarke in North America. With the establishment of the psychiatric clinic and with the indefatigable Ernest Jones at his side, how could C.K. Clarke, the most influential Canadian psychiatrist of his time, fail? But fail he did, and seventeen years elapsed before C.K. Clarke's dream was realized by the opening of the Toronto Psychiatric Hospital in December 1925. By that time, Clarke was dead and Ernest Jones, who left Toronto in 1913, had gone on to become one of Freud's closest disciples and Freud's official biographer.

Defeat or retreat?

In his study of Ernest Jones (1896–1913), Paskauskas provides an interesting analysis of the "Rise and Fall of the Clinic."[30] To explain what happened, some recapitulation is necessary.

Hanna, as provincial secretary, was responsible for prisons and hospitals, as well as the asylums of Ontario. In this role, he was subject to many competing and frequently conflicting demands. For example, he was persuaded by Clarke and supported by Sir Robert Falconer, president of the University of Toronto, to fund the building of a new psychiatric clinic.

At the same time, equally powerful voices forced Hanna to consider the merits of two rival enterprises. According to Paskauskas, the

$100,000 reserved for Clarke's psychiatric clinic was diverted to finance the building of the new Guelph Reformatory, which cost $1,200,000.[31] At about the same time, Sir Joseph Flavelle (1858–1939), one of Toronto's wealthiest and most influential businessmen, campaigned to re-build the Toronto General Hospital at a cost of $3,450,000. Flavelle, chair of the Toronto General board of trustees, was also chair of the University of Toronto board of governors. In this respect, Paskauskas observes that Flavelle: "far outstripped Clarke's relatively meagre place in the social, political, and economic arena of Toronto's influential elites."[32]

WOULD TPH BE TOO EXPENSIVE?

Criticism of C.K. Clarke's plan for a psychiatric clinic came from several sources. First there were the neurologists who feared that the upstart profession of psychiatry would occupy their turf. Clarke's *bête noire*, Donald Campbell Meyers (1863–1927), was a persistent critic. Having served as the staff neurologist at Toronto General since the 1890s, Campbell Meyers was responsible for a successful nervous ward where a variety of mental and nervous conditions were treated (see pp. 33 – 34 for details). He was convinced that a majority of these patients could be helped in a general hospital, thus avoiding the calamity of admission to an asylum. However, to Clarke, Campbell Meyers and his neurological colleagues were minor irritations. In 1912, he found an excuse for closing the nervous ward, and Campbell Meyers was compelled to leave Toronto General and retreat to his private neurological hospital at 77 Heath Street, Toronto.

The backbiting of Clarke's asylum colleagues was much more difficult. Years later, reflecting on this unhappy period, Clarke revealed that his disappointment was intensified by the malicious tactics of his medical colleagues in other mental hospitals.[33] Believing the proposed psychiatric institute threatened their prestige, hospital psychiatrists were relentless in their opposition. The medical staff of the Ontario Hospitals for the Insane feared that the new psychiatric clinic would not only receive more than its fair share of public funds, but would also filter off a better class of patients. Thus, in addition to being underfunded they would also be inundated with less desirable patients, turning provincial mental hospitals into second-class facilities. To counter this degradation, reception hospitals, dealing with acute forms of mental illness, were developed in several of the Ontario Hospitals. Ironically, the reception hospital idea was pioneered in Ontario by C.K. Clarke first at Rockwood Hospital, Kingston, in 1894 and then, in 1907, at the Toronto Asylum.

Ryan's revenge

A vindictive attack on C.K. Clarke's reputation, published in the October 1912 issue of the *Bulletin of the Ontario Hospitals for the Insane*, was deceptively titled "Seven Years' Advance in the Ontario Hospitals for Mental Diseases."[34] Its author was Edward Ryan, who succeeded Clarke as medical superintendent of Rockwood Hospital, Kingston, in 1905. Although Clarke's name is not mentioned anywhere in the article, those reading between the lines had no doubt that Ryan was settling an old score. (Years before, Clarke had referred to Ryan as a "political hireling.")

The main burden of Ryan's article was that until his appointment as medical superintendent at Rockwood, there was an entire absence of therapeutic measures. But he avoided stating that these disgraceful conditions applied specifically to Rockwood which, under Clarke's direction, was the flagship of the Ontario Hospitals.

> Absolutely nothing was done in the way of treatment. There was no laboratory, nor was there any attempt at laboratory work. Original investigation of any kind was entirely absent. Records of patients were very indifferently kept. In many cases no record could be found beyond the mere entry in a book that the patient was admitted on a certain date and sent to a certain ward. The disturbed patients, acute and chronic, were restrained by drugs, by locked door and iron bars. There was no attempt to diagnose, to treat, to nurse, to cure. No wonder then, that the disease became chronic or that a useful life was lost.[35]

Reviewing the progress at Rockwood, Ryan took special pride in the modified Kraepelinian classification adopted by all of the provincial hospitals in 1909. He also expressed approval of the development of laboratories, the appointment of pathologists, and the inauguration of a modern record keeping system. Other innovations at Rockwood included the Training School for Nurses (established by C.K. Clarke in 1887), treatment by continuous baths, electrotherapy, and provision of special diets.

The result of these innovations, Ryan claimed, was a 276 percent increase in the discharge rate between 1900 and 1911. This crude figure was produced by calculating the difference between 26 discharges in 1900 and 72 in 1911. Ryan added that restraint of every form had entirely disappeared from Rockwood. "Drugs are rarely used, and if at all for purely therapeutic purposes... The only restraint, in fact, is the kindly, soothing presence of a firm, tactful and intelligent nurse."[36] For an external appraisal, Ryan quoted a "prominent physician" who said, "the asylum was the last place to send a patient, but Rockwood Hospital is the first place and the only."[37]

Then, in carefully measured words, Ryan destroyed the argument for the psychiatric clinic which he, Clarke, and Willoughby recommended in their 1908 commission report. Instead, he concluded that the same treatment was being provided at Rockwood.

> We are getting a better class of patients and more satisfactory patients are seeking treatment in the early and curable stages of disease. We are breaking away from the old methods of admission and opening our doors to the sick seeking relief. With us certificates are no longer exacted. Voluntary patients are received, treated and discharged.[38]

Finally, in a barb obviously aimed at C.K. Clarke, who was deeply concerned about Canada's lax immigration policy, Ryan said:

> We are devoting much time and energy and literature, good and bad, to the question of heredity, to the marriage of human misfits, and to the degeneration in store for us in the days to come. Let us rather apply our efforts to the plain demands of our own day, and posterity will be most thankful.[39]

Ryan's rebuke to Canada's best known and most influential psychiatrist was, most likely, published in the hospital bulletin with the tacit approval of the inspectors, if not with the government's connivance.

It seems unlikely that Clarke's frequent comments on the evils of political interference, and his intemperate demands to spend scarce public funds on a psychiatric clinic, would make him popular with the Whitney government. Also, despite his high office as dean of medicine, professor of psychiatry, and superintendent of the Toronto General Hospital, Clarke lacked the support of his medical colleagues. Some of them, at least, saw Clarke's demand for the psychiatric clinic as little more than an opportunity for self-aggrandizement and the imposition of his will on a reluctant government.

Campbell Meyers and the nervous ward at Toronto General

As we have seen, another source of irritation to Clarke was his continued conflict with the neurologists. In 1906, Donald Campbell Meyers, neurologist-in-chief at Toronto General since the 1890s, had been authorized by the board to establish a nervous diseases ward, the first of its kind in North America. The ward, situated in the former medical superintendent's residence, had twelve beds, six each for male and female patients. The cost of renovations was covered by a $5,000 grant from the Ontario government. Meyers reported that, in the first 16 months of operation, 100 patients had been admitted: 24 for observation and 76 for treatment.

> Of the 24 observation cases, 16 were found to be insane and transferred to an asylum or taken home; three refused to obey instructions and were discharged in a few days after admission; two were cases of brain tumour, one cerebral syphilis, and two still remain under observation. Of these 16 cases of insanity, which had been recommended for treatment as cases of nervous exhaustion, the majority belonged to the class of chronic insanities, as they were suffering from Dementia Praecox or Paranoia.
>
> Of the 76 cases of Functional Neurosis under definite treatment, 64 suffered from Neurasthenia, two from Hysteria, two from Catalepsy, one from Epilepsy, and seven patients still remain under treatment, 26 recovered. Of the 69 cases whose treatment had terminated, 26 recovered, 35 improved and eight were unimproved by treatment.[40]

Campbell Meyers claimed these results supported his contention that insanity might be prevented by prompt treatment before the borderline between functional neurosis and insanity has been reached. "Further, he felt that similar results could be obtained in any general hospital."[41]

Other advantages of psychiatric units in general hospitals included the absence of legal constraints and of the stigma traditionally associated with admission to an asylum. Campbell Meyers also thought useful the opportunity for clinical instruction in the treatment of mental diseases given to nurses, students, and the house-staff. And, unlike Clarke's grandiose plan for a new psychiatric hospital, Campbell Meyers argued that the nervous ward was an exceedingly economical operation which actually saved the government many thousands of dollars.

Although C.K. Clarke and Ryan were antagonists, they united in opposition to Campbell Meyers. Ryan claimed that it made better sense to turn asylums into hospitals than to turn hospitals into asylums. The extent to which this view was shared by Clarke, as medical superintendent of Toronto General Hospital, can be observed in his annual report of 1912. Recording the closure of the nervous ward, Clarke wrote:

> In order to provide accommodation for pupil nurses, it was found necessary to do away with the ward for nervous cases. It is a matter of surprise to find so many patients suffering from mental disease in the general wards of the hospital. The public does not understand, apparently, that the institution is not equipped to deal with these people satisfactorily or with safety to the patients and nurses. Apparently, there is no adequate provision made for them in hospitals for the insane, and it is a matter of regret that no psychiatric hospital has been provided either by the city or government. In the meanwhile, if we must open our doors to patients suffering from various psychoses, we do so at very great risk, especially when patients are either homicidal or suicidal. No amount of foresight in a building not specially equipped will provide against a tragedy occurring in some of these instances, and that we have escaped during the past year has been largely a matter of good luck.[42]

Following his departure from Toronto General in 1911, Campbell Meyers' influence in Toronto languished. Even at the time of his death in 1927, little attention was paid to his pioneer work in being the first in Canada to introduce inpatient neuropsychiatry into a general hospital. However, in 1974, thanks to former Psychiatrist-in-Chief Robert Pos, the board of trustees of the Toronto General Hospital named the Department of Psychiatry, the "D. Campbell Meyers Memorial Department of Psychiatry." Clifford Scott, one of the first student interns at the Toronto Psychiatric Hospital in 1926, provided this touching, but somewhat ironic, postscript.

> Meyers remained the humanist: my last contact with him was when he was dying of cancer of the pancreas, I think, and asked me to take as many psychiatric books from his library as I wished and 40 were in the library of the interns' sitting room of the Toronto Psychiatric Hospital.[43]

The Symposium on Mental Hygiene

The Symposium on Mental Hygiene held on January 28, 1915, suggests the medical community's support for the work and ideals of C.K. Clarke. It was also an indirect response to Ryan's attack on Clarke published in 1912. The symposium, held under the auspices of the Toronto Academy of Medicine's section on state medicine, was chaired by Charles Hastings, medical officer of health, City of Toronto. In addition to C.K. Clarke, the main speakers were J.M. Forster, medical superintendent, Hospital for the Insane, Toronto; John McCullough, chief officer, provincial board of health, Ontario; John FitzGerald, associate professor of hygiene, University of Toronto; Harvey Clare, medical director, Toronto Reception Hospital for the Insane. The discussants of record were Donald Campbell Meyers and Bruce Smith, inspector of hospitals.

In his opening remarks, Clarke admitted that the onset of the (1914–1918) war made it virtually impossible to contemplate the building of the psychiatric clinic. Nevertheless, it was useful to reflect on the past. He said that Joseph Flavelle (chairman of the board of trustees of the Toronto General Hospital) had supported the establishment of a psychiatric hospital and persuaded the government to appoint the Willoughby Commission. He also said that inspector Bruce Smith warmly defended the scheme and gave it all the assistance he could. However, "...much to the surprise of those who expected better things, some of the authorities in the institutions of the province exhibited hostility, apparently thinking that it would interfere with their personal glory."[44]

After the government had allocated $100,000 towards the cost of the psychiatric clinic, an unsuccessful attempt was made to buy a site close to the new Toronto General Hospital on College Street. When this failed "the practical politicians," who did not understand the importance of the subject, lost their nerve.

> With the re-building of the new General Hospital commenced and a very large sum of money to be produced by this community, it was more than ever apparent that the Psychiatric Clinic would have to wait, because it was no longer possible to look for a half a million dollars from the Ontario Government. Perhaps this, of itself, was not an unmitigated evil because, if such a Hospital is [to] be established, it must be kept absolutely free from political control and the ideal arrangement would be to have it under the supervision of a dignified Board of Trustees of the same class as

those found in the General Hospital; men who are superior to the temptation of political exigency.[45]

Attributing the poor morale in the Hospitals for the Insane to persons without scientific knowledge controlling hospital policies, Clarke provides the following "glaring" case example:

> ...of one of my assistants [probably Ernest Jones] who would have been an ornament to psychiatry and who had before him the most brilliant possibilities. He understood how thoroughly collaboration between the clinical and laboratory sides of Psychiatry should be if any advance is to be made, and yet when he stood up for his ideals was bitterly condemned.[46]

Clarke concluded that:

> probably the real solution of the difficulty will eventually be found, and I think it will be discovered that this solution will have to be arrived at by cooperation between the government, city and private beneficence, with the accent on the private beneficence. We shall have to look for a Henry Phipps [who endowed the psychiatric clinic at Johns Hopkins University] to arise in our midst...[47]

The only discordant notes at the symposium were those introduced by Campbell Meyers and Bruce Smith. Donald Campbell Meyers, as might be anticipated, spoke of the benefits to be derived from the formation of neurological wards in general hospitals. He was followed by Bruce Smith, who denied the existence of "political interference." Condemning Clarke's pessimism, Smith said that:

> He looked forward to the time in the not too distant future when Ontario would have in Toronto a Reception Hospital for the Insane with a Psychiatric Clinic in connection therewith on lines broader and better than had ever been attained in any country, notwithstanding the discouraging and discordant note that, unfortunately, had been introduced in the evening's discussion which was uncalled for as it was unwarranted.[48]

Responding to this rebuke, Clarke denied being pessimistic and qualified himself as "a rather sceptical optimist, as his experience of the last seven years in connection with Government promises regarding the future had given him every reason to believe that 'all that glitters is not gold.'"[49]

THE RECEPTION HOSPITAL ACTS OF 1913 AND 1914

In the heat of the debate, Bruce Smith missed an opportunity to challenge Clarke's pessimism. He should have mentioned the strategically important legislation which the provincial secretary had introduced in 1913 and 1914. These two acts provided the legislative foundation for the development of the reception hospital in Toronto.[50]

Under the 1913 act, the ancient term "asylum" was abandoned and replaced by "hospital for the insane." Provisions were also made for voluntary admission. Voluntary patients, who were required to be legally competent, could not be detained for more than five days after giving written notice of their desire to leave.

Another part of the act made it illegal to commit or to detain an insane person in a gaol, lock-up, prison, or reformatory while the question of insanity was being determined. The ancient practice of confining "lunatics" in prisons was thereafter abolished in Ontario. Instead, municipalities were required to provide a suitable place where an insane person could be comfortably detained until the inspector and the superintendent of the hospital of the district could be contacted and admission to the hospital secured.

Finally, in order to prevent hospitals for the insane from being overcrowded with patients who might as well be cared for in a house of refuge, the act provided for the transfer of such patients. This included "quiet and harmless" patients who had recovered sufficiently to be cared for by friends, as well as those whose mental condition was due to senility. In these circumstances, the inspector could order patients to be removed to a house of refuge in the counties from which they were originally admitted. The "Board of Management and the Superintendent of such a House of Refuge shall admit such a patient and maintain him therein."[51]

As far as the City of Toronto was concerned, the noose was tightened on May 1st, 1914, by the *Act Respecting Reception Hospitals*. Although the act was permissive, the City of Toronto had no option except to agree to establish a reception hospital. To reduce the city's option, the government decided to close the reception hospital which had operated since 1913. Plans were also made to close the venerable Toronto asylum. The Queen Street patients would, it was proposed, be relocated to a completely new hospital for the insane being built, on the cottage plan, at Whitby. Meanwhile, to reduce overcrowding in the Toronto asylum, an advance party of 100 patients was sent to Whitby to assist with the construction. The patients lived in tents. The cottages, as they were built, were occupied by invalid soldiers.

Preoccupied with winning the "war to end all wars," the city and province could do little to improve the dreadful conditions which prevailed in the overcrowded and understaffed mental hospitals. Yet, had the City of Toronto fathers been vigilant they would have been shocked to discover the obligations which, under the *Reception Hospital Act*, the province had imposed upon them. The act obliged the city to "establish and equip" the hospital and be responsible for the cost of maintenance of patients. Under the same legislation, the government, through the lieutenant-governor-in-council, reserved the right to approve its location, design, and function. The staffing, operation, and control of the reception hospital would remain in government hands. Additional control over the governance and management of the reception hospital was provided for in the rules approved by order of the lieutenant-governor-in-council on July 28, 1914.

THE RECEPTION HOSPITAL

Reception wards, pioneered by C.K. Clarke at Rockwood in 1894 and at the Toronto Asylum in 1907, were established at the London Asylum in 1908 and at Brockville in 1916. The first separate reception hospital, an annex of the Toronto Hospital for the Insane, was opened in Toronto on July 4, 1913. Housed in an abandoned building, it was formerly used as the private patients pavilion of the old Toronto General Hospital, located on Gerrard Street East. The medical director was Harvey Clare, previously the assistant medical director at 999 Queen Street West. This building, far from ideal, was the only one available.

In 1916, the Toronto General building was requisitioned for war purposes and used as part of Riverdale Barracks. The reception hospital was then moved to the Bickford Home at the rear of Old Trinity College on Gorevale Avenue, Toronto (an even more unsuitable building). William McLean, resident physician of the reception hospital, provided a cheerful and insightful account of his work.[52] At the outset McLean states that the main purpose of the reception hospital was to admit and treat incipient cases of insanity. "It is a place where they can be admitted with the least possible delay, without the necessity of certification, and where the patients may be kept under observation of medical men specially trained for this work."⁵³ McLean continued:

> If the patient is found to require prolonged treatment, he is passed on as soon as convenient to the regular hospital for the Insane. If found to be normal or able to get along outside they are discharged back to their friends, after sufficient observation. If there seems to be a promise of recovery in a short while the patient is put under the proper rational treatment, and kept in the hospital if necessary, for as long as two months.⁵⁴

The reception hospital maintained an open-door policy, "refusing admission to no patient who seemed at all suitable for care or observation..."⁵⁵ The virtual elimination of admission formalities had some disadvantages, including the dumping of unsuitable patients by various public institutions, and the menace of infectious diseases among a closely confined population. McLean cites some examples of dumping:

> There was admitted to our wards within a few days, from three different public institutions or associations in the city, three patients. One aged lady, dying from a rodent cancer of the face; another, a young woman, in the last stages of tuberculosis; the third, a middle-aged woman, who came to our hospital so intoxicated that she fell down between the street and the door and had to be assisted into the hospital by our nurses. These three patients, admitted in quick succession to our female ward, presumably insane, but on short observation shown to have a mentality normal to their physical condition, almost discouraged those who desired to maintain the open door, and lead to a desire to increase the formalities of admittance...⁵⁶

Describing the social class and occupations of his patients, McLean stated:

> We have had medical men, ministers, lawyers, dentists, druggists and the wives of professional men. We have had the artisan, the railway man, the merchant, the man of wealth and leisure, and on through the whole gamut of social life, to the vagrant from the street. We have had the old man of fourscore years and two, and the boy of six.⁵⁷

According to McLean, the staff of the reception hospital were kept very busy. For example, between July 1914 and October 1915, 685 patients were admitted (roughly ten per week). Of these, 185 were admitted from the courts. The other 500 admissions were arranged by friends. After a short sojourn 360 (52 percent) were sent home. Two hundred and fifty (36 percent) were sent to the hospital for the insane. Fifty of them (20 percent) were paretics. Twenty-eight (four percent) died. Some of the remainder were discharged to other charitable institutions and 33 remained in residence.

These statistics provide a remarkable record of accomplishment for a war-time hospital, previously a private home, accommodating 35 patients. Reflecting on the inadequate accommodation, McLean hoped that the reception hospital idea could be "kept alive until a happier day shall arrive and, the war being over, attention can be again given to these problems, which are now quite properly given second place. Like the bear, we are, as it were, hibernating and awaiting our springtime."[58]

It is clear, however, that things were not going well at the reception hospital. In despair, Harvey Clare complained to W.W. Dunlop, inspector of asylums, prisons, and public charities. After pointing out that in January 1918, 45 patients were being housed in a building which had accommodation for 39, Clare reminded Dunlop that there is only one bathroom, with one tub and a common lavatory. This truly pathetic state of affairs is revealed by Clare's description of patients admitted in December 1919.

> Two acute tuberculous cases, three paretics, (these are syphilitic cases), three cases of acute alcoholism, eight imbeciles, two cases dying of acute heart disease, two cripples, two negroes, two shoplifters, three epileptics, eight cases of senility, four soldiers (two of whom were wounded in France), four puerperal cases (in each case the baby was less than two weeks old). One pregnant woman. Three cases who had attempted suicide. Two cases of paralysis from apoplexy, one Chinaman.[59]

Clare's letter continued:

> About one half the patients coming into this Hospital are women and men from good families, who have been accustomed to lives of refinement. In the Reception Hospital we have treated many women from the best homes in Toronto, and the purpose of my letter is to draw your attention to the almost impossible situation where we are compelled to recommend the Hospital to good, clean living, decent people, when we are admitting to the same room patients who will use the same bathroom and the same closet, and who are suffering from contagious diseases, such as syphilis, gonorrhea, tuberculosis, scabies, and all other forms of skin diseases.[60]

Clare concluded, "It may be that it is up to the City to provide a building suitable for this work, but it certainly is impossible to treat mental cases successfully under present surroundings."[61]

THE BATTLE FOR THE TORONTO PSYCHIATRIC HOSPITAL

More than 15,000 patients had passed through the old reception hospital before it was closed in 1920. During the war years, conditions at 999 Queen Street had also deteriorated to an alarming degree. For example, between 1912 and 1919 the patient population had increased from 952 to 1,269. The government seemed paralysed with indecision. It made no sense to renovate a building that was due to be abandoned and the new Whitby hospital was not yet available for occupation. This desperate situation was only relieved when the new hospital at Whitby, occupied by the militia from 1914-1919, was restored to the province. The officials wasted no time and, in 1920, 855 patients were transferred by train from Toronto to Whitby. However, during the following year, 635 patients were admitted to Queen Street. Price said that "this was the highest number of admissions in a single year ever recorded during the long history of Toronto Hospital for the Insane."[62] This deluge of admissions was obviously due to the closing of the reception hospital, which had functioned successfully as a filter.

Faced with the daunting task of rehabilitating the rapidly decaying Toronto Asylum building or investing in a new reception hospital, the provincial secretary chose the latter. In the end, because of the protracted negotiations with the City of Toronto and the University of Toronto, the province was forced to do both. However, under the terms of the *Reception Hospitals for the Insane Act*, 1914, the City of Toronto was compelled to establish and equip a reception hospital, which it clearly was reluctant to do. In comparison, as will be seen, the university's contribution to the reception hospital was civilized as well as modest.

Compared to the contortions of the City of Toronto, the University of Toronto's involvement in the establishment of TPH was exemplary. Under the 1910 agreement between the university and the Toronto General Hospital, the head of a university service became ex-officio head of the equivalent hospital service.[63] This arrangement provided a bridge between the university and the hospital and was designed to serve the interests of clinical research, teaching, and treatment. In this way, it was understood at the outset that the medical director of the new reception hospital would also serve as the professor of psychiatry. Until he fell into disfavour with the government, it was always assumed that C.K. Clarke would occupy this position. Although unpopular with the Ontario government, Clarke was not without influence in the university and medical communities.

Clarke's influence across Canada was enhanced by his appointment in 1918 as the medical director of the Canadian National Committee for Mental Hygiene (CNCMH), now the Canadian Mental Health Association. The objectives of the CNCMH included war work and the cross-Canada provision of facilities for diagnosing and treating mental disease. War work involved assessing the adequacy of care being provided to returned soldiers suffering from mental disabilities. In his reminiscences of C.K. Clarke, C.B. Farrar recalled the tours of inspection of the provincial mental hospitals across Canada undertaken at the request of the Dominion Department of Soldiers' Civil Re-establishment in 1919–20.

> It was desirable that one Inspector outside the government should be engaged; Dr. Clarke was the obvious choice, and it was my privilege, as chief psychiatrist for the Department, to be associated with him on this tour. Beginning with British Columbia, institutions in the four western provinces were comfortably surveyed, provincial and hospital authorities offering every possible assistance. In Winnipeg word reached us that Clarke would not be permitted to visit any of the Ontario Hospitals. In his home province which he had served so faithfully and so long and with such splendid results he was persona non grata as far as the government of the day was concerned.[64]

What Clarke felt about this exhibition of churlishness is not recorded. But it is unlikely that his enthusiasm was diminished by the Ontario government's embarrassing lack of civility. In fact, as will be seen, under Clarke's direction the Canadian National Committee for Mental Hygiene flourished. Together with Clarence Hincks, the associate medical director and secretary, and with Charles Martin, dean of medicine at McGill University, as president, a vast range of mental health activities was launched across Canada. Most notable were the mental health surveys undertaken at the request of the governments of Manitoba (1918), British Columbia (1919), and Saskatchewan and Nova Scotia (1920). Only the provinces of Ontario and Quebec refused to allow surveys to be undertaken in their facilities.

Hincks, who had worked with Clarke at the Toronto General psychiatric outpatients clinic from 1914–1918, had many skills. He was, for example, a gifted but sometimes intemperate orator. In a rabble-rousing address to the Ontario Education Association, Hincks blasted the Ontario government for their neglect of the mentally ill and said that he had enough scandalous information to "blow up the Parliament Buildings." Predictably, this florid statement made headline news in the *Toronto Star* on April 1, 1920. One scholar described what followed:

> Howard Ferguson was then the leader of the Opposition, and next day on the floor of the House he waved a copy of the Star at Premier Drury and demanded to know who this character was. "Probably an immigrant," he suggested, and if so "he should be deported." Drury indicated that for once he could agree with the Leader of the Opposition.[65]

Following this illuminating parliamentary exchange, Hincks arranged a private meeting with Premier Drury and Harry Nixon, provincial secretary. When Nixon admitted that the Hincks account of the wretched conditions in the Ontario hospitals was not exaggerated, Drury apologized and agreed to table Hincks' report without comment. Much to the satisfaction of Clarke and the CNCMH, the national press published the report and Hincks' reputation was vindicated. This event served, no doubt, to speed the faltering negotiations with the city concerning the establishment of the new reception hospital.

In addition to being a spell-binding public speaker, Clarence Hincks was an inspired fund-raiser. Seeking funds to support the ambitious research program initiated by the committee, Hincks approached the Rockefeller Foundation. In a very short time Hincks developed close friendships with several of the directors, including Edwin Embree, the secretary, who took a personal interest in Canadian mental health issues. As a result, five million Rockefeller dollars were used to support worthy Canadian projects, including the University of Toronto's faculty of medicine.

With the promise of a substantial grant from the Rockefeller Foundation, the University of Toronto established a committee to consider the requirements of the Faculty of Medicine. In March 1920, the committee made several recommendations. One of them was the erection of a psychopathic hospital of at least 85 beds in or near the grounds of the Toronto General Hospital.

The institution should include
 (a) An outdoor department with adequate staff for social work, parole, etc.
 (b) Adequate laboratories for research in metabolism and pathology and psychology.
 (c) Quarters for treatment by physical and occupational means.
 (d) A library.[66]

These recommendations were promptly accepted by the Rockefeller Foundation. On November 19, 1920, in a letter to Falconer, the university president, a $1 million grant to the University of Toronto was announced. This included "approximately $500,000 for the new psychiatric clinic."[67]

THE TOWN, CROWN, AND GOWN AGREEMENT

After months of negotiation, threats, and promises, in 1921 a formal agreement was reached between the town, crown, and gown. The object of the agreement was to secure the building of a reception hospital, to be called "The Reception Hospital of Toronto," on land owned by the University of Toronto. This agreement bound the City of Toronto to proceed with the erection of the hospital according to plans approved by the provincial secretary and the (university) governors and "equip it to the like satisfaction."

> The government of Ontario is required to maintain the hospital, provide for its upkeep and provide clinical facilities for the University of Toronto for the teaching of psychiatry by the regular staff of the hospital.[68]

The staff of the hospital would be selected and appointed after consultation with the university.

The city and the province reluctantly agreed to locate the reception hospital at 2 Surrey Place, a site owned by the university. Nevertheless, Inspector W.W. Dunlop had strong feelings about this matter. Writing to the provincial secretary on March 15, 1921, he said:

> I have come to the conclusion that if the government approves putting this building on a site offered by the University to the City of Toronto, it will damn posterity for all time to come.
>
> One needs no imagination to know that from Yonge Street to University Avenue will be business blocks before many years. The City has already started to tear down residences to accommodate the Terauley Street extension. What does that mean? It

means above College Street just what it means below College Street. Residences were turned into business houses, large blocks were constructed, and you will find in ten years from now that the whole line will be a business thoroughfare. Where will our hospital be at that time? Stuck like a wart in between the back yards and laneways of business blocks. It is not my intention to say anything in public against the site offered, but I wish to be on record that it is not acceptable to me, and that I disapprove of putting the building on any site that will be as cramped as indicated by these plans.

I might add that the only argument I have ever heard in favour of the University site was to save the time of the students, and the argument I think is very flimsy, but if it really did mean a loss of time to the student, it would be eminently better for the Government to agree to have at least two motor carryalls ready and at the disposal of the students who would attend the lectures on certain days in each week, but, with the means of transportation in this City, the easy methods we have of getting to and from different sections of the City, I doubt if it is good business to break down our whole system just for the simple idea that it is going to lose a little time for the students at college.

This hospital should have lots of space, and it wants to be on a site where there is no possibility of being surrounded by business blocks for the next fifty years.[69]

Dunlop's gloomy predictions were both right and wrong. The space at TPH was most inadequate and there was no room to expand. A chronic problem over the years was the lack of space for an outpatient department, which was a central feature of a psychiatric service. He was obviously wrong in assuming that the TPH would be shrouded by "business blocks." Except for the enlarged Woman's College Hospital and some new government and university buildings, the appearance of College Street between Yonge and University has changed very little since the 1920s.

There were two further sticking points. Both are interesting examples of the power and control exerted by the university. The university wanted an inclined floor in the lecture theatre. This made good sense from the student's point of view, but it made the room virtually useless for other activities, such as occupational therapy or a sitting room for patients and their visitors. The government representatives argued that since space was at a premium, public areas, such as the lecture theatre, should be designed to serve various purposes, but the university remained unconvinced and unmoved.

Appointing the medical director and the new professor of psychiatry also provided a battlefield for the exercise of power. The first sign of belligerence came with a seemingly innocuous letter dated December 8, 1923, from Goldwin W. Howland, chief of neurology at the Toronto General Hospital, to Ryan. Howland explained that he was a member of a university nominating committee for the medical director of the new reception hospital and professor of psychiatry to succeed C.K. Clarke. Ryan was invited to make a recommendation, in confidence. Instead, Ryan sent Howland's letter to W.W. Dunlop, the inspector representing the provincial secretary. A few days later, on December 12, Dunlop fired off this response to Howland:

> ...I gather that a Committee has been appointed, the status of which is not apparent to this Department but which, if the aims and objects mentioned in your letter were carried out, would appear to seriously endanger the entente cordiale which has heretofore existed between the signatories of the Agreement, between the Provincial Government, the University of Toronto and the Corporation of the City of Toronto, in the establishment of a Reception Hospital.
>
> I am sure you will appreciate that one of the outstanding features of the Agreement above referred to was to bring about harmonious working arrangements between the parties concerned and thus provide the only possible conditions under which this Institution could be established and operated.
>
> This department is most anxious that these relations between the various parties interested should continue, and views with apprehension the appointment of the Committee to which you state you belong, and the appointment of which this Department has not been advised.[70]

After assuring Howland that the government had no intention of delegating its control of all appointments, Dunlop concluded in a more conciliatory fashion. "I am sure that you will not misunderstand my object in writing to you, and should you at any time desire further information on the subject, do not hesitate to write to me."[71]

Goldwin Howland responded next day, December 13, with characteristic nonchalance:

Awfully sorry but you have got the wrong idea. The committee is to discuss the selection of a Prof. of Psychiatry, and is formed by the new Government regulations. It has no relationship to the Superintendent, or the staff of the Reception Hospital, and my meaning, so badly expressed, should have been, "in charge of the University teaching in Psychiatry probably at the Reception Hospital."

I do not even know whether it would be wise for the Superintendent and the Professor to be one and the same, that I suppose will later come before your Department, but I wrote a private letter to certain personal friends and I'm glad to say that they all apparently understood the situation as I have their answers. I am sorry that you were bothered by this misconception as I have no doubt that the relationship between the University, the Government and the City will always be as happy as it is now.[72]

Upset by Howland's unconciliatory letter, Dunlop lost no time in acquainting his boss, Lincoln Goldie, provincial secretary, with some other disturbing gossip. Considering the significance of the message, the flippant tone of Dunlop's first paragraph is surprising. His December 17, 1923, memo started:

Because of certain rumours emanating from a source which I have always regarded as a little bit too advanced for the demands of the people, I mean this hygiene and uplift organization, I am attaching certain papers which will give you a brief outline of the purpose of the Reception Hospital in Toronto, and how it should function.

I am doing this because you will shortly be called upon to hear a deputation from outside organizations, possibly including some of the faculty of the University, to entertain a proposal for the engagement of Dr. McFie [sic] Campbell, who is now Director of the Boston Psychiatric [sic] Hospital. The arrangement as rumoured is that the Rockefeller Foundation Fund would advance to McFie Campbell $5,000.00 through the Toronto University if he would take hold of the work in Toronto, the Government to supplement the plans and pay all expenses in connection with the hospital.[73]

Dunlop's main complaint was not with Charles MacFie Campbell, medical director of the Boston Psychopathic Hospital, but with what he regarded as the excessive cost of patient care (six to seven dollars a day) there. He was also concerned because the Boston Psychopathic, under

MacFie Campbell, was an ultra-scientific hospital which failed to meet the needs of ordinary people. Dunlop's preference was that,

> The Reception Hospital in the City of Toronto should be a mecca of scientific treatment for mental cases in the incipient form, for the teaching of psychiatry for the University, for the training of graduate nurses in the handling of mental diseases, and should be a clearing house for this great centre for every mental case coming within notice of its several branches.[74]

Dunlop concluded: "I have gone to some length to acquaint you with this matter, but I think it is my duty to arm you with this outline so that you will be prepared when the time comes."[75] However, MacFie Campbell was not interested in coming to Toronto, even with the inducement of a Rockefeller grant. Instead, after considerable negotiation, Clarence B. Farrar accepted the joint appointment as medical superintendent and as professor of psychiatry.

To tell the rest of this story coherently, we must move back and examine the part played by C.K. Clarke in maintaining the momentum for the complicated undertaking of the negotiations between the province and the city.

TOWN AND CROWN

Anticipating the closure of the reception hospital in January 1919, the provincial secretary instructed Dunlop to ask the law department what should be requested of the City of Toronto. Responding to the provincial secretary on February 14, Dunlop recommended:

> ...that the Council of the City of Toronto be informed immediately that on the first day of May, if the studies for plans for a Reception Hospital have not been submitted to the Department for approval and the site selected for such Hospital, the Department of the Provincial Secretary will close the institution so far as the government is concerned, requiring the City to make application for their patients to the regular Hospital for the Insane as any other municipality in the Province; also drawing the attention of the Council to the fact that the Toronto Hospital for the Insane will shortly be closed and all patients removed to Whitby, and that the Hospitals for the Insane Act requires that no insane person shall be confined in a Gaol or Reformatory.[76]

The province had taken this uncompromising stand when, despite years of negotiation, the City of Toronto still evaded its responsibilities for the reception hospital. For example, in 1912, an abortive attempt was made by the city to settle on a site at the foot of Dowling Avenue, on the lakefront in South Parkdale. In a letter to the provincial inspector dated August 16, 1912, George R. Geary, mayor of Toronto, explained that the site was rejected because "It appears to be held at much too high a price, and its selection moreover has aroused a great feeling of protest amongst the people of Parkdale."[77] Several other properties were considered and rejected for various reasons. This cat-and-mouse game continued for several years. At last, in desperation, the government established the reception hospital in the old pavilion of the Toronto General. The city's magnanimous contribution was 40 beds and bedding.

On the instructions of the provincial secretary, Dunlop threatened the City of Toronto with dire action. His letter of April 9, 1919, to D. Chisholm, property commissioner, described the perilous state of the reception hospital and concluded:

> The building has been condemned by every physician who ever visited it. It has been condemned by your own Health Officer, and now we condemn it and tell you frankly and plainly that on the first of May, if you do not have in our hands an undertaking to provide an institution that will be worthy of the name of a Reception or Psychopathic Hospital, the Government will close the doors and you will have to place the patients coming from the Courts in the Gaol, as we did five years ago.[78]

While the provincial government goaded the city into action, the government, in turn, was being coerced by C.K. Clarke and his colleagues. Their attack was both direct and indirect. For example, in his presentation to the Hodgins Commission (Royal Commission on the Care and Control of the Mentally Defective and Feeble-Minded, 1919) on May 1, 1919, Clarke complained that no progress was being made in building a reception hospital because the city and the province were playing "Battledore and Shuttlecock" with each other. Next day, Justice Hodgins sent an unsolicited transcript of Clarke's evidence to the provincial secretary.

On the day prior to his appearance before the Hodgins Commission, C.K. Clarke was part of an elite delegation to the City of Toronto Board of Control, which was considering the reception hospital. The next major step entailed a joint delegation meeting with William McPherson, provincial secretary; Isaac Lucas, attorney general; and Finlay McDairmid, the minister of public works. This meeting, which took place on May 27, was attended by three representatives from the board of control, the medical profession, local Council of Women and other bodies. The medical profession was represented by Alexander Primrose, Academy of Medicine; Charles Hastings, medical officer of health; and the ubiquitous C.K. Clarke from the Canadian National Committee for Mental Hygiene. Gordon Bates and Mrs. Archibald Huestis represented the Toronto Branch of the Association for the Care of the Feeble-Minded. Other distinguished deputants included Jean Gunn (superintendent of nurses, Toronto General Hospital), representatives from the Neighborhood Workers' Association, the Rotary Club, and the Social Services Council of Ontario. With one exception, all the deputants favoured the building of the reception hospital. The dissenting voice was that of Campbell Meyers. Once again, he opposed the psychiatric clinic and favoured the re-establishment of the nervous ward at the Toronto General Hospital. At the close of the hearing, a private meeting was held between the provincial secretary, Inspector Dunlop, and the two of the controllers.

Although the City of Toronto had agreed in principle to spend $400,000 on the reception hospital, the lengthy correspondence between Chisholm, property manager representing the city, and Dunlop, representing the provincial secretary, lacks enthusiasm for this decision. Two issues were particularly contentious. The city wanted to build the hospital on its property on the north end of Trinity Park, but this was unacceptable to the university. Next, although the city had agreed to build the hospital, it wanted the government to equip it. On more than one occasion, Dunlop referred Chisholm to the 1914 act which confirmed that the city council was obliged to "establish and equip a Reception Hospital." Yet Dunlop was willing to compromise without appearing to do so. For example, on February 17, 1920, he wrote:

> In my humble judgement I believe the word 'equip' means that the Municipality shall equip the Institution with the necessary therapeutic appliances, electrical fixtures, stove and cooking utensils, but not the actual furniture, which the Government has always maintained as better left at our discretion than outside interests.[79]

The latter comment seems ambiguous—perhaps deliberately so.

In order to prevent the city from reneging, a public meeting was held on March 29, 1920, under the auspices of the Canadian National Committee for Mental Hygiene in the medical building of the University of Toronto. A resolution was passed urging the government to build a reception hospital without further delay, in the vicinity of the Toronto

General Hospital. Those present also decided that three "spokesmen" should meet with the provincial secretary on April 7 at 11 a.m. and with the city council at a time to be arranged. As agreed, on April 7, a deputation met with Harry Nixon, provincial secretary, and Robert Grant, the minister of education. Their aim was to persuade the government to provide a more central site for the new reception hospital.

Curiously, attendees of the meeting at the medical building also recommended the immediate establishment of a temporary reception hospital. In retrospect, the deputation's request that the city should provide a temporary reception hospital seems puzzling. Nevertheless, such an arrangement would have served to relieve the pressure on the dangerously overcrowded Toronto Hospital at 999 Queen Street. Also, it was reported that cases of insanity or suspected insanity were being sent to the Toronto Jail, although this was illegal. For these reasons the CNCMH, headed by C.K. Clarke, had taken an option on renting the Spadina military hospital, which they offered to hand over to the board of control.

Was this merely a stratagem to spur the city into building the reception hospital on the university site without further delay? Stratagem or not, Clarke's proposal for a temporary reception hospital was ignored, and the bickering between the town and the crown continued for several years—even after the opening of TPH in 1925.

There is a striking resemblance between the exterior of the Toronto Psychiatric Hospital and Kraepelin's psychiatric clinic in Munich. Was this a coincidence or was the city architect encouraged to copy the Munich design? In the absence of documentary evidence, this question cannot be answered with confidence. For symbolic and sentimental reasons, it should be assumed that C.K. Clarke probably had a hand in the design. After all, the hospital's function and the tri-partite arrangement which governed the foundation of TPH was borrowed from Munich. And Clarke had the highest hopes for the future of Kraepelinian psychiatry.

In preparation for the building of the new reception hospital, in January 1922, Edward Ryan and James Govan set off on a tour of mental hospitals in Ann Arbor, Michigan, New York, and Boston. On February 2, 1922, the committee responsible for planning the reception hospital at 2 Surrey Place made its first report. Its members included Harvey Clare and Edward Ryan; G.F.W. Price, architect for the City of Toronto; James Govan, government architect; and W.W. Dunlop.

After considering the function of the hospital, the committee made five key recommendations. First, it should serve as a place for the examination and diagnosis of suspected mental illness. Second, it should provide early treatment of the incipient and mild cases. Third, it should encourage preventive treatment of mental cases; that is, the hospital to act as a centre whereby these patients could be treated, either in the institution or in their home. Fourth, it should provide for the teaching of nervous and mental diseases to the medical students of the University of Toronto. Five, it should act as a centre for research.[80]

The committee recommended that initially the hospital should have 60 beds (30 each for men and women), but that provisions should be made for 40 additional beds. The architect was also required to provide space for various functions, including preventive work, classrooms for thirty students, two small rooms for instructional purposes, and accommodation for medical and nursing staff. A sign of the times, it was recommended that the male and female staff quarters should be segregated.

Formal plans for the reception hospital were submitted to Sir Robert Falconer in March 1922. He, in turn, asked Duncan Graham, chief of medicine at Toronto General and professor of medicine, to look them over. In the same month, the City of Toronto formally agreed to make the sum of $400,000 available for the building. On May 29, 1922, contracts were awarded for building the reception hospital.

A RECEPTION HOSPITAL AT LAST

The four Toronto newspapers provided handsome coverage of the cornerstone laying ceremony for the Toronto Reception Hospital held on October 12, 1923. The ceremony, presided over by Mayor Maguire, was both brief and simple. Not more than 50 people were present, including C.K. Clarke and his son Eric Kent Clarke, also a psychiatrist. Representing the University of Toronto, Sir Robert Falconer spoke first. He said:

> The Institution was a monument to the enlightenment, intelligence and progressiveness of the efforts now being made to treat mental disease in the same skilful manner and scientific manner as other forms of disease. It was also a fine demonstration of what could be accomplished by friendly co-operation, for unless the city, the Government and the University had co-operated the

hospital could not have been built and the medical profession would have been unable to do their part in making the institution the success it was destined to become.[81]

Similar sentiments were expressed in brief addresses by C.K. Clarke, Alex Primrose, Harvey Clare, and Robert A. Pyne, former minister of education in the Whitney government. Rev. Edwin Henry, pastor of the Deer Park Presbyterian Church, asked for Divine blessing on the institution. Lincoln Goldie, provincial secretary, was present, but did not speak. Strange behaviour for a politician!

> Mayor Maguire, who had been presented with a silver trowel, spread the mortar and dropped the stone into position, at the same time declaring it to be well and truly laid. Deposited in the cavity of the stone was a copper box containing copies of the Toronto daily newspapers of the day, their reports on the Lloyd George visit, a typewritten report on the day's proceedings with the name of those taking part, and other souvenirs.[82]

In addition to its news report, the *Toronto Star* marked the occasion with an inspiring editorial in which the history of the reception hospital was traced. The editorial concluded: "there was never a time when so great a proportion of people lived at high tension, and mental and nervous disorders are the natural outcome. In many instances a cure is possible."[83]

A somewhat distorted version of this event was recalled almost 34 years later by Clarke's son Eric. In a letter (October 11, 1957) to C.B. Farrar, he wrote:

> I was particularly touched by your reference to his being persona non grata in the Ontario Hospital system during the last few years of his life. One of his last trips outside the house before his death was to the ceremony of the laying of the corner-stone of the new Psychiatric Hospital on Surrey Place. As you recall he was not on the platform of dignitaries for the ceremony—but stood in the crowd in the rain—a really pathetic disillusioned sick old man.[84]

This sad picture is, fortunately, contradicted by the contemporary press. For example, the *Globe* (October 13, 1923) published a picture of C.K. Clarke and reported that he made a brief speech. Pyne mentioned, "Dr. Clarke's long labour to have the reception hospital established here; for 25 years Dr. Clarke worked with this end in view."[85] So, while the stone-laying ceremony was obviously not designed to honour C.K. Clarke, to suggest that he was deliberately ignored is untrue. The strange tricks that memory plays on aging minds are intriguing but difficult to explain. Was it "wish fulfillment" that led Eric Clarke to remember his father as a "pathetic figure" standing in the rain? For according to weather records, it did not rain in Toronto on October 12, 1923.

C.B. FARRAR, PROFESSOR OF PSYCHIATRY AND MEDICAL SUPERINTENDENT

Except for the brief alarm about the prospect of MacFie Campbell coming to Toronto, there was only one candidate for medical director: C.B. Farrar, a friend of C.K. Clarke, who trained with Kraepelin and Alzheimer in Germany. Farrar had been in charge at Homewood for less than a year when rumours of his University of Toronto appointment started to circulate. Then, on February 1, 1924, his appointment as professor of psychiatry in the Faculty of Medicine was announced. Although the negotiations leading to Farrar's joint appointments took several weeks to complete, there are no records of the issues which had to be resolved. The negotiations with university president, Sir Robert Falconer, were probably straightforward. The negotiations with Lincoln Goldie, provincial secretary, were evidently much more difficult. This can be assumed because at one stage an impasse was reached and Farrar declined the appointment. Then, shortly after a third-party intervention, Farrar's appointment was formally announced on January 23, 1925 (see pp. 80–82 for further details).

We can only speculate about the nature of the differences between Lincoln Goldie and C.B. Farrar. My guess is that it concerned the power of the medical superintendent to hire and fire staff with the minimum of political interference. This hunch is, to some extent, supported by a confidential memorandum from Goldie to Dunlop dated January 20, 1925. Headed "Re: Reception Hospital," the memorandum reads: "Before any appointments are made to the above institution remind me to consult Col. Price."

Price, a former lieutenant colonel and MPP for Parkdale, was the treasurer of Ontario from 1923–26 and attorney general from 1926–34. Since in those days patronage appointments were quite common, it seems reasonable to assume that, in addition to his other cabinet duties, Price was responsible for vetting government appointments. Support for this view is provided by Clifford Scott, the doyen of psychoanalysis in Canada, who was one of the first student interns at TPH. Recalling those days (1925–26), Scott said,

Politics were important when the Toronto Psychiatric Hospital was opened. Farrar was sad to tell me a couple of days before I was supposed to come in as a student intern that the appointment was out of his hands, and "political." I wanted the job so much that I spent two days (for the only time in my life) politically lobbying and luckily got the job.[86]

Discussing this recently, Scott remembered seeking his father's advice. He, in turn, recommended a talk with the minister of his church. The minister, who was well connected, promptly arranged for Scott to be catechized by a senior member of the government at Queen's Park.

TORONTO PSYCHIATRIC HOSPITAL OPENS

The first patients were admitted to the Toronto Psychiatric Hospital on December 18, 1925. Except for a tour of the facility by Ontario Medical Association (OMA) members, there was no formal opening ceremony. The opening, planned for July 1, was deferred because the government architect complained that the refrigeration unit and the kitchen equipment were improperly installed. Due to these and other differences of opinion as to whether the building was properly completed, according to contract or not, relationships between the city and the government were strained.

Evidence of these tensions was, however, carefully concealed from the OMA annual meeting held in Toronto on May 6, 1925. Farrar welcomed the OMA members and cordially invited them to the new hospital. They were addressed by Lincoln Goldie and by Henry J. Cody representing the university board of governors. Although present, the mayor did not speak. While not inspiring, the remarks of others were predictable. Goldie stated "the Government would take over the Psychiatric Hospital as soon as Mayor Foster turns it over to us." Cody said,

> This new hospital is unlike any other in the province, because it is not only for those who we call insane, but will also be a teaching place for training medical men. It marks the new attitude of the scientific world towards insanity.[87]

Farrar, whose talk made headlines in the *Toronto Star,* said that, "One of the features of the Toronto Psychiatric Hospital will be the study of criminals."[88] This was the first step in the development of forensic psychiatry in Canada. Farrar also explained that he wanted the atmosphere of TPH to be in every way just like an ordinary hospital. "It will be a place where a patient's relatives can call upon him, just as if he were at the General Hospital, and a place into which he is admitted in just the same way."[89] It is clear that those present believed that a new era in the history of psychiatry in Canada was about to begin. Tragically, C.K. Clarke was not present to savour the fruits of his labour.

Endnotes

[1]C.K. Clarke.
[2]Clarke, as cited in Cyril Greenland, *Charles Kirk Clarke—A Pioneer of Canadian Psychiatry* (Toronto: Clarke Institute of Psychiatry, 1966), p. 8.
[3]*Annual Report of the Inspectors of Hospitals for the Insane*, 1915.
[4]*Annual Report of the Inspectors of Hospitals for the Insane*, 1925.
[5]John Scott, as cited in Gifford C. Price, "History of the Ontario Hospital, Toronto: The Development of Institutional Care and Treatment of the Mentally Ill in Ontario As Revealed Through the History of the Ontario Hospital" MSW thesis, (Toronto: University of Toronto, August 1989), p. 40.

[6]Ibid, p. 41. Price reports that on two occasions Scott was "'severely censured and admonished' by the Board who considered him to be indiscrete and lacking in judgement."
[7]Greenland, p. 10.
[8]T.J.W. Burgess, as cited in *Dominion Medical Monthly* 29 (3): 136 (September 1907).
[9]C.K.Clarke, "Annual Report of the Medical Superintendent for the Insane, Kingston, for the year ending September 30, 1893" in *The Report of the Inspector of Lunatic and Idiot Asylums* (1893).
[10]Ibid.
[11]Ibid.
[12]Ibid.
[13]*Bulletin of the Ontario Hospital for the Insane*, 9 (1): 3-9 (October 1916). This issue of the *Bulletin* has generated discussion as the date for the issue 9 (1) follows that of 9 (2) printed in January 1916 and evidently the publication ceased with volume 9 (4), dated July 1916.
[14]Archives of Ontario RG 8 1-1-A Box 39. "Provincial Secretary Correspondence 1916-1919."
[15]Ibid.
[16]Ibid.
[17]"A Psychiatric Clinic," *Bulletin of the Toronto Hospital for the Insane*, 1 (1): 6 (1907).
[18]Ibid.
[19]C.K. Clarke, "The need of a Psychiatric Clinic," *Bulletin of Ontario Hospital for the Insane*, 8 (3): 108 (April 1915).
[20]See Edward Shorter's chapter on Farrar (Chapter 3).
[21]*Dominion Medical Monthly* 29 (3): 1 (September 1907).
[22]Ontario Legislative Assembly, *Report of Commission on the Methods Employed in Caring for and Treating the Insane* (Toronto: L.K. Cameron, 1908). The report of the commission, probably written by Clarke, consists of twelve printed pages, addressed to W.J. Hanna, M.P.P., provincial secretary.
[23]Ibid.

[24] Richard Andrew Paskauskas, "Ernest Jones: A Critical Study of his Scientific Development (1896-1913)," PhD. Thesis (Toronto: University of Toronto, c1985), p. 182.
[25] Ibid, p. 182.
[26] C.K. Clarke, as cited in Greenland, pp. 18-19.
[27] Paskauskas, p. 183.
[28] A. Ross Diefendorf, *Clinical Psychiatry: A Textbook for Students and Physicians*, Abstracted and adapted from the Seventh German Edition of Emil Kraepelin's *Lehrbuch der Psychiatrie*, New edition, revised and augmented (New York and London: Macmillan, 1907); and Emil Kraepelin, *Psychiatrie: ein Lehrbuch für Studierende und Aertze*, as cited in Paskauskas, p. 177.
[29] *University of Toronto Monthly* 8: 139-41 (1907-8).
[30] Paskauskas, pp. 183-99.
[31] Ibid, pp. 191-92.
[32] Ibid, pp. 193-94.
[33] Greenland, p. 15.
[34] Edward Ryan, "Seven Years' Advance in the Ontario Hospitals for Mental Diseases," *Bulletin of the Ontario Hospitals for the Insane* 6 (1): 3-11 (October 1912).
[35] Ibid, p. 3.
[36] Ibid, p. 7.
[37] Ibid, p. 7.
[38] Ibid, p. 7.
[39] Ibid, p. 9.
[40] Donald Campbell Meyers, as cited in Robert Pos, Allan Walters and Frank Sommers, "The History of Psychiatry, the Toronto General Hospital," confidential, unedited, unabridged working draft dated October 1972. QSMHC Archives.
[41] Pos, p. 21.
[42] C.K. Clarke as cited in Pos, p. 35-36.
[43] Pos, p. 36.
[44] C.K. Clarke, *Bulletin of the Ontario Hospitals for the Insane* 8 (3): 104 (April 1915).
[45] Ibid.
[46] Ibid, p. 106.
[47] Ibid, p. 107.
[48] Ibid.
[49] Ibid, p. 108.
[50] Ontario Legislative Assembly, "An Act Respecting Provincial Hospitals for the Insane and the Custody of Insane Persons," assented to May 6, 1913; and "An Act respecting Reception Hospitals for the Insane," assented to May 1, 1914.
[51] Act of May 6, 1913.
[52] W.J. McLean, "The Reception Hospital," *Bulletin of the Ontario Hospitals for the Insane* 9 (2): 47 (January 1916).
[53] Ibid.
[54] Ibid.
[55] Ibid.
[56] Ibid.
[57] Ibid.
[58] Ibid.

[59] Archives of Ontario RG 10-107-0-1010. "Psychiatric Hospital" Box 161.
[60] Ibid.
[61] Ibid.
[62] Price, p. 90.
[63] Pos, p. 34.
[64] C.B. Farrar, "I remember C.K. Clarke," draft for publication in *American Journal of Psychiatry*, 1957. QSMHC Archives.
[65] J.D. Griffin, *In Search of Sanity: A Chronicle of the Canadian Mental Health Association, 1918-1988* (London, ON: Third Eye, 1989), p. 25.
[66] "Report of the committee appointed to consider the requirements of the faculty in view of a possible grant of money from the Rockefeller Foundation", dated March 21, 1920. QSMHC Archives.
[67] George Vincent (president of the Rockefeller Foundation) to Sir Robert Falconer (president of University of Toronto). QSMHC Archives RFRG.1/s.427/s.s.Canada/Box10/Folder 79.
[68] Archives of Ontario RG 10-107-0 -1010. "Psychiatric Hospital" Box 161.
[69] Ibid.
[70] Ibid.
[71] Ibid.
[72] Ibid.
[73] Ibid.
[74] Ibid.
[75] Ibid.
[76] Ibid.
[77] Ibid.
[78] Ibid.
[79] Ibid.
[80] Ibid.
[81] *Toronto Star* October 13, 1923.
[82] Ibid.
[83] *Toronto Star* October 13, 1923.
[84] Farrar private archive.
[85] *The Globe*, October 13, 1923.
[86] See Clifford Scott's chapter (Chapter 7).
[87] *Toronto Star* May 7, 1925.
[88] Ibid.
[89] Ibid.

3

C. B. Farrar: A Life

Edward Shorter

Clarence B. Farrar figures in our story because he was the first director of TPH, opening the hospital in 1925 and leaving it in 1947 the premier institute for training psychiatrists in English Canada. Yet Farrar matters in the history of psychiatry for other reasons as well. He lived to be 95. His life spanned an enormous stretch of psychiatric history, encompassing most of the good, and some of the bad, in North American psychiatry in the fist half of the twentieth century.

Thus we should not recreate Farrar's life for reasons of marginal importance. Its significance lies not in the fact that he edited the *American Journal of Psychiatry*, one of the world's leading psychiatric publications, for more than three decades. Nor does Farrar claim our attention as a major academic psychiatrist, for he wrote no big book and virtually ceased doing hands-on research after he came to Canada. He is interesting as a symbolic figure; his long life reached across not one but two sea changes in world psychiatry: the eclipse of biological psychiatry by psychoanalysis, and the reassertion of biological psychiatry towards the end of his life. He participated intimately in these events and left us a full record.

Early Life

Farrar was born November 27, 1874, in Cattaraugus, New York, an upstate village with a population then of around 900. His mother, Marie Hawkins, was a homemaker; his father, Thomas Jefferson Farrar, was a small businessman who sold insurance locally and directed a mining company whose head office was located in Cattaraugus. The ambience in which Farrar grew up, an ambience in which he remained immersed throughout his life, was that of upper-middle-class gentility. A photograph shows a large Victorian frame house, built around 1890, with an

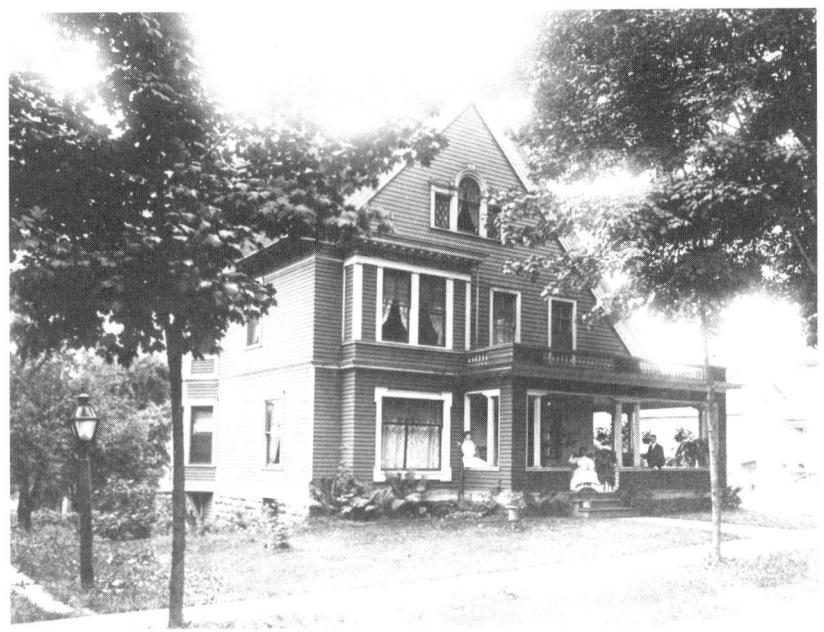

C. B. Farrar's childhood home in Cattaraugus, N.Y., c. 1890.

extensive front porch and ladies sitting in long dresses. Farrar, who must have been in his late teens when the photo was taken, stands pencil-thin in the background. (He was five feet nine inches tall and weighed about a hundred and thirty pounds.)

It is interesting that, although he had an apparently happy childhood, he later looked back upon Cattaraugus as something of a snakepit, at least from a psychiatric point of view. In this village of 900, he later noted, there were "43 disturbed families...ca. one family in five involved, adding unrecognized cases, probably at least one in three."

"M.," a female member of one family tree, was said to be of "poor stock, lack judgment, extravagant, no management, later religious insanity."[1] He drew in other similarly burdened family trees. From early on in life, Farrar was interested in afflictions of the mind and brain, and even when growing up he paid close attention to the issues that filled the psychiatric textbooks of his day.

Farrar did the "classical" program of studies at Cattaraugus high school with emphasis upon languages and saw himself as bound for medical school. In 1891, the year of his graduation, the state of New York issued him a "medical student certificate."

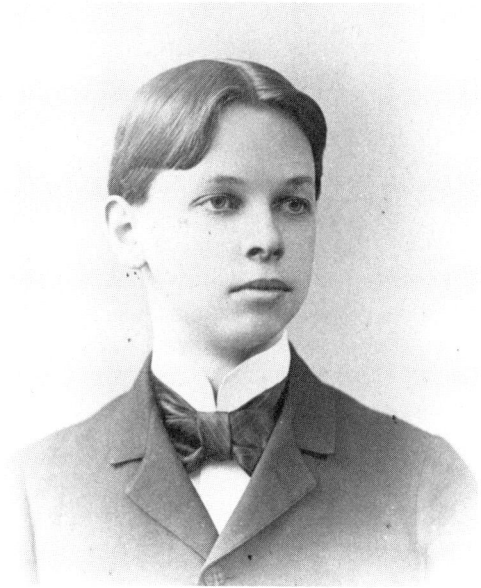

Clarence B. Farrar as a boy.

But Farrar did not enroll in any of the many little medical schools that would have accepted him immediately from high school. He spent the next two years as an undergraduate at Allegheny College in Meadville, Pennsylvania, transferring then to Harvard for his last two years. It was at Harvard that Farrar, a student of such famous professors as the philosopher George Santayana and the psychologist William James, began to experience the excitement of learning. "To one coming to Harvard, as I did, from a small college where the curriculum was in the main prescribed, there opened an almost boundless horizon, a vast garden of learning where one might pluck the fruits..."[2]

Graduating from Harvard College in 1896, Farrar spent the next year at Harvard medical school, then decided to transfer to the new Faculty of Medicine, just opened in 1893, at Johns Hopkins University in Baltimore. Modelled on the German medical schools, the Hopkins medical "department" emphasized basic science in connection with bedside contact ("clinical research"). It admitted only students who had already completed a B.A., and was loathe to accept transfers from other medical schools. William Welch, dean of the Hopkins medical school and one of the famous "four horsemen" of Hopkins (the others being William Osler, William Halsted, and Howard Kelly), responded in 1897 to Farrar's request for admission: "Our faculty is reluctant to admit students to advanced standing upon the basis of work done elsewhere, and, as you will observe, the requirements for such admission have been made stringent."[3] (It is interesting that Welch took the time to respond personally with a longhand note of two pages: could one imagine the dean of a medical school—who happened as well to be, as Welch was, an internationally-known microbiologist—doing this today!) Farrar would have to pass exams. He took them and was admitted to the second-year class at Hopkins.

Farrar seems to have relished everything he experienced at Hopkins, but of special influence for his later development was his contact with William Osler. Osler, who had been born in Bond Head, Ontario (receiving in 1872 a B.A. from Toronto's Trinity College), was at the time the best-known physician in the United States. In 1892, he had published a textbook of medicine which, on account of its grounding in science and straightforward commonsensical style, immediately became the standard work.[4] In 1889, Osler came down from the University of Pennsylvania medical school to become chief physician of the Johns Hopkins University Hospital, and with the opening of the medical school he was, of course, the professor of medicine. Osler was widely remembered for his habit of careful observation at the bedside, scientific diagnosis, and interest in the patients' lives and problems. One of Osler's aphorisms was, "the good physician treats the disease but the great physician treats the patient who has the disease."[5]

Although Osler never used the term, he in fact practiced with great success an informal kind of psychotherapy, and this is what Farrar learned from Osler. Farrar learned the therapeutic benefits of taking a sympathetic interest in patients, which became a leitmotif for his later career in psychiatry. But Farrar learned this kind of psychotherapy not in Osler's formal lectures but rather by osmosis, on ward rounds.

> Osler could examine the patient, talk to him and about him, perhaps crack a joke at the expense of the houseman [intern] and introduce other pleasantries to make every one feel comfortable. Osler at the bedside, and a dozen of us standing around, were just a little family party and the patient could feel that he was a pretty important member of that family party.[6]

> So it was in this context of the gentle family party at the bedside that Osler practiced psychotherapy. He never used the word. There were no courses in psychotherapy. He didn't talk about it. He lived it. He oozed it, you might say. Every contact with patients, every word, every tone of voice, every facial expression, was psychotherapeutic.[7]

This bedside apprenticeship was important because Farrar himself took extraordinary pains with his patients, giving them great amounts of time, never referring to them as patients but as "friends," and noting in their medical records, or charts, the problems of their lives, even passages of dialogue, in great detail. Farrar graduated from Hopkins with an M.D. in 1900.

HEIDELBERG

After graduation, Farrar worked for two years as a clinical assistant at the Sheppard and Enoch Pratt Hospital, a private psychiatric hospital on the outskirts of Baltimore,[8] then went to Europe. Although he traveled widely, attending lectures and meeting scientists in cities from Munich to London, he spent most of his time (from October 1902 to May 1904) in Heidelberg, at Emil Kraepelin's psychiatric clinic.

How did this European trip come about? Although it was indeed common for American physicians with ambitions towards specialty practice to do postgraduate work in Europe (no fewer than 15,000 of them studied in Germany, for example, between 1870 and 1914[9]), such a trip required money. Farrar had little. How could he possibly take off from work for two years?

The answer lies in the political ambitions and intellectual aims of a gentleman-scholar and psychiatrist named Stewart Paton. Paton was around 35 when Farrar would have first known him in 1900. Having received his medical degree from Columbia in 1889, Paton had come to the Sheppard in 1899 as the director of the new laboratory. Paton also had a faculty appointment at Hopkins as an associate in psychiatry. This was an era when psychiatric hospitals were just beginning to realize that they needed laboratories, partly in order to do postmortems in the increasingly organic search for the causes of mental illness, partly to do routine tests on the blood and cerebrospinal fluid, such as the Wassermann test for syphilis (described in 1906). Edward Brush, the superintendent of the Sheppard, had charged Paton with "organizing and directing the scientific work of the hospital."[10] Farrar was Paton's first trainee.

It was a time of exploding interest in the microscopic study of the brain. Neurohistology occupied the same intellectual position and radiated the same excitement that brain imaging does today. In psychiatry in particular, the microscope seemed to offer the key to understanding the causes of mental illness. Analogizing from the model of neurosyphilis,

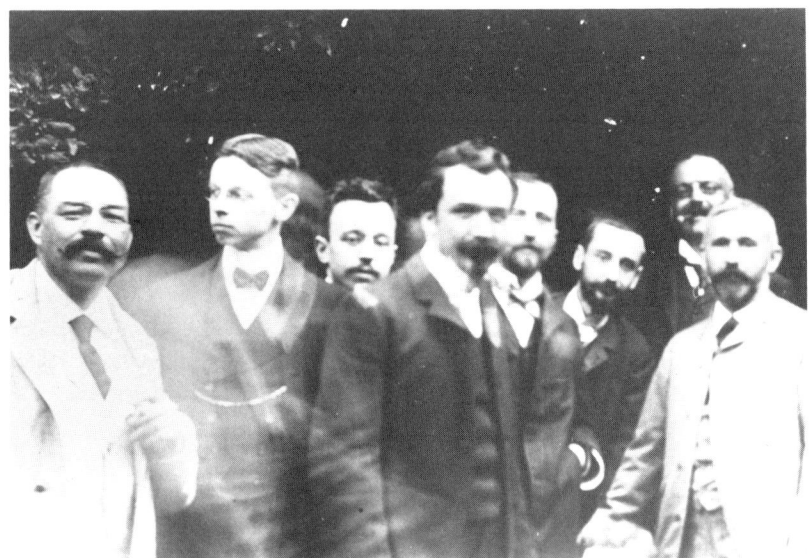

Farrar, second from left, at Kraepelin's psychiatric clinic in Heidelberg, 1902-1904. On far right is Kraepelin; Aloys Alzheimer is standing behind him.

where demonstrable anatomical changes were responsible for psychiatric symptoms, neuropathologists decided to search the brain's microscopic anatomy for the key to manic-depressive illness and to schizophrenia, then called dementia praecox. That was Stewart Paton's field of research. Because Hopkins at that point had no psychiatric clinic, Paton was trying to make the case for setting one up. He wanted to glamorize psychiatry as a new kind of fast-lane, organically-based science in order to persuade such powerful internists as Osler and Welch. "You had better plan for a few talks on the advances that have been made in clinical psychiatry," Paton wrote to Farrar in 1903. "Get together facts that would serve to arouse the interest of Drs. Welch and Osler."[11] In his letters to young Farrar, Paton returned again and again to the need to impress Osler, urging Farrar to get in touch with Osler directly. Osler, said Paton, was "quite enthusiastic" about Farrar's being trained in "psychological work" in Heidelberg. Paton said, "Be sure to write to Drs. Osler and Welch. They often ask for you and are very anxious to know how you are getting along."[12]

Also, Paton was working on a psychiatry textbook that would stress German contributions, especially of a histological nature, to research.[13] He was therefore avid to network, wanting to stay up to date on the latest findings in these laboratories at Heidelberg or Strasbourg, the most

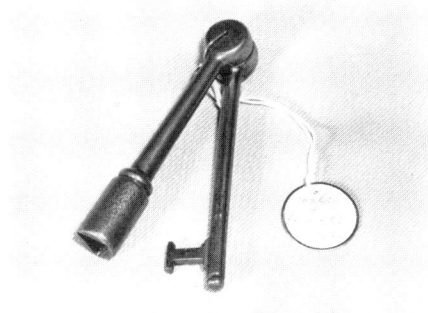

Keys to the wards of the Heidelberg Psychiatric Clinic, c. 1902-1904. Farrar brought them back from Germany, and referred to them as "the keys to knowledge."

famous of their kind in the world. His letters to Farrar were filled with long lists of people whom Farrar must see. Go to Breslau and see Carl Wernicke, Paton urged in 1904. "If Breslau does not appeal to you how about Berlin. Can you not get [Franz] Nissl or [Ludwig] Edinger to give you introductions to the different men. Have you yet met [Albrecht] Bethe. I will drop a line to Professor [Christian] Bäumler in Freiburg and he will introduce you to [Alfred] Hoche."[14] These were all the big names in Central European neuropathology. On another occasion Paton prodded Farrar to look up the famous Frederick Mott, director of the pathological laboratory of the London county asylums at Claybury: "You must not forget to stop and see Mott, so that we can keep ourselves in touch with the work in England."[15] Thus Farrar's European trip was born of Paton's enthusiasm. Paton apparently persuaded superintendent Brush of the need for the trip, and Brush persuaded the hospital's trustees. The trustees formally requested Farrar to spend the year in Germany, "for the purpose of studying there the advanced methods prevailing in the most modern institutions, for the treatment of the acute insane; also the scientific investigations as to the causes and prevention of mental derangement."[16] The hospital gave Farrar a thousand dollars and promises of a job upon returning.

The trustees were so pleased with Farrar's progress at Heidelberg that they later extended the trip by another year.[17] During this second year, the trustees especially wanted Farrar to take a look at the new psychiatric clinic in Munich. (In 1904, Kraepelin moved from Heidelberg to Munich to become director of this clinic.)[18]

Heidelberg 1902: It was "the new era," as Farrar later put it, of the microscopic study of brain disease, and two associates of Kraepelin's, Alois Alzheimer and Franz Nissl, were right at the center of it.[19] The new

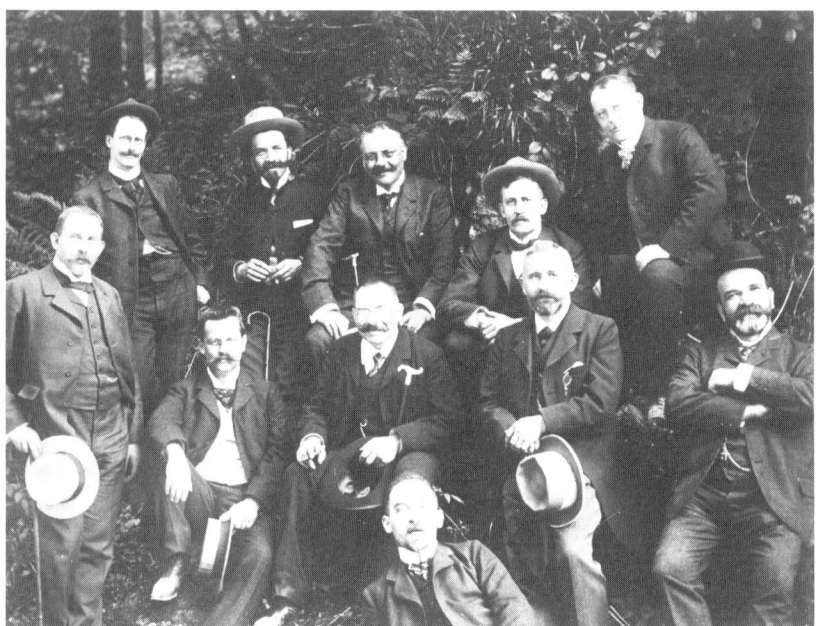

Taken by C. B. Farrar some time during his stay at the Psychiatric Clinic of the University of Heidelberg, 1902-1904. The photograph captures the members of the Clinic on a picnic. Second from right, hat in hand, is Emil Kraepelin, head of the Clinic. Franz Nissl is in the top row second from left. Next to Nissl in the center is Aloys Alzheimer. The others are unidentified.

era had begun in 1880, when the Austrian physiologist Sigmund Exner succeeded in making individual nerve "fibres" (neurons) stand out distinctly under the microscope. Nissl was among those who picked up the baton, and, by 1900, Nissl's own work had made him the single most important shaper of the discipline of neuropathology.[20] Alzheimer would shortly discover the characteristic changes in a kind of dementia named after him. At the clinical level as well, Heidelberg had a reputation for intense organicism, meaning the desire to reduce disease of the mind to disease of the brain. Schizophrenia, in the Heidelberg doctrine, counted as an organic brain disease.[21]

Farrar divided his time in Heidelberg between working in Nissl's lab (where he soon developed enough competence that he could instruct other visitors) and seeing patients in the psychiatric hospital ("clinic").[22] Although he counted merely as a voluntary assistant (*Hospitant*) and graduate student, Farrar seems to have taken part in patient care as well, and soon had acquired enough German that he could interview patients

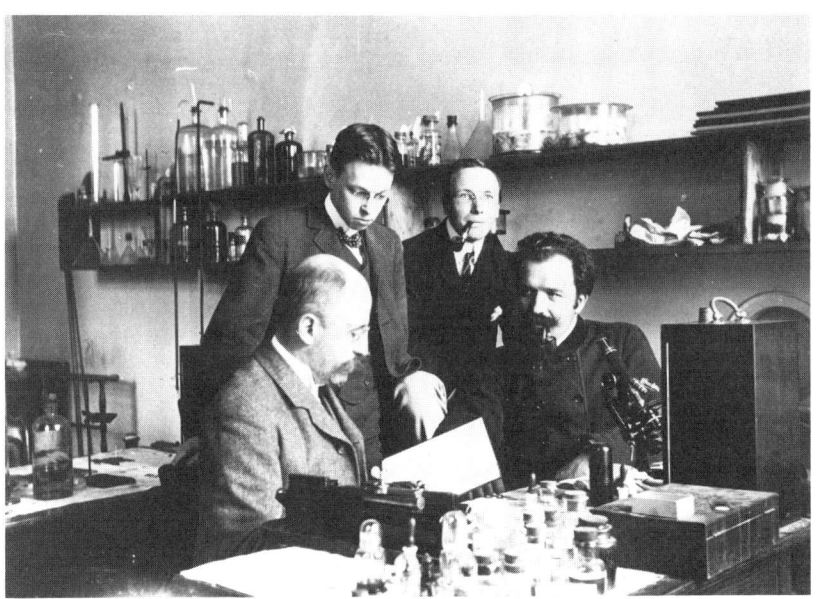

In Nissl's laboratory at Heidelberg, c. 1902-1904.
Upper row: C. B. Farrar, C. Macfie Campbell.
Lower row: Alfred Devaux, Franz Nissl.

and attend rounds.[23] He passed the time with several other foreigners who also had come to Nissl's lab to learn the techniques of the new discipline—notably Albert Devaux of Paris and Charles Macfie Campbell than of Edinburgh.[24] (After finishing at Heidelberg in 1904, Campbell went to the United States.) It was part of the charm of Heidelberg that these young outsiders socialized together with clinic staff and took excursions together. For example, Farrar accompanied Nissl on an excursion to Paris, where Paton evidently joined them. (On this trip, Nissl reduced Parisian psychiatrist Valentin Magnan almost to tears by insisting that a patient with one of Magnan's pet diagnoses, "délire chronique à évolution systematique," was actually "a quite typical case of dementia praecox.")[25] In this manner, over a two-year period, Farrar got to know just about everybody who was anybody in the scientific study of the nervous system in Central Europe.[26]

When Farrar returned to Baltimore in the summer of 1904, he counted as one of the most promising members of the young generation of American neuroscientists. He fired off a series of articles on the new techniques and ideas he had learned[27] (not always sparing the sensibilities of his laggardly senior colleagues). As Farrar, the 31-year-old cosmopolite, preached in 1905 to the provincial dullards he had left behind,

> psychiatry as a science, loved and cultivated, exists in but a few living centres in each country. In multitudes of hospitals and asylums it is a dead letter; the number of staff physicians is small and composed perhaps largely of men who have no aptitude or liking for laborious research. A meagre routine examination recorded possibly on a stereotyped printed sheet...may constitute the entire history of the case. Under such circumstances it is useless to expect illuminating scientific investigations to be carried through. We have thus to do with the lamentable situation of *the most difficult problems which science has to present being left in the hands of men the least able to solve them.*[28]

The slight sense of superiority with which Farrar returned from Heidelberg communicated itself in his social relations as well. As a female friend in the days at Heidelberg teased him much later in life, "you weren't so frightfully grown up with all your superior knowledge!"[29]

The important point is that, as Farrar returned to Baltimore, he was well placed to become one of America's leading psychiatrists. As his friend Paton had written him in 1904, "your connection with the Sheppard, Carnegie [a grant], and the university should in a few years lead to some enviable position."[30]

A FASHIONABLE YOUNG PHYSICIAN

In the seven years from 1906 to 1913 that Farrar spent as an assistant physician at the Sheppard-Pratt Hospital, he became very much a "fashionable" man, in that he was showered with offers to come elsewhere, and was therapeutically fashionable as well. Of course, the two go together, and Farrar would later go "out of fashion" as well.

Farrar's reintegration in American psychiatric life began just as soon as he stepped off the boat in the summer of 1904. For the next two years, though nominally a staff physician at the Sheppard and director of the laboratory, he would mainly eat and sleep there, for he had a research grant from the Carnegie Institute in Washington for work in "physiological psychology."[31] From 1906 to 1913 Farrar continued to direct the laboratory and supervised one of the women's wards as well. After his return, Farrar also had a part-time staff appointment at the Hopkins Faculty of Medicine, becoming in 1909 associate professor of psychiatry.

Thus, by 1909 Farrar had accumulated several prestigious posts and was situated squarely at the epicentre of the American psychiatric establishment.

Job offers poured in. In 1903 he had received a tentative inquiry from Yale.[32] Paton alluded to it in a letter of March 1903, delighted that Farrar would be staying at Hopkins. The new "psychopathic ward" of the University of Michigan in Ann Arbor (the first "psychopathic hospital" in the United States at a place then so obscure that Paton kept referring to it as "Ann Harbor") tried in 1905 to hire Farrar.[33] In 1908 the Georgia State Sanitarium at Milledgeville, assuring Farrar that he would be "fac[ing] the sea-coast negro in a state of aberrant felicity," expressed interest in making an appointment.[34] In that year William Allanson White, director of the Government Hospital for the Insane in Washington, tried to entice Farrar to come as clinical director.[35] It would be fair to say that Farrar had become one of the most sought-after young psychiatrists in the country.

And fashionability of ideas? Some of the charts of Farrar's patients at the Sheppard have survived, giving us an idea of what he believed about diagnosis and management.[36] Put simply, he believed what everybody else in his time believed. His ideas about the causes of mental illness and appropriate treatments reflected the conventional wisdom of the day.

For example, Silas Weir Mitchell's "rest cure" was still much in vogue.[37] Mitchell, the well-known Philadelphia neurologist, had elaborated a cure for "nervous disease," or psychoneurosis, the principal element of which was the enforced isolation of the patient from family and from the rest of the ward (secondary features involved a milk diet, massage, and electrotherapy). It became the standard treatment for troubled women from families sufficiently well-off to afford private rooms. Farrar routinely ordered isolation and bed rest for the agitated or emotionally uncontained female patients of his ward. Mrs. Mary M. had a "depressive hysterical condition." In his nursing orders, Farrar instructed that the

> patient remain in bed and isolated so long as, and whenever, these various symptoms are present. She should not be allowed to discuss her symptoms or unpleasant happenings in the past... *No visitors.* It is especially prescribed that [the] patient shall not see her husband or receive any letters from him; also not to write to him.

Mrs. Mal., for example, a chronic invalid with "constitutional neurasthenia," was ordered to "rest in bed" on a liquid diet "til patient has grown very tired of same." Mrs. R., admitted in 1910 for depression in "consequence of longstanding conjugal infelicity," was "absolutely forbidden to discuss family affairs with anyone, patients or nurses... Must go to bed at once if she loses control or continues to weep." Thus Weir Mitchell's spirit hovered over Farrar's ward.

Then there was psychotherapy. The teachings of the Bernese psychiatrist Paul Dubois, who described the psychotherapy of "rational persuasion," were still much abroad. Dubois emphasized rational discussion with patients as the highroad to abolishing symptoms, the goal being the restoration of the patient's sense of self-control.[38] This theme runs as well through Farrar's management of his patients. His comments about Miss R.'s "reactive depression from domestic unhappiness," for example, were very Duboisian: "December, 1910: chief symptom to combat—insomnia. Patient should be made to feel that as this is gradually corrected, the other symptoms will in turn disappear." This was the essence of Dubois' own treatment strategy: calling the attention of the patient to minor successes in the hopes that unconscious suggestion would lead to major ones.

There was a curious contradiction between German views of cause and French-Swiss views of treatment. What was somatogenic in the former view was psychogenic in the latter. One should not be able to abolish supposedly organic symptoms so easily by psychotherapy! This implicit tension, never resolved anywhere, remained unresolved in Farrar's mind as well. For example, Mrs. J., now 30, had had recurrent attacks of "worry" for the past eleven years. Farrar admonished the nurses to emphasize

> the fact that she is *ill*—and not in this state because of 'foolishness' or 'wickedness.' Must be made to realise that she will not be considered well, and cannot go home till she is convinced of the above. At same time she must know that she is not considered *very* ill, and that she can easily and fairly quickly recover.

One may distinguish between Farrar's genuine and lifelong interest in psychotherapy, and his willingness to apply the formal tools of psychology in the analysis of mental illness. Because he had worked in Kraepelin's psychological laboratory in Heidelberg, Farrar might have attempted to use this new discipline systematically.[39] Yet his few efforts to apply "psychology" to his Sheppard patients sound clumsy and uninsightful.

Miss R., for example, was hypochondriacal and "pseudo-suicidal." She suffered, Farrar said, from "subharmonious mental development— imperfect adjustment between the real and the ideal." Indeed Farrar seems not to have relished the psychological side of his stay in Heidelberg, as one infers from one of Paton's letters to him: "From a reference you made you do not seem to have enjoyed your psychological wanderings [in Heidelberg]. What is the trouble?"[40]

In another way as well, in the years before the First World War, Farrar reflected the soon-to-be-outmoded psychiatry of the day: attributing mental illness in women to the menstrual cycle. This was a late echo of the "reflex" theories of earlier generations, assigning psychiatric illness to the menses, menopause, and menarche. For decades the view had prevailed that uterus and ovaries, "irritated" by the menstrual cycle, reflexly affected other organ systems including the brain, causing "menstrual madness."[41] In the years before the First World War, Farrar believed wholeheartedly in the phenomenon of "menstrual psychosis." For example, at the Sheppard, Mrs. H.'s chief diagnosis was "menopausal psychosis,"[42] in association with the "shipwreck of the husband" and "recurrent family changes contributing to loneliness." To take another example, Farrar thought that Mrs. Mul.'s "indeterminate hysteriform paranoid complex [is] probably associated with a precocious menopause." But it was the "last phase of climacteric psychosis" that had caused Mrs. Mur., now 57, to become "'impossible' to live with," he thought. Comments on the menses are present in many of the 49 charts that have survived from this women's ward.

Finally, Farrar reflected the psychiatry of the day in adhering to the doctrine that psychiatric illness was biologically determined. He especially believed in the influence of heredity. Perhaps Farrar absorbed these views initially from Brush, and from Henry Hurd, who was then the professor of psychiatry at Hopkins as well as being the superintendent of the Johns Hopkins Hospital.[43] Perhaps Farrar's Heidelberg experience further strengthened his conviction that mental illness resulted primarily from inherited "constitutional" weakness.[44] Constitutional in those days meant approximately what later would be called "genetic." Thus, Farrar thought that Miss F. suffered from a "constitutional neurotic state with perverted 'fixed' emotional reactions." Mrs. Mul. displayed a "constitutional jealous tendency apparent throughout married life," and Miss R.'s "increasing nervous irritability" was attributed, in the first instance, to "psychopathic heredity especially on paternal side."

While the biological psychiatry of a later era would rely heavily upon psychoactive medications, Farrar was sparing in prescribing sedatives and hypnotics for his patients. In this entire series only Miss Ros. received anything to be taken internally; Veronal, a barbiturate, was prescribed to calm persistent "excitement" at the time of her menses. She was later put into a "resting jacket."

Farrar, 36 in 1910 and a rapidly rising star, made no claim to be an original thinker in psychiatry. He believed what the physicians of his day generally believed and as their ideas changed, so did his as well, for better or worse. Up to this point Farrar had shown virtually no interest in his patients' bowels or teeth.

TRENTON

Farrar's great success hitherto makes the next chapter in the story all the more difficult to understand, for in 1913 he left Hopkins and the Sheppard to become third assistant physician at the New Jersey state asylum in Trenton. The move is the more baffling in that he landed right in the middle of the therapeutic craziness of Henry Cotton.[45] In 1913 Cotton was 37, two years younger than Farrar. Like Farrar, Cotton had been scientifically trained, graduating in 1899 from the University of Maryland, then going to the Worcester State Hospital in Massachusetts as an assistant of Adolf Meyer (Worcester had been one of Meyer's previous posts before he became the professor of psychiatry at Hopkins in 1910). In 1903, Cotton took a post at the Danvers Insane Hospital in Hathorne, Massachusetts, briefly going on leave for a year in the spring of 1905 to study with Kraepelin and Alzheimer in Munich.[46] In 1907, Cotton was catapulted at a young age into the directorship of the asylum at Trenton, a previous kind of psychiatric Sleepy-Hollow that Cotton was determined to tug into the modern era. The problem was that Cotton, as Farrar to some extent, had fallen under the influence of the "reflex" ideas of his day, the view that irritation or toxicity at certain points in the body is able to produce symptoms in far-distant organs, specifically in the brain. Borrowing from the English surgeon William Arbuthnot ("Willy") Lane,[47] Cotton acquired the idea that constipation caused "autointoxication": as feces stagnated in the intestines, fecal toxins leaked into the bloodstream and madness was the result. Autointoxication was treatable

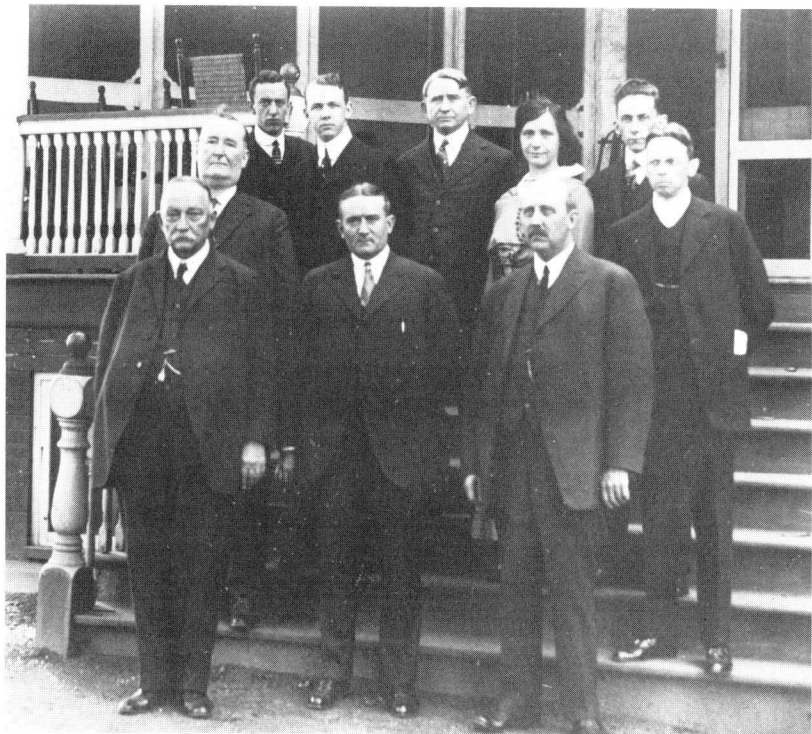

C. B. Farrar (on far right) at the Trenton State Hospital in 1915. Front and center is Henry Cotton.

with colectomy. Cotton's contribution to this growing body of lore on autointoxication was the view that infected teeth could also cause insanity. Pulling out all the patient's teeth therefore became a cure for mental illness at Trenton, in addition to removing colons and uteruses. (It was said that Cotton had all of his wife's teeth removed.[48])

The exact chronology of the growth of Cotton's theories is a bit obscure. Yet the point is an important one, because just as Farrar was contemplating a move to Trenton, Cotton seems already to have been in the grip of autointoxication theory, and it is inconceivable that the two men did not discuss these matters before Farrar accepted the job. Cotton had already written Farrar on several occasions, telling him, for example, in 1907 about his work at Munich on "[cerebral] cortex histology."[49] Whether the two men were close friends by the time Cotton took the superintendency at Trenton is unclear, but in 1908 Cotton invited Farrar to come and lecture at Trenton.[50] Already by 1911 Cotton must have been hatching his autointoxication theories, for in that year he added a fully-equipped dental office to the asylum, and hired the following year a full-time dentist, "the care of the patients' teeth having proved so beneficial."[51]

Why would Farrar have left his post at the center of psychiatry at Hopkins to move to the obscurity of this run-down asylum (which admittedly Cotton was rapidly fixing up)? Was Farrar himself a reflex theorist? No. Aside from his imputation of psychosis to the menses, he seems to have been not at all interested in irritation or autointoxication, and almost never commented in the patients' charts on the state of their bowels or teeth.[52] Did he become embroiled with Meyer, the new professor of psychiatry at Hopkins? To be sure, there had been some bad feeling in 1906, as Meyer, editing a special issue of some scholarly journal on neuropathology, thought that Farrar had already published elsewhere a book review that Farrar submitted to the issue in question. Meyer was wrong. The journal's main editor apologized profusely.[53] The incident might have left bad feeling with Farrar, who had a very refined sense of personal honour. Yet the two men seem to have had a harmonious relationship at Hopkins, or at least there is no sign of acrimony in the few letters that Farrar wrote Meyer.[54] But then, Farrar was almost never acrimonious with anyone.

Or were there family considerations? In 1911, Farrar married Evelyn Linwood Lewis, a nurse in training at the Sheppard, who graduated four months before their wedding. Children did not come along until four years later, yet perhaps new family responsibilities made Farrar think he simply needed a job that paid more money.[55]

Finally, there is the question of Stewart Paton. Independently wealthy, in 1904 Paton was able to resign his posts at Hopkins and the Sheppard and move with his family to Berlin. From Berlin, the Patons went on to a zoological research station in Italy where he stayed for four years. In 1909, Paton returned to the States, taking a job as professor of abnormal psychology at Princeton University.[56] Paton also became one of the trustees of the Trenton asylum. Did Farrar want to follow Paton? It is not unreasonable to speculate that Farrar, who became a part-time lecturer in abnormal psychology at Princeton as well, may have been following his mentor. The issue cannot be resolved with the documents at hand. We know only that in 1913 Farrar left the Sheppard for Henry Cotton's asylum in Trenton.

The story of Farrar's three years at Trenton seems to be that, after encountering Cotton's plans for doing abdominal surgery on patients,

Farrar fled in horror. When Farrar arrived, no operations to cure mental illness were as yet being carried out. The hospital's new operating room, installed sometime after 1907, went almost unused.[57] Yet while Farrar was still there, the initial patients were being readied for surgery. First to be operated on was Florence P., a patient of Farrar's. She was 25, a married housewife of English descent who half a year previously had lost her mother. The mother had opposed Florence's marriage; Florence was now pregnant, and after the sister had scolded her, Florence had what she called "a hysterical spell." In January she became depressed and anxious, attempting suicide by turning on the gas. "Asked her husband to shoot her, saying she had nothing to live for." Admitted February 26, 1916, she came onto Farrar's ward. Now in this case as in virtually no other, Farrar felt impelled to note the patient's bowel status: "no constipation" before her pregnancy. "During the first week in January there was very severe constipation." In the category "treatment" Farrar advised, "Attention to nutrition and intestinal condition."[58] Farrar must have been told by Cotton to pay attention to these kinds of symptoms and treatments, for the comments are completely anomalous in the context of Farrar's usual approach. Florence P. was the first patient to be colectomized at Trenton, apparently by Cotton's consulting surgeon John W. Draper of New York. She died after the operation.[59]

Farrar fled Trenton in 1916. In the face of such massive looming malpractice, he was probably desperate to get out. He told Paton of his misery and Paton began searching to find his friend a job. Paton wrote, for example, to Elmer Southard, the distinguished head of the Boston Psychopathic Hospital, a Kraepelin-style clinic of great scientific visibility. Southard mentioned to Farrar that, "Dr. Paton, in his letter about your leaving Trenton, suggested that state hospital conditions were not favorable for you." Unfortunately Southard had little to offer but concluded his letter, "By the way, there is another opportunity due to the provision in the will of a dead Canadian captain which might interest you. It is for a sanatorium for mental and nervous wrecks produced by the war, to be laid down upon an island somewhere in Canada."[60]

Farrar's Canadian sojourn was about to begin.

World War I

Why did Farrar come to Canada? Was it merely to escape the nightmare of autointoxication? Or were there other considerations? Farrar's widow, Joan Farrar (Farrar remarried after his first wife's death in 1964), suggested that he might have wished to join the Canadian army, then at war in France. "C.B. came to Canada to see if he could enlist. He came to Ottawa. But they wanted him to do psychiatry."[61] If any insight emerges from the mountain of material that Farrar left behind, it is that he had an interesting and complex mind, that he was not motivated solely by career considerations, and that, although an ambitious man, he saw himself perhaps more as a gentlemen or an intellectual than as a ladder-climber. Maybe in the summer of 1916 he saw himself as a patriot. In fact he did have other job options, but he evidently wanted to serve in the cause of what he considered to be right.[62]

Farrar had come that summer to an impromptu convalescent camp for cases of "shell shock" that Agnes Richardson had erected on the grounds of her family's estate, "Fettercairn," in the Rideau Lakes. Farrar later said he had taken the post "for experience," given that he had no previous connection with military matters or shell shock.[63] In November 1916, Farrar enlisted in the Canadian army and was certified as ready for overseas service in a hospital unit based in Kingston, Ontario.[64] A month later the army realized that it was short of psychiatrists for the treatment of men who were being invalided back to Canada, either because they had a pre-existing mental illness before joining up or because they had acquired one during military service, and Farrar was transferred to Ottawa for duty with the military hospitals commission. Like all medical officers, he had the rank of captain. Farrar and his family thus lived in Ottawa during the war, Farrar going back and forth between Ottawa and the military hospital at Cobourg, Ontario.

Between April and December 1918 he was at Cobourg full-time as president of the standing medical board. This was precisely the period during which his marriage was breaking up, and the beginning of a long period of peregrination that would end only with his arrival in Toronto in 1925.

In December 1918 Farrar changed employers, from the Canadian Army Medical Corps to a civilian bureaucracy, the Department of Soldiers' Civil Re-establishment, or department of veterans' affairs, where he became the chief psychiatrist.[65] It is not our purpose to rehearse the bureaucratic minutiae of those years. The significance of Farrar's wartime service from the viewpoint of the history of the Toronto Psychiatric Hospital is that in these years he met C.K. Clarke, the professor of

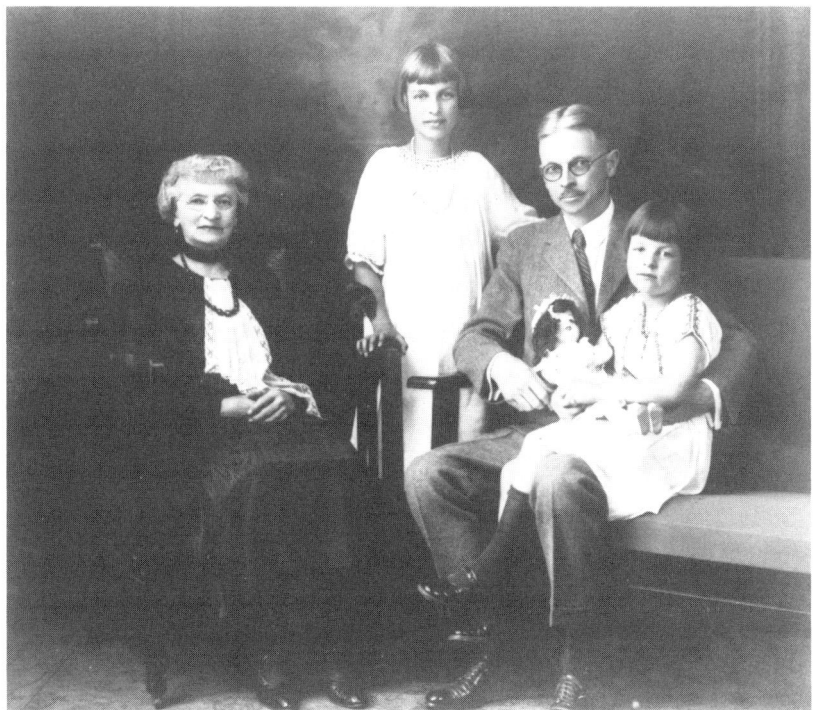

C. B. Farrar as a family man, c. 1920,
with his two daughters and his mother.

psychiatry in Toronto. Each man developed great fondness and admiration for the other.

Farrar had doubtlessly met Clarke before, if only because in 1904 Clarke was elected associate editor of the *American Journal of Insanity*, the forerunner of the *American Journal of Psychiatry*, edited by Brush and based in Baltimore. Farrar was "very thick with the American Journal crowd," as Joan Farrar put it, and would in 1931 become its editor. During his first month on the job in December 1918, Farrar went with Clarke on tour of Canada's western provinces to inspect arrangements made for hospitalized servicemen at the various asylums. Each seemed ghastlier than the next.[66] At Clarke's suggestion, the two of them agreed to collaborate on an article.[67]

Until this time, Clarke had been more or less the only internationally known figure in Canadian psychiatry. He was evidently delighted that Farrar, 17 years his junior, had now come to stand alongside him. In 1919 Clarke was already 62 and feeling poorly. Farrar was 45 and at the top of his career. Clarke must immediately have glimpsed his successor in the younger man, which explains why Clarke bent over backwards in 1920 to try an obtain an Ontario medical license for Farrar. As Clarke told John Argue, a member of the executive of the Ontario Medical Council, Farrar was "one of the most brilliant of the young group of psychiatrists in the United States. I regard him as the best man they have. He has had a most brilliant career at Harvard, Princeton, and Johns Hopkins, and is such an eminent man that we all regard him most highly."[68]

Farrar by contrast seems to have had no further Canadian plans. He had in fact agreed to become chief psychiatrist at the U.S. Treasury Department's "Bureau of War Risk Insurance" in Washington, but declined at the last moment when the proposed salary was dropped from $6,000 to $5,000.[69]

Homewood

In 1923, Farrar left the Department of Soldiers' Civil Re-establishment to become superintendent of a private asylum in Guelph, Ontario, called the Homewood Sanitarium.[70] This move, yet another jump away from the world of academic psychiatry at Hopkins, was probably the result of his desire to escape a flagging marriage (for once Farrar left Ottawa, his wife moved back to Virginia) and to improve his economic circumstances.

The Homewood asylum had been founded in 1883 as the "Homewood Retreat," the first purely private asylum in Canada. Stephen Lett, a quite conventional psychiatrist for his day, had been its first superintendent. But upon Lett's retirement in 1901, the board of directors chose a man of very different orientation, a surgical activist and believer in reflex theory named Alfred T. Hobbs. Hobbs, a graduate of the University of Toronto in 1890, had previously been an assistant physician at the public asylum in London, Ontario, and there (in combination with the asylum's superintendent Richard Bucke) proceeded to conduct extensive pelvic surgery on the female patients.[71] By 1901 Hobbs had become internationally notorious for these gratuitous mutilations of female psychiatric patients.[72] At Homewood, Hobbs continued to perform pelvic surgery for mental illness, although apparently on a somewhat reduced scale. As late as 1920 he tried to cure depression in one patient by repairing her prolapsed uterus.[73]

Thus the aura of "science" had not clung to Homewood in the past. It is no wonder that in 1923 Edward Barnes, the former assistant director of Homewood, expressed to Farrar the opinion that the now-ailing Hobbs should have stepped down long ago: "... He had been there long enough—too long, in fact, for his own good."[74]

Farrar's contact with Homewood began in 1919, when Barnes had asked him to come over and assess "a deteriorating D.P." [dementia praecox patient], in order to save the family a trip down to Meyer's clinic in Baltimore. The families of such patients at Homewood were often very wealthy, and of course Barnes promised Farrar "a reasonable fee."[75] This would have been among the first occasions that a hitherto rather impecunious Farrar sampled the financial rewards of private psychiatric consulting.

Then Hobbs fell ill, and, in November 1922, the president of the Homewood's board of directors, Frederick C. Jarvis, a prominent Toronto businessman, offered Farrar the job of superintendent. Farrar would have Hobbs' house and a salary of $7,000 a year.[76]

There was only one problem: Farrar did not have a license to practice medicine in Ontario. What could be done? What in fact was done is interesting because it shows how much medicine in general, not just psychiatry, in those years was very much an old boys' network. Those who had connections could arrange just about anything they wanted, in contrast to the internationally renowned German and Austrian refugees from the Holocaust, who had no connections, and who could not get a foot in the Canadian door.[77] If one requires a medical license in Ontario (or anywhere else), one normally sits the exams of the licensing body of that jurisdiction. Yet this course would have meant going back and relearning all the medical-school information that most physicians forget upon graduation. Farrar, at 48, had spent all his life in psychiatry and could not have passed the Ontario exams without an inordinate and totally disruptive expenditure of effort. He appealed to Clarke for help.[78] Clarke had every reason for wishing to be forthcoming. He was already thinking of Farrar as his successor to the professorship in Toronto (as he mentioned to H. Wilberforce Aikens of Toronto, the registrar of the licensing body, the Ontario College of Physicians and Surgeons).[79] Hobbs, who hoped to be retained as consultant psychiatrist in Homewood, helped as well. From his convalescence in Florida, he barraged by mail members of the College's executive committee, all of whom he knew personally.[80] Under such pressure, Aikens agreed to give Farrar a special, pro forma exam, which the College had apparently never done before.[81] Farrar was to appear before two members of the executive committee—John Fotheringham and George Young—at 2:30 on Friday, January 19, 1923.[82] We do not know if the "examination" of one of the continent's most brilliant psychiatrists by two local Toronto doctors consisted of anything more than a handshake. But Farrar "passed," and became licensed to practice in Ontario. Clarke, in fact, was somewhat embarrassed that it had been necessary for a man of Farrar's stature to jump through even these hoops. "I am international enough in spirit to feel that such difficulties should never be thrown in the way of a man of your reputation and accomplishment, but, as you have long ago realized, Canada is yet a *very* little nation."[83]

For the first time, Farrar was in charge of running an institution. In his two years at Homewood, he was determined to introduce modern, scientific psychiatry. He asked Meyer, for example, for copies of all the forms the Phipps clinic in Baltimore used, so as to apply them at Homewood.[84] Farrar was responsible for building a new nurses' residence. And generally Farrar tried to communicate the spirit of progressive psychiatry to the family doctors of Canada who would be making referrals.[85] Then in 1925 Farrar moved to Toronto.

TORONTO

From 1925 until 1947 Farrar was the director of TPH and professor of psychiatry at the University of Toronto. He continued to edit the *American Journal of Psychiatry* until 1965 and was further active in professional interests until his death in 1970 at age 95. His life in Toronto therefore covers almost half a century, during which Canadian psychiatry developed from a stunted appendage of the United States and Great Britain to a major contender in international scientific circles. Much of Farrar's activity in these years is covered in other chapters. Here we single out two aspects: his efforts to hook up young psychiatrists with the same kinds of international contacts from which he himself had greatly profited, and the maturing of his ideas about diagnosis and treatment.

Farrar's journey to Toronto began in October 1923, when Clarke wrote him asking if he would like to become professor of psychiatry at the University of Toronto. There was some urgency: "As you are well aware, I am tired of hard work, having done my share of it, and more than my

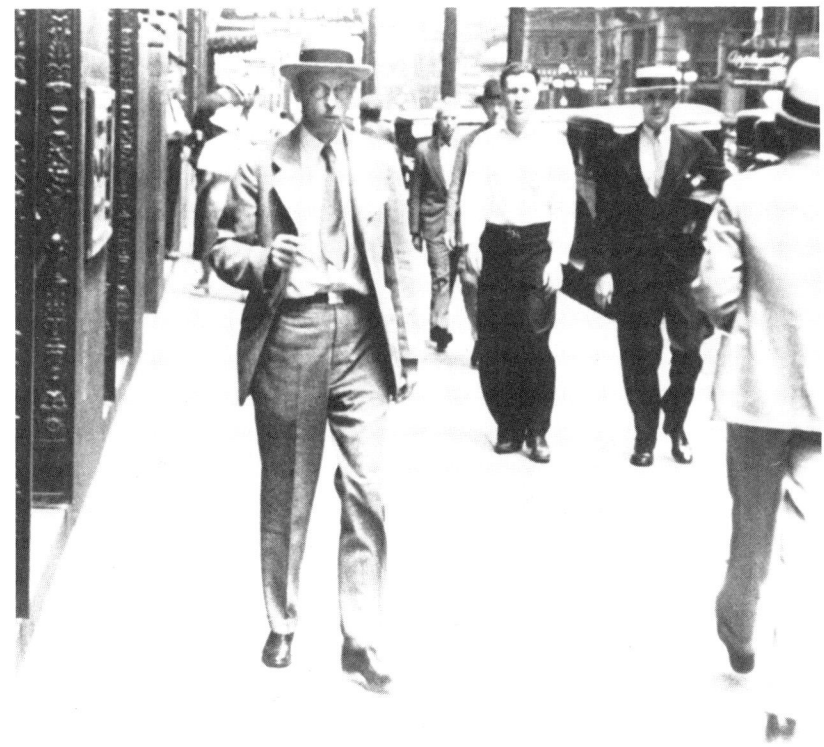

C. B. Farrar photographed on a Toronto street, c. 1930.
(Yonge Street at Queen Street West.)

share of it for the price paid. The psychiatric department is becoming a big thing in the University, and will require more activity than I now possess." Clarke added, "now tell me frankly exactly what you think of such a situation, as we have to get busy before the paid hirelings of the Ontario Government get on the job."[86] At this point Farrar was scarcely nine months into his post at Homewood. Within months, rumours would start to circulate that Farrar was leaving.[87] There was only one other candidate for the Toronto chair, an unnamed easterner.[88] In February 1924, University of Toronto President Robert Falconer offered the job to Farrar, at a salary of $5,000, plus the opportunity of supplementing it through private consultation and government grants.[89] Some negotiating ensued[90] and Farrar finally started his professorship as of February 1, 1925.[91]

The only sad note was that in the meantime, in January 1924, C.K. Clarke had died. It was clear that Farrar was Clarke's designated successor. Clarke's daughter Emma told Farrar just after the death, "He felt so secure in leaving in your hands the work dearest to his heart."[92]

Farrar saw that a major objective must be the building of a new generation of scientifically oriented Canadian psychiatrists. In addition to the training program he established at TPH, he also hastened his prize students off to Europe, to the great clinics of Munich and Heidelberg, London and Zurich. In the 1930s in particular, a whole camp of Canadians established themselves on the "far side of the pond," their way eased by Farrar's numerous letters of recommendation.

Archibald ("Archie") Kilgour, for example, a psychiatrist at Kingston who had graduated in medicine in 1922 from the University of Toronto, undertook his grand tour at the age of 41. From London he wrote in March 1934 of the spellbinding debates over psychoanalysis then raging. Kilgour said, "It's the story of Mesmerism all over again." Kilgour had also seen young John D. ("Jack") Griffin, then 28, and William Line. Griffin went on to become a prominent Canadian psychiatrist, Line a psychologist.[93] Then Kilgour and his wife were off to Munich, where the psychiatric research institute founded by Kraepelin was now, a year and a half after Hitler's seizure of power, in the hands of Walter Spielmeyer. It was all so exciting, Kilgour enthused, and Spielmeyer had recommended an article by Farrar to read![94] Six months later Kilgour was considerably less excited about what he had seen of Nazism in Germany, but now was in Zurich, where he had a flurry of interesting activities to report. Finally Kilgour returned to London, where he bumped into J. Clifford Richardson, later to become a well-known Toronto neurologist. Kilgour told Farrar he understood that John Dewan would be coming over shortly.[95] Dewan, having graduated in medicine from the University of Western Ontario three years previously, had been studying psychology at the University of Toronto and working in provincial asylums. Dewan would later become medical director of TPH following Aldwyn Stokes. Thus, Kilgour had wandered in his travels through the young psychiatric and neurological elite of English Canada. His letters breathe a sense of astonishment at all the science he was discovering on his grand tour. Kilgour committed suicide in 1937.

Ruth MacLachlan Franks, to take another example, went in 1931 to the Zurich university psychiatric clinic at the Burghölzli asylum. After acquiring an M.D. from the University of Toronto in 1926, she had trained at TPH and done postgraduate work in psychology. She was now writing a Ph.D. thesis on suicide and was working up her German so as to collect material, first in Munich, then in Zurich.[96] She wrote Farrar in stilted but correct German: "The number of patients here is very large, and the diversity of the cases most instructive. Most of them give the impression of being taken from [Eugen] Bleuler's textbook.[97] Dementia praecox seems almost not to be present. Schizophrenia plays the most significant role."[98] Farrar might have smiled with pleasure at reading these lines, having encouraged this young scholar to acquire a solid international basis for her work. (Kilgour, whom Ruth Franks had tried to cheer up about mastering the German language, wrote Farrar when he himself reached Zurich, "I had thought she pulled my leg on this language business and am sure of it when I meet this 'Swiss Deutsch!'"[99]) Farrar's efforts to give the next generation the same international exposure he had received came to an end in the late 1930s.

What did Farrar actually teach these young psychiatrists? In his later years he got away from some of the diagnostic and therapeutic trendiness that had dogged him before World War I, becoming much more his own man, indeed espousing ideas that were downright out-of-step with the dogma of the 1940s and 1950s. One past burden that Farrar abandoned was "menstrual psychosis." In an article that he and Ruth Franks wrote in 1931, the two authors agreed that no causal relationship existed between the menopause and psychiatric illness, and that women who became symptomatic during their menopause were likely also to have been ill before. It was indeed the duty of psychiatrists to help female patients to disabuse themselves of these old folkloric notions and to "promote a more wholesome mental-hygiene outlook upon what is, after all, among women a universal phenomenon."[100]

Farrar was equally cool to other reflex ideas. When in 1938 a Toronto G.P., still in the grips of autointoxication fantasies, proposed nasal surgery for the relief of "mental illness and epilepsy," Farrar was bidden by the government to respond. The physician had been doing it for 14 years and proposed now that Ontario adopt the procedure in its asylums.[101] Farrar first consulted with a baffled ear-nose-and-throat surgeon, then suggested that "further consideration" would be unnecessary.[102]

As for Farrar's previous ironclad credence in the organicity of psychiatric illness, one might distinguish between belief in the presence of a brain lesion every time a patient has mental symptoms, and belief in heredity as a predisposing cause (in that if one is not genetically disposed, one will not develop schizophrenia or manic-depressive illness regardless of the stress to which one is subjected). By the time that Farrar attained his psychiatric maturity at TPH, he had moderated his adherence to both, without abandoning them entirely.

In terms of organicity, Farrar often called himself a "neuropsychiatrist," a term itself in the tradition of the Berlin psychiatrist Wilhelm Griesinger, who believed that mind disease was reducible to brain disease.[103] In 1929, Farrar told the nurses at Toronto General Hospital, "plainly speaking, there is actually no difference between a nervous disorder and a mental disorder. Every single nervous disorder is a mental disorder, and every mental disorder is a nervous disorder."[104]

Nor did Farrar's belief in the driving force of heredity weaken much. In 1937, he told the fourth-year medical students at the University of Toronto that heredity was the "first" cause of mental illness, and that they must be tactful enough to deal with the "embarrassing question of anxious relatives."[105] Just after arriving in Toronto, Farrar advocated at a meeting of the Children's Aid Society "the complete sterilization of mental deficients to prevent procreation of mental defectives."[106]

There is, however, evidence that in the 1930s and 1940s Farrar modified this strong reductionism. His mature views became subtler and more complex. For example, his contribution to the 1944 edition of the *Physician's Hand Book* positively radiates the spirit of social psychiatry, displacing the emphasis from the organic to the communal: "In general terms mental derangement can properly be considered as a dislocation of the social relationship. In a word, behaviour, both normal and pathological, is an expression of a group situation..." He gave the example of jealousy. "Is there such a thing as 'normal' jealousy? At what point does jealousy become morbid or delusional? Obviously this type of response cannot be cleared up by studying the patient alone." One would have to study the family, the community, the culture in which the patient's notion of jealousy is situated. Madness was, in other words, highly relative (and not solely brain-driven).

> It is useful to reflect that there are no absolute standards in psychiatry. There is no ultimate measuring stick by which to judge the normality of a psychic event. Not one but many arbitrary norms must always be kept in mind,—norms of age, sex, race, occupation, social status, educational and cultural level, and even of the historical epoch... Above all, it is necessary to hold in check our inevitable tendency to estimate an individual as normal or abnormal by comparing him with ourselves.

And the Heidelberg inheritance? In this manual for psychiatrists-in-training at TPH and elsewhere, Farrar turned his back upon Kraepelin, though perhaps not 180 degrees. To be sure, "We are still in the Kraepelinian era." But he warned against overpreoccupation with classification:

> There can be no question that the actualities of many a mental patient have been missed through zeal for strict definition and delimitation of his "disease" — through adherence to the view that [here he quoted Gustav Aschaffenburg's textbook] "each disease-type is an independent, self-bound entity, distinguishable from other diseases."[107]

Farrar closed by indicting the very organicist school with which he had once closely identified himself. "It is hardly more to be expected that a cellular change would show the basis of a delusion or of a return of insight, than that the flash of genius which gives birth to a great poem or haunting melody should be registered in the cortex for observation post mortem."[108]

Probably the greatest contribution Farrar made in his mature years was his advocacy among family physicians of informal psychotherapy, a psychotherapy based not upon rigid doctrinal systems but upon the intrinsic healing power of the doctor-patient relationship. Of course Farrar had learned from Osler that the physician possesses the power to do great good just by talking with the patient and by the laying-on of hands. These insights Farrar developed in later years to a specific notion of psychotherapy. In 1938 he wrote, "We may define psychotherapy...as the scientifically controlled influence of one mind upon another in the direction of health." How was the physician to achieve this influence? "The nucleus of psychotherapy is suggestion... It is obvious that the treatment begins with the first contact with the patient and with history taking." Therefore, the physician should discuss at length with the patient his or her "somatic, ecologic and personal" history. In aiming this advice towards family doctors, Farrar risked it falling upon deaf ears, for this approach requires lots of time, but it also gives the patient the impression of the physician's interest, the sense of being cared for, and the chance to achieve a catharsis, all of which Farrar (the good Oslerian) was well aware.

On the subject of psychosomatic illness, Farrar cautioned that one should never challenge the patient's own illness views. There can be no talk of "imaginary." "If a person thinks he is sick, he *is* sick. The circumstance that the illness is located in his thinking does not make his disability less real."[109] These words could stand today as the quintessentially humane approach to psychosomatic illness.

Later, Farrar argued that "psychotherapy of a single common sense type is applicable throughout the field of medicine." The family physician's objective is to confer upon the patient a sense of empowerment: "The objectives are first to give the patient a better understanding of his case, and then to show him how, with more or less help, he can do something about it."[110] Of course this was merely a restatement of the therapy of rational persuasion of Paul Dubois and Jules Dejerine, but Farrar recalled it to mind for a North American audience that had long forgotten those names, an audience being inundated with a radically different sense of what constituted psychotherapy: namely psychoanalysis.

Farrar despised psychoanalysis. In public, his critiques gave off an air of moderation and judiciousness. Freud's contributions, conceded Farrar in 1940, "were not inconsiderable," even though the basic idea of psychoanalysis (namely that disorders of adult life are to be sought in anomalies of early childhood socialization) "may be rejected by the builders of the future." Psychoanalysis had "engendered not a little charlatanism in the practice of healing," Farrar concluded, although sounding quite positive about Freud himself.[111]

In private Farrar was scathing about analysis. His wife Joan, unbeknownst to him, wrote down some of his shafts: "the shadows of Freud linger as the last touch of mysticism in medicine... It will take a long time to clean this scourge out of psychiatry." On another occasion, Farrar said that the four horsemen of the Apocalypse were: Communism, Catholicism, Unionism, Psychoanalysis.[112]

Of course, it was no secret to the Toronto psychoanalysts that Farrar scorned them. Having ridden high on the wave of fashion before the First World War, he would be pommelled by it after the Second.

FAREWELL

After the Second World War a wholly new spirit began to blow through American psychiatry. Ideas stressing brain biology and heredity became outmoded, and those emphasizing the psychogenesis and sociogenesis of psychiatric disorder rushed onto center stage. Chief among these new ideas was psychoanalysis. "In 1946," writes historian Gerald Grob, "the

American Board of Psychiatry and Neurology gave its stamp of approval to psychodynamic principles; this anticipated the emergence of a more psychoanalytically oriented psychiatry." By the 1950s the chair of virtually every psychiatry department in the United States had become psychodynamically oriented.[113] It greatly galled the few Canadian psychiatrists sympathetic to analysis that progress here was so slow. And among the obstacles to the onsweep of their doctrines they identified Clarence B. Farrar. Denigration of Farrar's reputation on the part of the psychoanalysts became one of the chief reasons for the silence that becalmed Farrar's ideas after his retirement from the professorship in 1947.

Among his principal detractors was Brock Chisholm. Chisholm, who had graduated in medicine from the University of Toronto in 1924, had turned first to general practice. Then in the early 1930s, he did a training analysis in London, England, returning in 1934 to open a psychotherapy practice in Toronto. During the Second World War Chisholm became the director of medical services of the Canadian army. He now had the power to begin setting his ideas through. He made a start by bringing analyst Lawrence Kubie up from New York for a group of weekend seminars, held at various military medical establishments from London to Montreal, and intended to reorient army psychiatrists towards psychoanalysis.[114] In 1944, Chisholm became Canadian deputy minister of health.[115] Thus, when in May 1945 Chisholm wrote to Sidney Smith (the new president of the University of Toronto) on the subject of Farrar's replacement in the chair of psychiatry, the letter came truly from the commanding heights of medicine. "There is a good deal of concern from many directions about the succession to the position of Professor of Psychiatry at the University of Toronto," Chisholm said.

> I think you will have known for some time that the psychiatric faiths prevalent and official at Toronto have been perhaps the most important factor in the prevention of the development of psychiatry in Canada in tune with that in Britain and in the United States.

Chisholm meant, of course, that Farrar's long tenure in Toronto was keeping psychoanalysis from acquiring in Canada the same entry it had gained elsewhere. "The holding to concepts which have been regarded as obsolete almost everywhere else, has produced an attitude in other countries which very strongly discounts all education in the psychiatric field in Toronto."

Chisholm proceeded to list all the great psychiatric moguls that had "indicated to me over a period of several years their concern about the stasis in psychiatric education in Toronto... It has been generally recognized that as long as Dr. Farrar occupies his present position there is no hope of a progressive or enlightened point of view developing."

So who should succeed Farrar? Chisholm thought first of England, recommending Aubrey Lewis or Ronald Hargreaves. Lewis, who was clinical director of the Maudsley Hospital at the time and opposed to psychoanalysis, was an interesting choice. Chisholm had probably thrown his name in to give the impression of balance, for there was not a chance in the world of getting Lewis to come to Toronto. Lewis became professor of psychiatry in the University of London in 1946.[116] There was one further problem with Lewis. "The fact that he is Jewish, though not Orthodox, and married to a non-Jewish wife might conceivably be somewhat of a handicap in Toronto." Chisholm moved on to possible American candidates. Here the list became more serious. He recommended William Menninger, O. Spurgeon English, and his old friend Lawrence Kubie. All were psychoanalysts. Menninger, who had been analyzed by Franz Alexander, was an authority on ego psychology.[117] Spurgeon English at Temple University, who had co-authored two years previously a standard text on psychosomatic medicine, was a member of the American Psychoanalytic Association.[118]

Chisholm created the impression that every enlightened psychiatric department in the world was watching events in Toronto with bated breath.

> The matter of this succession has been discussed with me in England and in the United States many times. The future of psychiatry in Canada, the necessary development of psychosomatic medicine in which Toronto is so far behind, and the fitting of doctors generally...to deal adequately with a very large part of their practices, will depend on the choice that is made.

Chisholm concluded histrionically, "This appointment will decide whether Toronto will remain in the psychiatric Middle Ages or will develop in a way that will make the knowledge of modern psychiatry of real service to the people of Canada."[119] Smith replied noncommittally.[120] In fact, Aldwyn Stokes, the recently appointed medical superintendent of Maudsley Hospital, was chosen: a man sympathetic to psychoanalysis, but not an analyst himself.

Chisholm's efforts to diminish Farrar's accomplishments were a straw in the wind. Farrar spent his last years in Toronto intellectually isolated from his colleagues who were riding upon the new wave, and was increasingly seen, as Chisholm had intended, as a representative of a mercifully overthrown old regime. Later generations would remember Farrar mainly for his editorship of the *American Journal of Psychiatry*, neglecting Farrar's efforts to produce well-rounded psychiatric graduates and to bring the principles of informal psychotherapy to the front lines of medicine where psychosomatic illness was encountered in primary care. Robert Pos, a historian of psychiatry, wrote in 1992 that as Stokes took over at TPH in 1947, "He was taken aback by the outdated limited physical facilities of the TPH itself, where nothing had been changed since 1926."[121] Farrar was made to appear a troglodyte.

If we try to place the accomplishments of the mature Farrar in perspective, he emerges as an important bridge figure between the first and second "biological psychiatries." The first biological psychiatry dominated the last decades of the nineteenth century and the first two of the twentieth, and was characterized by the themes that ran through Farrar's life until perhaps 1930: an emphasis upon heredity and upon brain biology as the causative factors in mental illness. This first biological psychiatry was then suspended in a hiatus of half a century in which psychoanalysis acquired the upper hand. Then from the 1970s onward biological doctrines returned with a vengeance, bolstered by the discovery of receptors in the brain for medications that were effective in psychiatric illness, and by the discovery of powerful genetic mechanisms in some of the commonest psychiatric disorders.[122] This was the "second biological psychiatry," which, it would be fair to say, is now in ascendancy. Did Farrar, a historic figure in establishing intellectual continuity between the two psychiatries, ever feel vindicated as he witnessed the triumph of this second biological psychiatry? He never said.

ENDNOTES

[1] Papers in Farrar private archive, 20 Oriole Road, Toronto, labelled "C.B.F's notes re Cattaraugus, N.Y. The residents and his family." All subsequent manuscript material in this chapter, unless otherwise identified, is taken from this archive.

[2] C.B. Farrar, *Portraits: After-dinner Address Delivered January 20, 1958 at the First Canadian Mental Hospital Institute in Toronto, Ontario* (Washington, DC: American Psychiatric Association, 1958; reprinted by University Microfilms, Ann Arbor), p.2. Surprisingly, Farrar did not do well at Harvard. Although he had ranked close to the top of his class at Allegheny College, at Harvard his marks were generally B's and C's. He took mainly languages, art and philosophy, receiving in English a D+ at

midterm and a C as final mark. This must have been a curious comment upon the English course, for Farrar loved books all his life, accumulating a vast library, and wrote elegant prose. Records of marks in Harvard University Archives.

[3] Welch to Farrar, September 18, 1897.

[4] William Osler, *The Principles and Practice of Medicine* (New York: Appleton, 1892).

[5] Cited in Farrar, "The Four Doctors," *Proceedings of the Seventh Annual Psychiatric Institute, Held September 16, 1959* (Princeton: New Jersey Neuro-Psychiatric Institute, 1959), pp. l05-16, quote p. 110.

[6] Ibid., pp. 110-11. See also Farrar, "I Remember Osler, Psychotherapist," *AJP* 121: 761-62 (February 1965).

[7] Ibid., p. 111. On Osler's use of psychotherapy, see also William B. Spaulding, "Osler—As Much Heart as Head," *Canadian Family Physician*, 38: 1617-21 (1992).

[8] Endowed in 1853 by Moses Sheppard, a Baltimore merchant, the Sheppard Asylum opened its doors only in l891. Edward Brush, formerly at the Pennsylvania Hospital for the Insane in Philadelphia, was its first superintendent. When in l896 Enoch Pratt, a Baltimore banker, willed the asylum more money, it was renamed The Sheppard and Enoch Pratt Hospital. See Edward N. Brush, "The Sheppard and Enoch Pratt Hospital," in Henry M. Hurd, ed., *The Institutional Care of the Insane in the United States and Canada*, 4 vols. (Baltimore: Johns Hopkins Press, 1916-17), vol. 2, pp. 558-70. Farrar started there at a salary of $50 per month. See letter of Joseph Grape, secretary of the Board of Trustees, to Farrar, June 30, 1900.

[9] See Thomas Neville Bonner, *American Doctors and German Universities: A Chapter in International Intellectual Relations, 1870-1914* (Lincoln: Univ. of Nebraska Press, 1963), p. 23.

[10] C.B. Farrar, "I Remember Stewart Paton," *AJP* 117: 160-62 (August 1960).

[11] Paton to Farrar, October l0, 1903.

[12] Paton to Farrar, letters of November 28, 1902 and January 11, 1904. In fact, Paton could not have been disappointed with the results of Farrar's trip. Welch did become convinced of the importance of psychiatry, leading Henry Phipps to donate large sums of money to Hopkins for the establishment of the Phipps Clinic in psychiatry. Paton was offered the chair, but turned it down in favour of Adolph Meyer. See Paton's obituary, *Princeton Alumni Weekly*, February 13, 1942.

[13] Stewart Paton, *Psychiatry: A Text-Book for Students and Physicians* (Philadelphia: J.B. Lippincott, 1905). To put Paton's textbook in the context of American psychiatry, see Gerald N. Grob, *Mental Illness and American Society, 1875-1940* (Princeton: Princeton University Press, 1983), pp. 118-19.

[14] Paton to Farrar, January 11, 1904.

[15] Paton to Farrar, October 10, l903.

[16] Hospital president George Pope to Farrar, March 18, 1902.

[17] Pope to Farrar, May 13, 1903.

[18] Pope to Farrar, December 30, 1903.

[19] C.B. Farrar, "On the Methods of Later Psychiatry," *AJI* 61: 437-66 (January 1905), esp. p. 451.

[20] On Nissl see Hugo Spatz, "Franz Nissl (l860-l919)," in Kurt Kolle, ed., *Grosse Nervenärzte*, 2nd ed. (Stuttgart: Thieme, l970), vol. 2, pp. 13-31; Joachim-Ernst Meyer discusses Alzheimer on pp. 32-38.

[21] See on this Heidelberg tradition, L. Hermke, "Karl Wilmanns (1873-1945)—biobibliographische Betrachtung einer psychiatrischen Ära," *Fortschritte der Neurologie und Psychiatrie*, 56 (4): 103-10 (April 1988), esp. 107-08.

[22] See the "*Zeugnis*," or certificate, that Nissl later drew up for him, dated June 27, 1905.

[23] From a notebook of Heidelberg case histories that survives, it is clear Farrar was at the bedside as well as the laboratory.

[24] See Farrar, "Student Days at Harvard and Heidelberg, *University of Toronto Medical Graduate* 12 (2): 2-4 (Spring, 1966).

[25] C.B. Farrar, "I Remember Nissl," *AJP* 110: 621-24 (February 1954), quote p. 623; "tears" from oral account Farrar give to Joan Farrar.

[26] Farrar's journal of his travels in 1904 bristles with references to (and gossip about) the greats of neuropathology.

[27] Between 1903 and 1909 Farrar published fifteen scientific papers, the most widely cited of them being the report of his research in Nissl's lab: "On the Phenomena of Repair in the Cerebral Cortex: A Study of Mesodermal and Ectodermal Activities Following the Introduction of a Foreign Body," in Franz Nissl, ed., *Histologische und Histopathologische Arbeiten* (Jena, 1908), vol. 2., pp. 1-70. The others appeared for the most part in the *AJI*.

[28] C.B. Farrar, "On the Methods," p. 438.

[29] F. C. (née L.), December 28, 1920.

[30] Paton to Farrar, March 8, 1904.

[31] Paton wrote Farrar on February 28, 1904, "...You are no longer a Sheppardite... the Carnegie has appointed you a Research Fellow in experimental psychology at a salary of $1000.... You are to live at the Sheppard which will board and lodge you and do your work in the hospital which is to supply you with instruments and the current literature and have most of your time for research work."

[32] Paton alluded to it in a letter of March 26, 1903, delighted that Farrar would be staying at Hopkins.

[33] V.C. Vaughan to Farrar, June 1, 1905.

[34] J.W. Mobley to Farrar, January 1, 1908.

[35] White to Farrar, April 6, 1908.

[36] At Farrar private archive, Toronto.

[37] Mitchell first articulated his rest cure in 1875. See his "Rest in Nervous Disease: Its Use and Abuse," in [E.C. Seguin, ed.] *A Series of American Clinical Lectures* 1 (4): 84-102 (April 1875).

[38] Paul Dubois, *The Psychic Treatment of Nervous Disorders*, trans. and ed. by Smith Ely Jelliffe (New York: Funk, 1905). The first edition was *Les Psychonévroses et leur traitement moral* (Paris: Masson, 1904).

[39] In Farrar's appreciation of the role of psychology in the "study of mental disease," Kraepelin occupies center stage. Yet Farrar refers also to the work of Robert Sommer, Theodor Ziehen, and Gustav Aschaffenburg, all prominent German psychiatrists of the day. See Farrar, "On the Methods," pp. 460, 465.

[40] Paton to Farrar, November 1, 1906.

[41] See Shorter, *From Paralysis to Fatigue: A History of Psychosomatic Illness in the Modern Era* (New York: Free Press, 1992), pp. 40-68.

[42] "The menstrual curve," he wrote in 1906, "often furnishes valuable indications as to the nature of the psychosis." See Farrar, "The Making of Psychiatric Records," *AJI* 62: 479-509 (1906), quote pp. 491-92.

[43] In 1897 Brush, for example, had indicted "stress and heredity" as the two principle causes of insanity. In eighty cases of "pure melancholia" seen at the Sheppard Asylum, "Presumed hereditary predisposition... is shown in 32 percent." "An Analysis of One Hundred Cases of Acute Melancholia," *British Medical Journal* 2: 777-79 (September 25, 1897), quote p. 778. Brush was once asked by a Congress of Religious Education to lecture on "Moral Degeneracy in the Light of Medical Science,"

also on "Moral Imbecility." He asked Farrar in Heidelberg, "Can you give me any points?" Brush to Farrar, January 17, 1904.

[44] Emil Kraepelin was by no means a biological determinist and rejected Bénédict Auguste Morel's doctrine of "progressive degeneration." Yet Kraepelin conceded that "the general significance of heredity in the etiology of psychiatric illness is without doubt." Kraepelin, *Psychiatrie: Ein Lehrbuch für Studirende und Aerzte*, 5th ed. (Leipzig: J.A. Barth, 1896), p. 86. See p. 87 for Kraepelin's rejection of Morel.

[45] On Cotton's arrival at Trenton see James Leiby, *Charity and Correction in New Jersey: A History of State Welfare Institutions* (New Brunswick: Rutgers University Press, 1967), pp. 119-22; also Andrew Scull, "Desperate Remedies: A Gothic Tale of Madness and Modern Medicine," *Psychological Medicine* 17: 561-77 (1987), esp. pp. 562-63. On the extent to which Cotton's doctrines resonated through the American psychiatric establishment, see Gerald N. Grob, *The Inner World of American Psychiatry, 1890-1940: Selected Correspondance* (New Brunswick: Rutgers University Press, 1985), pp. 108-23.

[46] Scull offers a slightly different chronology. These details are from the *American Medical Directory 1906*, and from Hurd, *Institutional Care of the Insane*, vol. 2, p. 709. On Cotton's sailing for Europe, see his letter to Farrar of November 6, 1905.

[47] W[illiam] Arbuthnot Lane, *Operative Treatment of Chronic Constipation* (London: Nisbet, 1904).

[48] As Farrar told his wife Joan Farrar, interview of July 10, 1992.

[49] Cotton to Farrar, February 27, 1907.

[50] Cotton to Farrar, June 8, 1908.

[51] Hurd, *Institutional Care of the Insane*, vol. 3, p. 79. Scull situates Cotton's embrace of autointoxication theories in 1916. Scull, "Desperate Remedies," p. 563.

[52] Farrar retained copies of his patients' charts; those from the period 1909-16 are at the Farrar private archive in Toronto.

[53] H.C. Warren (editor of the *Psychological Review*) to Farrar, August 8 and 11, 1906.

[54] Farrar to Meyer, January 18, 1912 and January 30, 1913, both on trivial subjects, in the Johns Hopkins University Archives.

[55] How much he was paid at Trenton is not known. None of the documents for that period have survived in the mental hospital's archives.

[56] These details have been reconstructed from the Paton-Farrar correspondence and from Paton's personal file in the Princeton University Archives.

[57] See *Annual Report of the New Jersey State Hospital at Trenton, 1913*, p. 26, for a list of the operations for the year, which appear to be for routine abdominal indications. A table of "existing causes" of mental illness in the patients made no reference to autointoxication (p. 44).

[58] Trenton asylum chart no. 15524. Farrar private archive.

[59] Cotton wrote Farrar November 4, 1919. "Our surgical work at the present time is developing very nicely. Drs. Draper and Lynch, who I consider know more about intestinal pathology than anyone in the country, come to the hospital from New York once a week and we have operated on about forty cases." Cotton continued, "Our first case was one in which you were interested, that of Florence P.... She never got any better, in fact got very much worse and it was the first case on which we operated, resection of the colon. Unfortunately her physical condition was so bad and her heart so weak that she did not survive, although she lived a week. It served to confirm my opinion, however, that her trouble was largely in the intestinal tract."

Cotton concluded the letter, "I think our statistics show conclusively that the manic depressive and dementia praecox groups are toxemias due to chronic infections..."

We have not space to consider the subsequent public outrage over conditions at Trenton, especially over Cotton's operations in which 180 patients died. According to a letter to the *New York Times* by a former staff member (and former patient) named Henry Gibbons, the orgy of surgery did not commence until October 1918. (*New York Times* August 21, 1925, p. 12.) Yet already in 1916 the whistle was being blown. Walter Stewart, an official in the state of New Jersey's Department of Charities and Corrections, had written Farrar around September 1916, asking what Farrar knew about "conditions at the State Hospital." In a follow-up letter of September 19, 1916, Stewart charged that Cotton was neglecting public patients for his private practice, that patients were beaten, and that operative instruments were not sterilized. A coup against Cotton mounted by Dr. George Tracy, on the hospital's board of trustees, failed. See Tracy to Farrar, September 1, 1918. Paton was by this time no longer a member of the board.

[60] Southard to Farrar, June 28, 1916.

[61] Interview of July 10, 1992. Whatever patriotic or martial motives might have inhabited Farrar's breast in the First World War had vanished by the Second. He gave Toronto psychologist Roger Myers an earful "for being such a stupid ass as to get mixed up in this damn war!" Transcript of interview with Myers (1976). QSMHC Archives.

[62] Farrar also had feelers from the Manhattan State Hospital on Ward's Island in New York City (see George Kirby to Farrar, August 12, 1916), and from Frederick Tilney, who ran a neurological laboratory and service at Columbia's medical school. (See Tilney to Paton, June 23, 1916; Paton forwarded the letter to Farrar).

[63] See his testimony in *Returned Soldiers: Proceedings of the Special Committee...Evidence Taken...February 7th to July 17th, 1917* (Ottawa, 1917), pp. 692-93.

[64] General R.J. Gwynne gave a summary of Farrar's wartime service in a letter to the president of the Selection Board, February 15, 1919.

[65] For the larger picture, see Desmond Morton and Glenn Wright, *Winning the Second Battle: Canadian Veterans and the Return to Civilian Life, 1915-1930* (Toronto: University of Toronto Press, 1989).

[66] See their joint report on the Battleford Hospital for the Insane in Saskatchewan, sent to F. McKelvey Bell of the Department S.C.R., December 23, 1918, or on the Selkirk Hospital for the Insane in Manitoba, report of December 30. In Archives, Department of Veterans Affairs, R.G. 38.

[67] See Farrar to Clarke, January 22, 1919. See C.K. Clarke and C.B. Farrar, "One Thousand Psychiatric Cases from the Canadian Army," *Canadian Journal of Mental Hygiene* 1 (4): 313-17 (1920). Among other important publications from Farrar's World War One experience was "Neuroses among Returned Soldiers: Types and Indications," *Boston Medical and Surgical Journal* 179: 615-22 (November 7, 1918).

[68] Clarke to Argue, October 16, 1920.

[69] See Farrar's telegram to Haven Emerson of the Bureau, May 30, 1921 and the attached correspondence.

[70] For the previous history of the sanitarium see Cheryl Krasnick Warsh, *Moments of Unreason: The Practice of Canadian Psychiatry and the Homewood Retreat, 1883-1923* (Montreal: McGill-Queen's University Press, 1989).

[71] See S.E.D. Shortt, *Victorian Lunacy: Richard M. Bucke and the Practice of Late Nineteenth-Century Psychiatry* (Cambridge: Cambridge University Press, 1986), pp. 141-46.

[72] See George Henry Noble, "Traumatisms and Malformations of the Female Genital Apparatus and Their Relation to Insanity," *Journal of the American Medical Association* 35 (9): 531-34 (September 1, 1900). Refers to Hobbs as one of the leaders in operations for pelvic reflex insanity (p. 531). Hobbs told Noble, "organic lesions of the inflammatory type are the most prominent factors among pelvic diseases in exciting mental alienation and displaced organs rank next in importance..." (p. 534). In 1912 Josef Peretti, a reforming German psychiatrist,

singled out Hobbs especially for criticism, "Gynäkologie und Psychiatrie," *Medizinische Klinik* 8 (46): 1857-62 (November 17, 1912), esp. 1858.

[73]Warsh, *Moments of Unreason*, pp. 57-58.

[74]Barnes to Farrar, March 5, 1923; Barnes was now superintendent of the asylum in Selkirk, Manitoba. A report from Clarke had documented scandalous conditions at Homewood. See Clarke's letter to Jarvis, March 17, 1923, in the Homewood Archives. Clarke singled out "the Bungalow" in particular as a latter-day snakepit.

[75]Barnes to Farrar, August 25, 1919.

[76]Jarivs to Farrar, November 9, 1992.

[77]Unusual among Canadian physicians, Farrar was greatly preoccupied with saving Jewish-German colleagues threatened with death. Farrar exerted himself in particular on behalf of a distinguished Viennese psychiatrist named Erwin Stransky. Even though Farrar failed to get Stransky out, Stransky miraculously survived the war in Vienna (possibly because he had a non-Jewish wife) and in 1945 resumed his correspondence with Farrar. The thick file is at the Farrar private archive. In Stransky's manuscript autobiography, on file at the Vienna Institut für Geschichte der Medizin, he mentioned Farrar (p. 626).

[78]Farrar to Clarke, November 21, 1922.

[79]Clarke mentioned that he had used this argument on Aikens in a letter to Farrar of November 23, 1922.

[80]See, for example, Hobbs to Farrar, December 12, 1922. "I have sufficient influence with the men on the Council Board of Ontario, who would put you through pro forma so long as they know your name which could be arranged for." Hobbs went on to remind Farrar of Farrar's previous promise that Hobbs be kept on "as a consultant to the Board [of directors of Homewood]." Hobbs was, in fact, not kept on.

[81]Aikens to Farrar, November 30, 1922.

[82]Aikens to Farrar, January 16, 1923.

[83]Clarke to Farrar, January 29, 1923.

[84]Meyer's secretary replied that "Dr. Meyer does not favour the extended use of forms to be filled in." Letter of August 7, 1923. It is interesting that Meyer himself included no personal note to Farrar.

[85]See Farrar's "Dear Doctor" flier that he sent out sometime in 1923. Homewood Archives.

[86]Clarke to Farrar, October 9, 1923.

[87]Jarvis, in his acceptance of Farrar's resignation, dated November 12, 1924, said that ever since May, Homewood had been hearing the rumours.

[88]"A.T.H." [Alfred Thomas Hobbs] to Farrar, November 17, 1924, in University of Toronto Archives. Hobbs flattered himself that information he had given to the provincial secretary settled the job for Farrar.

[89]Falconer to Farrar, February 6, 1924. University of Toronto Archives.

[90]See Greenland chapter for further details.

[91]Mouré to Farrar, January 23, 1925.

[92]Emma Clarke to Farrar, January 31, 1924.

[93]Kilgour to Farrar, March 24, 1934.

[94]Kilgour to Farrar, June 30, 1934.

[95]Kilgour to Farrar, October 15, 1935.

[96]See Ruth Franks, "The Pathogenesis and Prevention of Suicide," University of Toronto Ph.D. dissertation, 1936.

[97] Eugen Bleuler, *Lehrbuch der Psychiatrie* (Berlin, 1916; 5th ed. 1930); Bleuler had retired from the Burghölzli in 1927 but was still a presence at the time of Ruth Franks's visit.

[98] Franks to Farrar, January 27, 1931. "Dementia praecox" was the older term for what Bleuler baptized "schizophrenia" in 1908. Perhaps she was making a terminological point, reminding Farrar, who often referred to "D.P.," that up-to-date Europeans had shed the older term.

[99] Kilgour to Farrar, January 6, 1935.

[100] Clarence B. Farrar and Ruth MacLachlan Franks, "Menopause and Psychosis," *AJP* 10: 1031-44 (May 1931), quote p. 1044.

[101] See Dr. F.J. Bell to R.C. Montgomery, director of the Hospitals Division of the Ontario Department of Health, January 13, 1938.

[102] Farrar to Montgomery, March 7, 1938.

[103] For Farrar, the modern period of the discipline of psychiatry began with Griesinger. See Farrar, "Some Origins in Psychiatry," *AJI* 66: 277-94 (1909): "With Griesinger the reins of Hippocratic teaching were at last fully recovered. Again came recognition that mental disease and brain disease are synonymous." (p. 291).

[104] Quoted in the *Toronto Telegram* March 5 (or 6), 1929.

[105] Manuscript lecture notes, March 11, 1937. "Psychiatry IV."

[106] *Toronto Telegram* May 19, 1926. The language is the reporter's. However, Joan Farrar believes that her husband was misquoted.

[107] Farrar, "Technique of Mental Examination and Classification of Mental Diseases," in *Physician's Hand Book* (n.p.: Lange, [1944?], pp. 5, 7.

[108] Ibid., p. 23.

[109] C.B. Farrar, "Psychotherapy in Medical Practice," *Proceedings of the Inter-State Post Graduate Medical Assembly of North America...1938, Philadelphia, Pennsylvania* (n.p., n.d.), pp. 2-3.

[110] C.B. Farrar, "Psychotherapy in Medical Practice," *Canadian Medical Association Journal* 57 (6): 519-22 (December 1947), quotes p. 521.

[111] C.B. Farrar, "Sigmund Freud, 1856-1939," *University of Toronto Medical Journal* 17: 97-99 (1940), quotes p. 99. On another occasion he criticized psychotherapy today as having "developed into a highly artificial technique and as complicated as the Ptolemaic system," in contrast to Osler's psychotherapy. Farrar, "Osler at Johns Hopkins," *University of Western Ontario Medical Journal* 20 (1): 127-35 (January 1950), quote p. 131.

[112] Joan Farrar's notebook. Farrar private archive.

[113] Gerald N. Grob, "Origins of DSM-III: A Study in Appearance and Reality," *AJP* 148: 421-31 (1991), quote p. 429.

[114] Kubie described his Canadian travels to Dr. Jack Griffin in a letter of October 24, 1973, on file at the Museum of Mental Health Services (Toronto).

[115] The facts of Chisholm's career are set out in Alan Parkin, *A History of Psychoanalysis in Canada* (Toronto: Toronto Psychoanalytic Society, 1987), pp. 58-67. At the request of Chisholm, "Jack" Griffin, Clarence Hincks and William Line, in 1946 Kubie played a signficant role in the development of postwar psychiatry in Canada by coming weekends to Toronto to hold seminars for demobilized Canadian military psychiatrists who now felt somewhat out of touch with the field. When Farrar learned of these efforts, he asked Griffin and Line, "Why in the world did you get a man like Kubie to come up here? Why didn't you get somebody respectable like [Gregory] Zilboorg?" Griffin interview, August 18, 1992.

[116] See his entry in Gordon Wolstenholme, ed., *Lives of the Fellows of the Royal College of Physicians of London, continued to 1975* (vol. 6 of Munk's Roll) (Oxford: IRL Press, 1982), pp. 284-86. Hargreaves had been at the psychoanalytically oriented Tavistock Clinic in London.

[117] See Lawrence J. Friedman, *Menninger: The Family and the Clinic* (Lawrence: University Press of Kansas, 1990), pp. 65-66, 83, 90.

[118] Edward Weiss and O. Spurgeon English, *Psychosomatic Medicine: The Clinical Application of Psychopathology to General Medical Problems* (Philadelphia: W.B. Saunders, 1943).

[119] Chisholm to Sidney Smith, May 25, 1945. QSMHC Archives.

[120] Sidney Smith to Chisholm, May 31, 1945.

[121] Robert Pos, "A History of Psychiatry at the Toronto General Hospital," p. 29. QSMHC Archives.

[122] See, for example, Herbert Pardes, et al., "Genetics and Psychiatry: Past Discoveries, Current Dilemmas, and Future Directions," *AJP* 146: 435-43 (April 1989).

4

THE LIFE OF THE TORONTO PSYCHIATRIC HOSPITAL

ROGER BASKETT[*]

Institutional histories, an important facet of any historical field, risk by their very nature being narrow and uninteresting to all but a select few. This chapter is not intended to be an exhaustive study of the day-to-day activities of the Toronto Psychiatric Hospital. It aims at a broader picture of the hospital and its significance as an institution.[1]

TPH always fit into a larger picture. In 1925, the idea of a separate psychiatric hospital, distinct from the old mental hospital asylum tradition, was in keeping with developments in Europe. In fact, TPH was inspired by the Munich Clinic of Emil Kraepelin, which as we saw had been visited by C.K. Clarke, Edward Ryan, and W.A. Willoughby in 1908. Yet, over the years the trend in Ontario, as elsewhere, was away from separate institutes for psychiatry and towards the integration of psychiatry with mainstream medicine in general hospitals. This integration had begun in Toronto as early as 1905 with Donald Campbell Meyers' nervous ward at the old Toronto General Hospital. In 1930, the newly created provincial Department of Health established six community-based psychiatry clinics in an attempt to reduce admissions to the Ontario Hospitals.[2] Later, in the 1940s, as the newly established federal Department of Health and Welfare began to play a role in mental health, travelling clinics and clinics in general hospitals were established and funded by Ottawa.[3] After some forays into community mental health clinics in the early 1930s and early 1940s, psychiatrists favoured the expansion of general hospital wards.

---

[*]Roger Baskett, M.A., History, University of Toronto, 1992, is currently finishing medical studies at Dalhousie University.

Yet the care of the mentally ill in Ontario remained dominated by the entrenched interests of the Ontario Hospitals. The Royal Commission on Health Services remarked in 1966, the year TPH closed:

> Unfortunately because of Ontario's larger investment in plant than any other Province, and its more strongly entrenched tradition, those who are responsible for its psychiatric service are more likely to encounter serious difficulties in making radical change.[4]

This observation about mental health in Ontario was even more pronounced in the first four decades of this century.

Thus psychiatry in Ontario was mainly characterized by isolation: lagging behind in research, education, and funding.[5] To be sure, the leaders of the profession tried to overcome this isolation. In a brief to the House of Commons Special Committee on Social Security, the director of provincial mental health services and the professors of psychiatry at the three Ontario medical schools stated that the most important step toward integrating medical fields was to establish full psychiatric services in general hospitals.[6] They sought the larger goal of the scientific and medical legitimacy for psychiatry that the hospital setting could provide.[7] In 1948, this aspiration was partly achieved with the establishment of the National Health Grants program. The 1952 *Ontario Health Survey* recommended that the size of the mental hospitals be reduced, and that the system be integrated with the rest of medicine by establishing wards in general hospitals.[8] Advances after the 1930s, such as insulin coma therapy, electro-shock, and neuroleptics, did a great deal to advance the medical model of psychiatry. As the 1966 Royal Commission on Health Services observed,

> Because the Mental Hospitals are large and isolated, difficulty keeping contact with the public they serve and with general hospitals the need for such contact is generally recognized, but there is no agreement as to how it can be sustained.[9]

Although general hospital wards and outpatient departments increased steadily, psychiatric care was still dominated by the Ontario Hospitals right into the 1950s.[10] The public health department tried to establish control over mental health services while the profession was pushing for integration with mainstream medicine via the wards in general hospitals. Yet, by the mid-1960s the battle was over and community mental health care was based in general hospitals.

TPH was the first real effort to bridge the gap between psychiatry and mainstream medicine. As the years went by, however, it became somewhat of an anachronism. Even though Clarke had envisioned TPH as the future of health care, it fit into neither the asylum, the community clinic, nor the general hospital model for psychiatry. Its chiefs had tried to drag psychiatry into mainstream medicine. C.B. Farrar noted in a *Toronto Telegraph* article in May 1925, "We want the atmosphere of the institute to be in every way just like an ordinary hospital."[11] However, its peculiar relationship to both the university and the government made achieving this goal difficult.

Established as a centre for treatment and teaching, it was in research that TPH made its major contribution. By the mid-1950s, a dozen hospitals and institutions in Toronto provided teaching facilities for the Department of Psychiatry.[12] In education, TPH itself really only served as a facility for formal lectures and the office of the department chairperson. Nor was it of great clinical significance; with only 60 to 80 beds, in 1961 TPH provided only a fraction of the province's inpatient psychiatric beds for its 20,398 patients.[13] Instead, as time went by, TPH became renowned for its contributions to psychiatric research, particularly in biological psychiatry. At a time when psychoanalysis and social theories of mental illness dominated elsewhere, the tradition of the belief in the essentially organic nature of mental illness persisted at TPH.

Unlike other Ontario Hospitals or general hospitals, TPH arose from scratch. For that reason the hospital was hailed as the new scientific approach to mental illness. As Sir Robert Falconer, president of the University of Toronto, said in 1923,

> The institution is a monument to the enlightened intelligence and progressiveness of the efforts now being made to treat mental diseases in the same skilful and scientific manner as other forms of disease.[14]

In 1925, however, this scientific side was as yet obscure, and, initially TPH was regarded as a new reception hospital and was treated as such.

Farrar went to significant lengths to explain how TPH was unique. Interviewed by a journalist in May 1925 soon after assuming his appointment, he set out his philosophy for TPH.

> The hospital will cooperate closely with all allied health and welfare activities. Our paramount aim will be to maintain a close touch with the medical profession so that the milder forms of mental trouble may be early recognized and dealt with... Our

work will also be carried on in close touch with the General Hospital.

Establishment of services

The story of TPH may be seen through the prism of steadily expanding services. First, came the outpatient department, beginning in 1926 as a weekly clinic conducted on a voluntary basis by Edmund P. Lewis of the Mental Hygiene Division of the city Department of Health. In September 1931, Lewis became the full-time director of the outpatient department. Its staff included a supervisor, a social worker, a psychologist and a number of voluntary postgraduate physicians, who helped with clinics and received instruction.[15]

Next came occupational therapy, becoming a separate department in 1927. Student interns were appointed as summer assistants and postgraduates were assigned for six months of experience. By 1932, over 80 percent of TPH inpatients received regular occupational therapy.[16] Other disciplines followed shortly thereafter.

The first social worker, Marion E. Stewart, a registered nurse, was appointed in 1930. Working through the outpatient department, she soon established links with the various hospitals and social agencies in the city.[17] Psychology also began as a part of the outpatient department. Jean Brown was the first psychologist and her work at this time was largely devoted to intelligence testing and teaching.[18]

Initially there was a good deal of confusion surrounding the role of TPH, stemming from the ambiguous nature of the agreement between the province, the city, and the university. It was never entirely clear which aspects of the hospital were run by the government and which by the university. TPH was an Ontario Hospital subject to the rigidly centralized administration of the Department of Health, criticized in 1937 by the Ontario Mental Health Survey as being cumbersome and politically corrupt.[19] Although some staff were paid by the province, others were paid by the university, and still others by both. There was also supplementary money from the Canadian National Committee for Mental Hygiene.

The original agreement of March 31, 1921, between the city, the province, and the university, was very brief and rather short on details.[20] The existing legislation (the *Reception Hospital Act* of 1914) was also inadequate. Under this act, a patient could only be admitted if his or her sanity was determined in advance: i.e., the patient was certified. But this was difficult in court cases.[21] As Deputy Provincial Secretary H.M Robbins wrote in a letter to Lincoln Goldie, provincial secretary:

> Patients admitted to the Reception Hospital [TPH] are not necessarily insane, and one of the main points to be considered in the operation of this class of institution is that the person being nervous, hysterical or otherwise in a disturbed mental state receive treatment which will correct the condition and which will obviate the necessity of treatment in a mental hospital.[22]

On December 23, 1925, a conference was held between representatives of the three institutions to discuss the function of the new hospital. A few months later, Robbins explained that:

> It was clearly realized by the conference that new legislation was required to properly cover the activities of the hospital and it was felt that a new Act should be passed relating exclusively to the Psychiatric hospital, and making all necessary provisions without reference to other existing legislation.[23]

In this legal obscurity, it was not entirely clear who could be admitted.

In the interim some informal arrangements were made regarding admissions. Indigent patients residing in the city were eligible for ten-day stays covered by the city at a fixed rate of $1.50 per day. Yet it was the city that determined who was eligible. In a similar fashion, court cases had to be approved by the city, but it was noted at the conference that "such a remand or committal does not constitute responsibility on the part of the city for maintenance."[24] The hospital was unable to refuse admission to any of these cases, even though payment was uncertain. Two-fifths of all cases admitted to TPH in the early years were referrals from the courts, and it soon became apparent that there was a problem.[25] It was agreed as a temporary measure that individuals picked up by the police would be examined by one or two city doctors and then, if necessary, transferred to TPH. This failed to resolve administrative tensions. On January 14, 1926, an exasperated H.M. Robbins (who dealt with the day-to-day problems of the hospital) wrote to Lincoln Goldie: "Some of the police and court officials seem to rather foster the idea that the Reception hospital should be a dumping ground for all the misfits who may be picked up in a city of this size."[26]

The *Psychiatric Hospitals Act* was passed into law on April 8, 1926, replacing the *Reception Hospital Act* of 1914.[27] It was a progressive piece of legislation designed to allow expedient admission and discharge.

The necessity of a certificate of insanity was removed, and in its place a patient could be admitted upon the certificate of one medical practitioner. The form would not state that person was insane, but rather that:

> The proposed patient is a person who is likely to benefit from treatment such as may be secured in an institution of this type and will furnish legal authority to the superintendent to detain such person until cured or until such time as the question of his or her sanity has been determined.[28]

Farrar was not entirely happy with the arrangements for court cases. In the original draft bill that Farrar prepared, "The final authority as to admissibility of a patient shall rest in the hands of the director of the institute rather than in the hands of the Medical fraternity in general."[29] The province was uneasy about the director's authority, although Robbins conceded that this was better than the police or the magistrates who "seem to be obsessed with the idea of using this institute as a dumping ground for all the derelicts which are picked up in the streets of this city."[30] Farrar was concerned about his own lack of control. "Our Hospital," he explained to the *Toronto Star* in 1926, "is relatively very small, and already we have had applications for the admission of a great many more patients than we could possibly accommodate."[31]

The new legislation of 1926 cleared up much of the ambiguity and many of the legal technicalities that initially hampered TPH, but trouble with the city persisted. The new act stated that anyone apprehended by the police who appeared to the judge to be possibly insane could be remanded to TPH for further observation. The act went on to say that the cost of maintaining the patient, "shall be payable by the city in which the patient was a resident at the time of his arrest."[32]

Many of the patients from court were not residents of Toronto. As a result, the city refused to pay their maintenance. The provincial secretary's office wrote a number of letters of complaint to the city relief officer, Thomas Rooney, and cited another section of the act which stated that: "If a person is unable to pay at the rate of $1.50 per diem...the municipal corporation shall be liable to the hospital at the said rate."[33] Robbins explained that it was the intent of the act, though not explicitly stated, that the city should pay for all court cases. He concluded by threatening further legislation.[34] The city remained firm, was very slow to pay, and frequently refused payments on a number of different grounds. The province accused the city of sending many cases that were sane.

Carrying out his threats, in 1927 Robbins drafted amendments to the 1926 *Psychiatric Hospitals Act*. He was particularly anxious to clarify the term "residence." For general purposes, a resident of Toronto was defined as anyone living there for three months or more. But in court cases it was often very difficult to ascertain a person's place of residence. Therefore all court referrals were deemed to be residents of the municipality where they were arrested. The province maintained that the amendment would impose no hardship on the city and that the intent was to make the courts more careful about who they sent.[35] Robbins added mistakenly that he thought none of the amendments would be contentious.

Although Farrar and the provincial solicitor were consulted, apparently the city was not. The city and the relief officer, in particular, took exception to what they saw as yet another attempt by the province to saddle them with the costs of TPH.[36] Rooney sent a memorandum to the members of the legislature with examples of cases for which they had refused payment. He enlisted the support of MPP Russell Nesbitt and asked the other city members to oppose the amendment.[37] The effort failed and the amendments were passed in April 1927.

Payment squabbles still dragged on. In November 1928, with the city obdurate, Robbins again complained to his boss in a memo.

> To put the matter plainly, the city Relief Office seems to be a law unto itself, disregarding the terms of the statute as relating to this institution and either paying or refusing to pay, largely according to the whim of the official in charge.[38]

The city continued to take the position that the amendment was a contravention of the initial 1921 agreement between the city and the province. It was not until December 1929 that the city finally agreed to pay the outstanding sum of $3,339 dating back to April 1927.[39] It is not clear how or why the impasse was ultimately resolved. The obvious answer is that when push came to shove, the province ultimately won out. Yet over the years, the city continued to be slow with payments and continued to complain. In March 1930 and again in 1931, the city attempted to draft a private bill to amend the *Psychiatric Hospital Act*.[40] Although the issue eventually petered out, the difficulties inherent in TPH's ill-defined role persisted, and it was certainly not the last incidence of government interference. The whole payment question illustrates the practical difficulty in making TPH work.

Teaching

From the beginning, teaching was an integral part of TPH's role. Any history of TPH is of necessity also a history of the Department of Psychiatry of the University of Toronto. In 1956, the Borden Committee noted:

> Because of the fact that the Toronto Psychiatric Hospital is the teaching unit in the field of psychiatry for the department of Psychiatry and, therefore, the University of Toronto, it is essential to consider the Toronto Psychiatric Hospital and its facilities...in dealing with the functioning of the department of Psychiatry in the University, and its overall relationship with the Faculty of Medicine.[41]

A solid teaching program was established early on at the hospital. Farrar in particular regarded the education of psychiatrists of paramount importance.[42] Instruction began in 1926 with lectures to fifth- and sixth-year students at the Queen Street hospital. The emphasis was on biological psychiatry and the relation of psychiatry to general medicine.[43] Final-year students were exposed to the more common and important types of mental disease at Queen Street, but only had one afternoon interviewing patients.[44] Beginning in 1927, the hospital offered clinical courses and doubled the clinical instruction given to final-year students. In addition, psychiatry was now introduced during the fourth year of medical school. Undergraduate training involved 150 hours of lectures, demonstrations, and clinics.[45]

In August 1928, Farrar, with the help of Edward Ryan, then director of medical services in the provincial Department of Health, established a weekly seminar on Saturday mornings called the Inter-hospital Psychiatric Society.[46] The seminar presented subjects in fields relating to psychiatry, and its object was to "demonstrate the vital interrelations between psychiatry and other disciplines such as biology, sociology, psychology, anthropology, law, as well as other departments in the medical sciences."[47] This seminar was intended to increase the exposure of psychiatry and help establish it as a legitimate medical science. Clearly, Farrar was organizing a department firmly grounded in science and biological psychiatry[48] and had already taken steps towards this by establishing medical consultants in neuropathology, ophthalmology, medicine, and neurology. Thus, while the Department of Psychiatry was not integrated with the general hospitals, TPH and the Department of Psychiatry were soundly based in scientific medicine.

In 1931, a one-year postgraduate course was established for junior doctors of the Ontario Hospital Service. Resident physicians became attached to TPH as full-time assistant physicians. This greatly augmented the staff at no cost to the government. To supplement the regular lectures and clinics given at the hospital, special courses were given in collaboration with various other departments including: anatomy, neurology, endocrinology, pathology, psychology, physiology, medicine, and ophthalmology.[49] In addition, there were four two-hour staff conferences a week. The report covering the period from 1926 to 1932 noted, "As a rule, one case is studied at each of these staff conferences which are calculated to furnish the foundation of the practical instruction."[50] Farrar noted in a later report that these conferences and the weekly seminars helped to integrate psychiatry with the biological sciences.[51]

In 1933, a Ph.D in psychiatry was established by enrolling the Department of Psychiatry in the School of Graduate Studies. The first student in the program was Ruth Maclachlan Franks, who was at the time in charge of the women's ward at TPH. In 1936, she was awarded her degree for a thesis entitled "The Pathogenesis and Prevention of Suicide." The study had been carried out between 1928 and 1935 on 350 cases of attempted suicide admitted to TPH.[52] It also marked the beginning of research at TPH.[53]

TPH was also active in training other specialists in the field of mental health. In March 1931, Nettie Fidler was appointed director of nursing and began to organize the nursing service and the teaching program at TPH. Starting in October 1931, the hospital offered a three-month affiliate course in psychiatric nursing. The experimental course stressed the importance of mental hygiene and psychiatry in general nursing, rather than qualifying psychiatric nurses. The following autumn, a six-month course was begun for nurses from general hospital training schools who wanted to qualify for public health work and other posts requiring psychiatric training.[54] In addition, the staff of TPH taught courses in social psychiatry for undergraduate nurses, as well as students in social sciences, occupational therapy students, public health nurses from the city Department of Health, and students of public health at the university. In 1934, a formal series of 12 lectures was initiated for the students of the one-year public health nursing course; 474 hours of instruction were being given annually by the nursing staff, in addition to 350 hours of staff conferences and 40 hours per week of seminars.[55]

Throughout this period, TPH teaching programs received a good deal of financial assistance from the Rockefeller Foundation. Established in 1913 by John D. Rockefeller, the foundation was intended "to promote the well-being of mankind throughout the world." From the beginning, the Rockefeller Foundation promoted psychiatry by funding the work of the (US) National Committee for Mental Hygiene. During the 1920s, Rockefeller support for psychiatry was largely directed towards acceptance by hospitals and medical schools as an important part of the medical sciences.[56] Beginning in 1924, the Rockefeller Foundation also assisted the Canadian National Committee of Mental Hygiene (CNCMH) by providing money for fellowships, a child study program, and, in the 1930s, training.[57]

A recipient of part of the foundation's five million dollar grant for medical education in Canada, Toronto benefited from the early support of the Rockefeller Foundation. One million dollars was given to the university's general endowment of the medical department.[58] As outlined in a previous chapter, the conditions of this grant were that the province and the university provide a number of additions to the medical faculty, including a psychiatric hospital.[59] Until the construction of TPH was assured, the principal of the gift was withheld and the interest paid quarterly beginning September 30, 1921. George E. Vincent, president of the Rockefeller Foundation, wrote Falconer in November 1920 explaining this decision.

> The withholding of the principal of the gift until you have secured the addition of the pathology laboratory and the new psychiatric clinic will, it is hoped, be of service to you in securing these essential features of your programme.[60]

Thus the university could use the promise of the Rockefeller money as leverage to get the government to provide the new facilities. Finally, when the city and the province reached agreement and construction began in spring 1923, the capital sum of one million dollars was paid to the university.[61]

In 1931 Clarence Hincks of the CNCMH offered Farrar a $7,500 annual grant to supplement salaries for five years.[62] As Farrar later told Harrison Spaulding, executive director of the CNCMH, the Toronto postgraduate psychiatry course had only been possible because the grant had enabled him to assemble a good core teaching staff.[63] From 1931 to 1937, TPH received $24,000 of Rockefeller money via the University of Toronto and the CNCMH for psychiatric education, nearly all of which went to supplement the meagre salaries paid by the Ontario Hospital Service.[64] This helped TPH through the Depression, when salaries in the Ontario Hospital Service were cut, in some cases by nearly 60 percent, and a third of the medical staff resigned.[65]

Perhaps the most important development in these early years was the establishment in 1934 of the Board of Psychiatric Examiners. Consisting of the psychiatry department heads at the three provincial medical schools, the board's task was to examine applicants for the provincial hospital service. Qualified graduate interns would complete the one-year TPH postgraduate course. At its end they would sit an exam set by the board of examiners, who could then recommend them for appointments as junior physicians in the service.[66] This was the first step towards establishing a specialty in psychiatry. By establishing the one-year postgraduate course at TPH as the prerequisite for appointment to the Ontario Hospitals, a higher and uniform standard for psychiatry was assured.

POLITICAL INTERFERENCE

The motivation behind the establishment of the board was largely political. In a letter to Dean of Medicine John FitzGerald, University President Henry Cody remarked:

> I am deeply gratified to learn that future appointments to the service will be made on the basis of competitive examinations and on the recommendation of the committee of psychiatric experts. The Minister in adopting this course will not only secure efficient service but will free himself from many embarrassments.[67]

In fact, the role of politics in the provincial hospital service was widely known. The *American Journal of Psychiatry*, commenting on the establishment of the board of examiners, remarked:

> At the instance of the Minister of Health, Dr. J.[ames] A. Faulkner, the government of Ontario has taken a decisive step the purpose of which is the elimination of even the shadow of politics in the constitution and maintenance of medical services in the provincial hospitals.[68]

Such interference had been constant in the Ontario Hospital Service since the beginning[69] and included Farrar's own appointment. It was no secret that C.K. Clarke had wanted Farrar as his successor and had lobbied to this end. As indicated in Shorter's chapter on Farrar, there was even a suggestion of help from A.T. Hobbs, Farrar's predecessor at the Homewood Sanitarium in Guelph. Even though Hobbs may have drifted into therapeutic byways, his claim to political pull may not have been that far-fetched.[70] The mere fact that he was able to see the provincial secretary, and apparently knew him, indicates a degree of political influence.[71]

Unhappiness with Farrar continued after 1925. Sometime in the late 1920s, a man named Stringer was sent down to Virginia by the Ontario government to see Farrar's estranged wife, in an effort to find something to use against the psychiatrist. Farrar, who was on good terms with his wife, explained in a letter to her:

> As I told you in my other letter there is an element here that was disappointed when their plans for running the new hospital were over-ruled and they have been using every means that sewer politics can command to hamper us and make trouble. This present incident is simply their latest and most contemptible attack.[72]

There are no other documents relating to this incident. According to the letter, Farrar took the matter up with Provincial Secretary Lincoln Goldie, who expressed amazement at the insolence of a government official prying into Farrar's private life. Farrar went on to explain to his wife that when the matter had gone further he would fill her in on the details. No further correspondence has been found. An interesting footnote to this story is that in 1930 the deputy provincial secretary, asking about the suitability of a TPH employee, mentioned that she had been seen by R.M. Stringer. Farrar replied curtly: "Dr. Stringer's opinion I think may be disregarded."[73] Robert Melbourne Stringer graduated from Queens in 1929 and was a junior resident physician assistant in the female service at TPH in September 1929. In 1930, he worked briefly at the Ontario Hospital London before moving to Hamilton and later doing anaesthesia.[74] Whether or not this is the same person is unclear; the point of the story is that Farrar had to endure a determined political attack on his position.

Even in 1934, Farrar was apparently insecure about his position. In responding to a request from Farrar for information about regulations governing civil servants in the Ontario government service, Bernard T. McGhie, deputy minister of hospitals, concluded, "I would hope it is quite well accepted in this province that if a superintendent keeps himself free of politics, he is not likely to be disturbed in the event of a change in the administration."[75] Obviously Farrar was nervous in the face of the newly elected Liberal government under Premier Mitchell Hepburn. The message from McGhie was clear—keep your nose out of politics and you will be all right.

An interesting case of internal politics and possible external interference includes the alleged involvement of Ontario Premier Mitch Hepburn.[76] The rumour that staff nurse Myrtle Foley, appointed in 1926, was Hepburn's mistress is merely hearsay, but her staff record and other related documents indicate that her career was rather unusual; and the events certainly illustrate the internal politicking of TPH. The rumour of an affair undercut her authority by suggesting she was not hired for her nursing skills. She served first under Nettie Fidler and then under Eileen Ditchburn. Under Ditchburn, Foley was assistant director of nursing. Her duties included supervision of nursing and housekeeping, and the care and education of student nurses—for a salary of $1,500. In contrast, Ditchburn, the director of nursing, was only paid a salary of $1,200 from April 1931 through July 1934. Although the steady annual pay increases given staff could explain the difference between Foley (on staff since 1926) and Ditchburn (newly hired in the early Depression), Foley's higher salary was grist for the hospital rumour mill. Furthermore, while she graduated in 1926 from the Toronto mental hospital nursing program, Foley's staff record noted she did not have the educational qualifications for her position. On the same record, Farrar indicated that she was not eligible for further promotion; while on Ditchburn's record he remarked that she "...should receive more than our increase in pay."[77]

Farrar was probably feeling generous, or guilty, because Ditchburn had resigned several weeks earlier. In her letter of resignation, Ditchburn listed a number of reasons for leaving, including a failure to get a promised salary increase and a decrease in pay following her assumption of Fidler's responsibilities. More interestingly, she mentions: "There is not sufficient or adequate assistance in teaching the nursing subjects. A properly qualified assistant was promised, nominated and refused in March 1933."

Apparently, Ditchburn was also unhappy with Myrtle Foley's qualifications and complained of political interference. "I cannot reconcile my personal and professional principles [with] political influences and demands." Her complaints were all directed at the Department of Health. Although she went out of her way to thank Farrar for his understanding and help, her only mention of the nursing staff was her appreciation of

Nettie Fidler and the lack of help from the Department of Health to improve the personnel.[78] Yet Foley went on to become director of nursing at TPH.[79]

By all accounts, Farrar found the interference and constraints of the Department of Health exasperating.[80] Opening up medical positions to competition was one thing, but all other positions in the hospital were still awarded by the provincial government. Appointments were made by the civil service commissioner on the recommendation of the minister. No examinations were held. Thus, a superintendent had very little say in who was on staff. Furthermore, he could only suspend an employee and recommend discharge, but had no authority to hire or fire. There were no boards of governors for the provincial hospitals; the Hospitals Division of the Department of Health maintained a highly centralized service.[81] This lack of power made it very hard for Farrar to build a capable and loyal staff. While this task was easier at TPH than at other provincial hospitals (since, as the centre of teaching and research, TPH attracted the best people), considerable difficulties with staff remained.

A memorandum found in Farrar's papers lists ideas for staff changes to be made at TPH. The first item reads: "gradual elimination of unfit members of staff and replacement by capable individuals who will be chosen purely on merit." The document is undated, but must be from before October 1930, because one of the proposals was to appoint Jason A. Hannah as neuropathologist. From this document and many comments on staff records it is apparent that many original staff of TPH were not qualified and were unsuitable for their jobs.

In August 1930, Farrar wrote to the deputy provincial secretary asking that he be allowed to dismiss Kathleen Robb, one of the occupational therapy nurses. Robbins refused, and Farrar was apparently quite annoyed by the constraints placed on him by the department.[82] In 1932, Robb was still director of occupational therapy, but in October 1933 Farrar did manage to have Helen P. LeVesconte replace her as director (although Robb remained on staff).[83] Farrar noted in his 1933 report to the Hospitals Division that LeVesconte was brought in to reorganize the department and make it more effective.

A number of staff members were dismissed in the early years of the hospital. An orderly, an attendant, and a nurse were all suspended for abuse or cruelty to patients. In each case, Farrar had to file extensive reports and even go through a number of hearings in order to secure their removal.[84] The point is that TPH was tightly controlled by the Department of Health and the politics of the government of the day.

Thus, the first decade of TPH was filled with many growing pains and political troubles. Nonetheless, the hospital established itself as an academic centre, with a strong emphasis on biological psychiatry. For teaching and patient care, it soon became obvious the facility was too limited. Two American doctors who surveyed the Ontario Hospitals in 1937 concluded of TPH,

> The building is too small for its purpose and not well arranged. Incoherent groups of patients must be in contact. Laboratory and occupational space is needed, quarters for officers, and a service for children.[85]

Even though the province believed TPH to be "...a structure which will adequately perform its functions for many years to come,"[86] by the late 1930s the hospital was already struggling to meet demands for patient care.

Physical therapies

Until the late 1930s patient care was very limited. Few effective medications existed and in reality there were no real physical therapies at TPH or any other mental hospital. John Dewan recalled in 1978,

> When I came in 1933, we had three continuous water baths practically going all the time. We didn't have any medication for the patients specifically. We used HMA's [Hyoscine Morphine Atropine] and HMC's [Hyoscine Morphine Codeine] to try and quieten them down. But the severe depressions were a real risk. And they might refuse to eat; and tube feedings went on all day long. Tube feedings and trying to keep them alive in the hope there would be a spontaneous recovery...... It was a different atmosphere altogether.[87]

A new wave of physical therapies began in the late 1930s with the advent of the various shock therapies. The first of these, insulin coma therapy, was the most important for the immediate future of TPH.

Insulin coma therapy, like many medical discoveries, was an accident. A Viennese physician, Manfred Joshua Sakel, began his career treating drug addicts at the Lichterfelde Sanatorium in Berlin. In 1930, Sakel inadvertently gave an overdose of insulin to a diabetic morphine addict. This resulted in a mild coma, but, when she recovered, her desire for morphine had abated. Soon, Sakel was giving insulin to all the drug addicts and claiming spectacular successes. Another accidental overdose of insulin produced a coma in a psychotic addict. Upon recovery his psychotic symptoms had improved. After some initial animal experiments to establish a safe method of administering an insulin coma, Sakel began treating schizophrenics at the hospital.[88] In the early 1930s, Sakel left Berlin (an inhospitable place for a young Jewish doctor) and returned to Vienna, where he continued his experiments at the Neuropsychiatric University Clinic.[89] In 1933, he published a short paper reporting the success of his method. Word of his discovery soon spread to the United States through the interest of a number of young American doctors studying in Vienna. In 1936, Sakel came to the United States and instructed 25 psychiatrists from New York state hospitals in the new treatment.[90]

It is hard to imagine the excitement and expectation that accompanied the advent of this therapy. The usual overcrowding and under-staffing of mental hospitals had become even worse because of the Depression. The new wonder cure was greeted in the press by spectacular and inaccurate claims.[91] The medical profession was also guilty of uncritically embracing the new therapy, which almost immediately came into extensive use. Sakel's explanation of how insulin shock worked was vague and unsustainable.[92] Other theories were equally fanciful and speculative at best. Yet, in a wave of enthusiasm, insulin coma therapy was widely tested and used with few dissenting voices.[93]

In early 1937, Norman L. Easton, a psychiatrist from the New Toronto Hospital, together with a nurse from the hospital, was sent to Bellevue Hospital in New York for two months to learn how to administer insulin coma therapy.[94] In May of the same year, Farrar attended the annual meeting of the American Psychiatric Association in Pittsburgh. Sakel presented a paper at the meeting; insulin therapy was obviously the hot topic. On May 19 and 20 respectively the *Toronto Telegram* and the *Toronto Star* ran extensive articles on the subject. Both Deputy Minister of Health McGhie and Farrar were anxious to stress the highly experimental and uncertain nature of the new therapy. The *Toronto Telegram* concluded,

> Dr. Farrar emphasized these dangers [changes to the brain, and hypoglycaemia] in order to show that the treatment was still in the experimental stage, that it was much too early to pass a definite opinion on the value of the treatment, and that undue optimism could not be supported by clinical facts.[95]

Farrar always stressed that insulin shock was not a specific treatment but an accidental finding with no real explanation of how or why it worked. Yet the public was greatly interested in these developments and there were many desperate pleas from relatives for the treatment. Farrar later told the press,

> Naturally hope is immediately raised everywhere among relatives of patients suffering from dementia praecox. Everyone wants the treatment used on their relatives, looking for great results.[96]

While Farrar and McGhie were cautious in public, they were eager to begin work on the new treatment. The first treatment in Ontario was administered on May 31, 1937, as part of an initial study of 12 patients. Six closely matched pairs of young women suffering from the same general mental disorder were selected for the treatment, one in each pair as a control. This study was carried out at the New Toronto Hospital with close cooperation from the insulin specialists at both the Connaught and the Banting laboratories.[97] Studies continued over the next two years in collaboration with the Department of Medical Research at the university.[98]

In the meantime Farrar was trying to interest the Rockefeller Foundation in funding a comprehensive study of insulin shock. While the foundation had been an indirect supporter of TPH since the beginning, its money had chiefly been devoted to improving teaching. In 1933, under Alan Gregg, the Rockefeller Foundation's emphasis in psychiatry was shifted to research and the advancement of knowledge in the field of "psychobiology."

> For the next twenty years the medical Sciences Division concentrated most of its programs in this broadly defined area focusing mainly upon psychiatry and neurology—and to a lesser degree physiology, endocrinology, and genetics—to investigate the biological causes of mental and nervous diseases.[99]

In fact, over the next decade three-quarters of all Rockefeller money for medical sciences went to psychiatry.[100]

On November 22, 1937, Gregg met with Farrar and Sir Frederick Banting in Toronto to discuss the study. Gregg summarized in his diary that a lack of space was hampering the study (which had been underway since April of that year). Farrar expressed confidence that an addition of 12 more beds and laboratory space could be secured from the province. Regarding the treatment, Gregg did note that "Farrar would not describe the results as overwhelmingly convincing thus far," and that "Banting was not enthusiastic for insulin shock, but is very keen for studying carbohydrate metabolism in mental patients." Nevertheless, Gregg concluded: "The development looks promising because Banting's direct interest is assured...and a careful long term study of carbohydrate metabolism of the brain would be practicable."[101] The foundation was evidently impressed by Banting's involvement.

In October 1936, Farrar had asked Gregg to fund an interdepartmental study of select mental cases at TPH which would involve anthropology, genetics, psychology, and constitutional studies at the children's hospital.[102] In late November, Farrar sent Gregg a detailed written proposal requesting $15,000 per year for three to five years.[103] In the weeks between Farrar's two requests, C.M. Hincks had visited with Gregg in New York City. During the course of the interview, Hincks described Farrar as having "no clear idea of investigative work" and stated that he did not know how to surround himself with superior personnel.[104] In December 1936, Robert A. Lambert of the Rockefeller Foundation sent a memorandum to Gregg detailing his objections to the TPH proposal. He felt the program was essentially a number of unrelated activities in various departments and saw the grant as a fluid research fund administered by Farrar, of whom he concluded: "He is a scholarly gentleman and a competent teacher but not a real scientist. I am a little disturbed that he should be so sanguine in his expectations of RF aid."[105] It seems the request for funds was refused largely because of Farrar's own abilities.

A month after his initial meeting with Farrar and Banting, Alan Gregg met with Deputy Minister of Health B.T. McGhie and informed him that if the provincial government would undertake the necessary additions to TPH, and pay for the maintenance of the patients under study, that: "He would be prepared to recommend that a five year grant be made to research on effect of use of insulin in mental diseases." But by this time, the emphasis of the study had shifted. "The essence of the undertaking is not properly understood as concerning merely the insulin shock treatment, but more generally the nature of carbohydrate metabolism in mental patients." This change in approach seems to have been due to Banting's interest. In reality, Banting had not had any real contact with research for many years and it is highly unlikely that he had any interest or involvement with the project at all. But his name on the proposal was what mattered, and Banting was no doubt happy to have his name used to secure funding for medical research at the University of Toronto.[106] Gregg again indicated how important the involvement of the Nobel laureate was: "Sir Frederick Banting would I understand take an active part in selection of personnel."[107]

Finally in January 1939, the Rockefeller Foundation granted $104,000 to the University of Toronto for the period January 1, 1939, to June 30, 1943. The money, split roughly fifty-fifty between TPH and the Department of Medical Research, went mostly toward salaries.[108] The province was slow to come through with the promised expansion of facilities and nursing staff. In early 1939, Easton, who the previous year had been appointed director of research in the Ontario Hospitals, was moved to TPH and retained as consultant for shock therapies. Burdett McNeel was put in charge of the unit, which was up and running by the summer of 1939.[109]

The timing of the establishment of the research unit was unfortunate, as the onset of war soon took its toll on TPH staff. Farrar wrote to the Rockefeller Foundation in the summer of 1940 explaining that staff changes due to war service had significantly slowed down the research.[110] Animal experiments related to the study were discontinued at the Banting Institute due to lack of personnel.[111] But in spite of these setbacks, insulin-shock research continued at TPH.

In these first two years, the study was to compare schizophrenic patients under routine psychiatric hospital care and under insulin therapy. Staff had to develop methods to assess accurately the psychological, psychiatric, and physiological changes inpatients experienced when undergoing the treatment.[112] At this time, it was decided to concentrate on glucose tolerance administered both intravenously and orally (using close biochemical and physiological testing of carbohydrate metabolism). It was established that glucose levels were abnormal in schizophrenics and returned to normal as the patient recovered from the symptoms.[113]

Then in February 1941, Banting died. Farrar quickly sent a handwritten note to Alan Gregg, assuring him that it was business as usual with research.

> Doctor Lucas, with whom next to Doctor Banting our group has been most closely in touch, replied to a letter of mine and I thought I would like you to see the correspondence since Doctor Lucas' letter gives assurance that collaboration between our two departments will continue without interruption just as Doctor Banting wished it to do.[114]

Thus research at TPH continued, in fact, expanding well beyond the original area of insulin therapy. Soon after the advent of insulin coma therapy, metrazol (a synthetic preparation with convulsive properties) began to be given in large doses to produce epileptiform seizures in schizophrenic patients. Conceived by Joseph Ladislas von Meduna of Budapest, the therapy was based on the erroneous assumption "a certain biological antagonism exists between the convulsive state and the schizophrenic process."[115] Despite the flimsy theoretical basis for the therapy (as in the case of insulin shock), metrazol shock was rapidly accepted.[116] Psychiatrists and the relatives of patients were desperate for anything that held out hope, regardless of how novel or untested it was. Toronto was no exception.

In January 1938, Richard Montgomery, director of the Hospitals Division of the Ontario Department of Health, received a letter from D.R. Fletcher, the superintendent of the Ontario Hospital at Whitby, asking that a metrazol program be established. Fletcher hoped that this would help his patients, or "if not by this treatment, at least by increasing the enthusiasm of my staff, which will in the long run be beneficial to our patients."[117] This illustrates the faute-de-mieux attitude towards all the new somatic therapies at the time: try anything, it has to be better than what we can now do.

The press also played a role, placing in the public mind the idea of yet another wonder cure for mental illness. "Drug Ends Dementia By Causing Convulsions Psychiatrists Claim" proclaimed the front page headline of the *Toronto Star* on November 3, 1937. "It causes convulsions similar to epileptic fits and literally snaps the patient out of his psychoses," stated the article. The paper quoted spectacular results from asylums in the United States and calculated impressive statistics for the potential savings to the people of Ontario. Despite the fact that Easton himself disagreed with its theoretical foundation, he was willing to go ahead with metrazol therapy. The presumed antagonism between epilepsy and schizophrenia became irrelevant in face of the growing confidence with which the treatment was being used.[118] Easton concluded: "To my way of thinking, the convulsion acts as a 'battering ram' to the psychosis and as such should have some favourable therapeutic effect."[119] Thus metrazol was quickly included in the armoury of treatments available in the Ontario Hospitals.

One of the advantages of metrazol was that it was cheaper and easier to administer than insulin coma therapy. The *Toronto Star*, in an article

"Cheap and Easy," wrote: "It is finding favour with the Ontario department of health because of its cheapness and ease of administration, as opposed to the insulin practice."[120] Furthermore, all the superintendents of the Ontario Hospitals, including Farrar, expressed enthusiasm for the new treatment.[121] Easton held a two-day course at the end of April 1938, and metrazol was soon being administered in a number of Ontario hospitals.

It quickly became apparent elsewhere that metrazol was not the wonder drug it had first appeared to be. Scarcely a year after its widespread introduction to Ontario, Easton, as director of research, received a letter from psychiatrist Joseph Wortis in New York warning that 25 to 50 percent of metrazol cases had shown up with spinal compression fractures. Easton was immediately instructed by the Department of Health to conduct a study of the treatment at the Ontario Hospitals.[122] Metrazol therapy was temporarily suspended. Yet, in June, a research committee concluded that:

> Despite the possibility of complications from metrazol therapy, and with the precautions which can be taken to minimize them, its use is justified in selected cases under careful controlled conditions as a scientific undertaking in experimental therapy.[123]

Some of these precautions involved x-raying all patients before and after treatment. By the spring of 1939, Easton was satisfied that the few cases found with fractures were not the direct result of the therapy.[124] In early 1940, the routine practice of x-raying all patients was no longer considered necessary. In addition, curare was now being used to paralyse the neuromuscular end organs to prevent injury during the seizures.[125] Despite a difficulty of supply in 1940–41, the use of metrazol continued in the Ontario Hospitals.[126] Initial comparisons of insulin and metrazol shock showed that metrazol was cheaper and easier, requiring a shorter stay in hospital. Quite often the two were used in combination. Thus, because of its ease and success rate, metrazol became the commonest of the shock therapies in Ontario during the war.

The last of the shock therapies to appear was electroshock, or electroconvulsive therapy (ECT). It is perhaps the most familiar of the three because it has today become the treatment of choice in major depression. It was first used in April 1938 by Ugo Cerletti in Rome. Like insulin and metrazol, electroshock soon rapidly spread to the United States and was in extensive use by 1941.[127]

Electroshock did not begin in Canada until 1941. In February of that year a bulletin prepared by the National Committee for Mental Hygiene recommended that experimental work should proceed with electroshock in much the same way as it had with metrazol. It warned that: "as yet very little has been published in the way of statistical data," and that "It is perhaps too early to call this technique a therapy."[128]

Electroshock was regarded as an alternative to metrazol rather than to insulin because it also produced seizures. It was another method of obtaining the desired convulsion without the unpleasant side effects associated with metrazol (fear, nausea, vomiting, and severe headaches) which often led patients to shun subsequent treatments.[129] At the request of Easton, who in October 1941 had visited various New England centres, an electroshock unit was set up at TPH under Lorne Proctor.[130]

The inherent simplicity of electroshock, its significantly lower cost, and lack of apparent side effects led to its extension to other Ontario Hospitals. Although the committee on shock therapies (set up to deal with the problems of metrazol) said that its introduction should proceed with caution, by the mid-1940s electroshock was being used extensively in all Ontario Hospitals.[131]

It is ironic that the three therapies represent the first real breakthrough in the somatic treatment of mental illness in an era when somatism was on the decline. From the summer of 1941 onwards, schizophrenia studies at TPH centred on electroshock in conjunction with insulin rather than metrazol. Catatonic schizophrenics were selected because they showed the greatest clinical change. This early work with electroshock centred on finding the best apparatus, current, voltage, and number of shocks. Particular attention was paid to developing reliable and accurate methods of 'scoring' a patient's progress in various psychiatric categories.

A typical course of treatment involved seven to ten grand-mal seizures induced by electroshock, followed by a week or so of observation. A note from a patient found in Farrar's case records describes the experience of electroshock.

> There is absolutely no pain but it is something like having one of those terrifying dreams where you are struggling to free yourself from something. I also had the impression that I was falling through bottomless space and all the time there was a sort of tattoo beating in my head very similar to the one experienced under anaesthetic. All this fortunately ends in complete obliv-

ion... When you become fully awake it is with the most delightfully refreshing feeling.[132]

If the patient failed to respond favourably after this week of observation, a course of about 25 treatments with insulin (including four or five full comas) was tried.

The patient's electroencephalogram (EEG) was used to monitor the effect of the electroshock and determine when it should be stopped. Electroencephalography, the reading of electrical brain activity, was also a new development of this time. The instrument was first used by German psychiatrist Hans Berger in 1929 to measure and record brain wave patterns. Although chiefly a diagnostic aid for head injuries, in research it also revealed functional abnormalities of the brain.[133] Thus EEG monitoring gave valuable information about the various shock therapies.

EEG's of psychotic patients showed only small differences from the normal acceptable range. But, in electroshock the EEG's changed dramatically, gradually subsiding after treatment ended. This was seen either as evidence of its effectiveness or an indication of possible dangers. Researchers at TPH were in agreement that there was a definite correlation between EEG results and improved mental condition after insulin or electroshock.[134]

By 1941 the demands of war service had made serious inroads into the effectiveness of the research unit. Charles H. Best, who had assumed Banting's role of figurehead, expressed grave doubts to Alan Gregg about the wisdom of continuing the grant. As Gregg noted in his diary in 1942,

> I told Best I thought that probably I would write to Farrar in connection with this whole enterprise and express my uncertainty of the desirability of going on a further year—no protest from Best at this suggestion.[135]

Yet Best continued, "Farrar is extremely keen to push ahead with it;" the psychiatric team seemed less affected by wartime demands. By 1942, the work had stabilized and Best was more satisfied.[136] Farrar felt vindicated for his perseverance and confidently reported to the Rockefeller Foundation:

> Our research personnel is now in a stronger, and I believe, more stable position than at any previous time. It has been possible to step up the work during the past year and some valuable findings have been recorded.[137]

Although from 1939–42 TPH had not required the full annual appropriation from the Rockefeller Foundation, the hospital did require the full $10,800 by 1943. Work in 1942 continued to focus on schizophrenia and expanded on earlier work with glucose tolerance. The main contribution of the research was the establishment of a correlation between improved mental state and glucose, insulin, and pyruvic tolerance (pyruvate is an important biochemical intermediary in metabolism). Psychological testing also confirmed these biochemical findings.[138]

Originally, the grant was to have ended in 1943. Because of the disruptions caused by the war, and the fact that not all the money had been spent, Gregg agreed to extend the period of the grant for another two years.[139] During this time TPH continued essentially the same work, enlarging the series of observations and confirming earlier work with statistically significant samples.[140] The work suggested a definite somatic basis for mental illness. Furthermore, it established TPH as a centre of biological psychiatry in a world leaning increasingly towards psychoanalysis.

Although the Rockefeller support for research at TPH ended in June 1945, Farrar arranged for the Banting Foundation and the Department of Health to continue some funding.[141] In other ways as well, TPH managed to continue its services and adapt to the exigencies of the war. In 1943, at the request of the Canadian Army Medical Corps, the hospital developed a course of psychiatric instruction for medical officers.[142] The many young Canadian psychiatrists who went overseas brought back ideas that would change the profession and TPH significantly.

TPH AFTER WORLD WAR II

John Dewan recalls that the war was a period of monumental change for psychiatry in Ontario.

> The war certainly hurt research in psychiatry. But in other ways the war years, of course, were a godsend to psychiatry in that it blasted us out of the thinking only of patients in hospitals into seeing people of all walks of life who showed difficulties under stress, it made it a more realistic and broader approach...[143]

The whirlwind of change began with the return of many physicians with new experience and new ideas, coinciding with the retirement of many of the old guard in Toronto psychiatry. Duncan Graham, chief of medicine at the Toronto General Hospital (TGH) and professor of medicine at

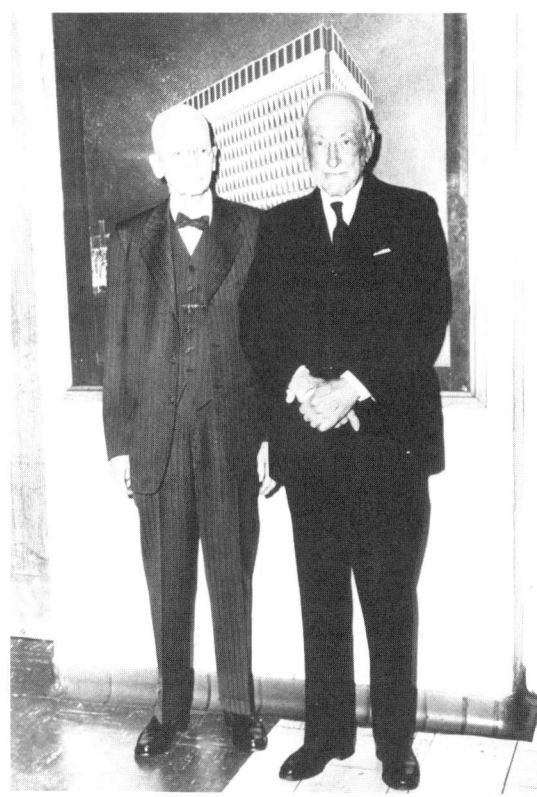

C. B. Farrar and Duncan Graham, head of medicine at the Toronto General Hospital, at TPH. It was one of the last occasions when Farrar appeared publicly. Farrar and Graham had great disagreements and almost never met.

the University of Toronto, retired in 1947. His tenure was slightly longer than Farrar's. Together, "these two men dominated the scene in Medicine and Psychiatry from the end of the first world war till the end of the second world war."[144]

Graham, the first full-time professor of medicine at the University of Toronto, was appointed in 1919 to the Sir John and Lady Eaton Chair. The only condition of this gift was that TGH have only one medical service. Following British tradition, neurological organic diseases were separated from mental illnesses. As noted in Greenland's chapter on the "Origins of the Toronto Psychiatric Hospital," the 1911 TGH act made the head of each service at TGH also the head of that department at the university. Psychiatry, not represented at TGH, was the only exception to this. It was C.K. Clarke, then dean of medicine and soon-to-be superintendent of the new TGH, who negotiated this separation. He wanted psychiatry to be separate from other medical teaching and remain based at Queen Street, with himself as professor of psychiatry at the university.

Clarke, resolutely opposed to psychiatry in the general hospital, was able to "consolidate a schism between alienists and neurology."[145]

This schism meant that the Department of Medicine (neurology) was left to carry on general hospital psychiatry, while Queen Street and TPH were the centres of psychiatry. TPH assumed the asylum tradition of psychiatry from Queen Street. Also, the administration of TPH by the provincial Ontario Hospital Service perpetuated the link with alienist psychiatry rather than with the teaching hospitals.[146] Major psychiatric disorders remained the exclusive domain of TPH and the Ontario Hospitals, while psychoneuroses continued in general hospitals under the aegis of neurology, a sub-specialty of the Department of Medicine.[147]

The retirement of both Farrar and Graham left the door open for a new generation to unite the two psychiatries. The shift towards general hospital psychiatry got a push from the recognition of psychiatry as a specialty by the Royal College in 1943. Under Farrar there had been no general hospital experience for those training at TPH, while those recruited to the Toronto General Hospital by Graham were all from a medical background.[148] Recognition by the Royal College required a reorganization of the training program and an expansion of facilities.

ALDWYN B. STOKES' APPOINTMENT

Politics had always been a part of events at TPH. The selection of a new professor of psychiatry was no exception. In 1947, Farrar was 73 years of age and had been trying to retire for several years, but had been prevented by the disruption and shortage of staff caused by the war.[149] In the late thirties and forties, and even more so in the postwar climate, Farrar was out of touch with the new trend in psychiatry. In an interview with Alan Gregg in 1936, Clarence Hincks remarked of Farrar: "... He has not passed much beyond Kraepelin or possibly Kretschmer—he is profoundly critical or ignorant of psychoanalysis."[150] Farrar's well-known opposition to psychoanalysis became an increasingly contentious issue.[151] Thus the matter of his replacement was of vital importance to the various factions of psychiatry in Ontario, and, indeed, in Canada.[152]

Farrar himself was very anxious to have Toronto alumnus Leslie R. Angus succeed him. Angus, who had moved to the United States, was a friend of Farrar's and had visited him in Toronto on a number of occasions. In May 1946, Farrar responded to the request of the new dean of medicine, John A. MacFarlane, for recommendations with a glowing

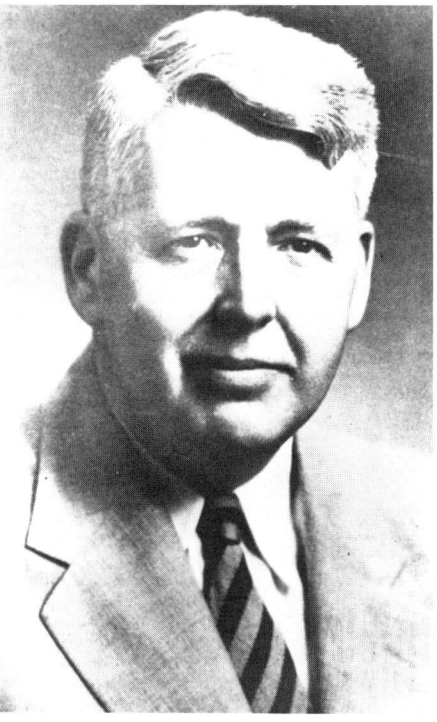

Aldwyn B. Stokes (1906-1978), professor of psychiatry at the University of Toronto, 1947-1966 and Farrar's successor as director of TPH.

reference for Angus.[153] Angus' own views on psychoanalysis were probably an important factor in Farrar's assessment of him. In one letter Angus said, regarding a return to Toronto, "... I should not like to see too many of our psychoanalytical friends established and making the public think that they speak for the profession."[154]

Over the next few months, Farrar pushed hard to have Angus chosen as his successor. The process itself seems to have been very much in the hands of the dean. Farrar was, however, able to have Angus included in the short list of candidates—the only Canadian considered. Farrar was at pains to convince MacFarlane that Angus, a Canadian who had spent most of his professional life in the United States, was eminently qualified for the job. He added: "The United States is at the present time the world centre in psychiatric teaching and research."[155] The dean, it appears, was of a different mind; he wanted a foreigner and preferred to look towards England.[156] The selection committee itself was small, consisting of MacFarlane; J.T. Phair, deputy minister of health; Trevor Owen; Ray F. Farquharson, chairman of medicine; and Sidney Smith, university president (ex officio). According to MacFarlane, they unanimously chose Aldwyn Stokes.[157]

Of the candidates on the short list, Stokes was undoubtedly the most qualified.[158] He also seemed to fit the bill politically. Any local candidate would have been on one side or the other of the psychoanalytical fence. Stokes was sympathetic to psychoanalysis, but had a strong organic background. His qualifications were diverse and included a physiology degree, a diploma in psychology, and extensive research work. Stokes' publications were also a testimony to his diverse interests in psychiatry.[159] His references attested to his broadminded approach to psychiatry: L.S. Maclay wrote, "...he has a balanced outlook towards the relationship of psychiatry to general and social medicine..."[160] Thus, Stokes was a candidate that both sides could live with.

According to John Dewan, there was some uncertainty about Stokes before he came. Yet, "Most of us, I think, were very pleased to find out that he was quite global in his approach."[161] Looking back Abraham ("Abe") Miller recalls:

> Stokes as a person: a man of quiet personal charm, reserved, frequently courteous, scholarly, a good listener... He had a capacity to use fine diplomatic skills in dealing with the powerful. A consummate clinician, skilled in interviewing, masterful therapist.[162]

Stokes seems to have been surprised by what he found in Toronto—unpleasantly so. "The teaching strength of the Department of Psychiatry needs considerable augmentation: the clinical material is limited to the administratively urgent problems of an acute reception hospital."[163] He detailed other areas that he felt were weak and set the agenda for his new department. His priorities were education and association with general hospitals, community services, and industry. In addition, Stokes wanted an open system of staff appointments, long-term financing, recruitment of higher calibre postgraduate students, and the fostering of research projects on a long-term basis. He concluded at the end of his first year:

> Some progress has been made in setting up the Department of Psychiatry as a centre of liberal psychiatric education, properly linked on the one hand to physical medicine and on the other to the social sciences.[164]

Postwar planning

In 1947, with the promise of federal government funding, an advisory committee on mental health was set up. It was agreed that more psychiatric beds should be established in general hospitals, that community mental health clinics be extended, and that more public education was needed.[165] This committee, and many others to follow, was a response to the severe overcrowding that developed in the decade after the war. In 1949, the province of Ontario was short 9,500 beds, with 1,500 of these shortages in the Toronto area.[166] TPH was also greatly overtaxed. The government attempted to introduce legislation to limit its use to residents of Toronto and York. The heavy opposition that defeated the bill indicates how serious the shortcomings of the hospital service were. The *Globe and Mail* noted that the "objection was based on a belief that the Toronto hospital was the only adequate psychiatric hospital in the province."[167] The Borden Committee, appointed in 1955 by the university to investigate the running of the Department of Psychiatry, also reached this conclusion and argued that, because difficult cases were sent from the rest of the province: "The hospital has been the foremost centre in the Province of Ontario for specialized clinical services."[168]

In 1951, the government initiated a ten-year program of construction. Three new hospitals were to be built: Toronto, Port Arthur, and Smith Falls. In addition, 300 to 600 beds were to be added when hospitals at Brockville, Kingston, Hamilton, and London were renovated.[169] Furthermore, only four travelling clinics (plus the outpatient department at TPH) had been able to continue during the war. The city's social agencies were particularly anxious to have these replaced by stationary clinics.[170]

Outpatient services were added too, which also stimulated interest in establishing psychiatric units in general hospitals. In 1952, the province offered grants of $8,500 per bed to supplement $1,500 per bed from Ottawa, to establish psychiatric units in general hospitals.[171] By 1960, there were 12 such units across the province.[172] But it was lack of money to train and pay people good salaries that produced the biggest shortage: a lack of trained personnel. In the existing Ontario Hospital system there was an estimated shortfall of 24 physicians and, as always, a great scarcity of nurses.[173]

Reordering of teaching in the Department of Psychiatry

In 1948 the federal government began funding psychiatry in Ontario through the National Health Program Grants. In February, the federal government announced that of the $30 million available for that year, $4 million would be spent in Ontario, of which $1,284,235 was to go towards mental health. "A major undertaking will be a mental health training programme at the University of Toronto, which will include $72,700 in fellowships."[174] In total, $170,000 of the federal grant money went to the university for the training of psychiatric personnel.[175] This enabled Stokes to expand the teaching staff and bring more postgraduate students from the Ontario hospitals. The enrollment in 1949–50 doubled over the previous year.[176] In 1946 undergraduate medicine was also reorganized and reduced to a four-year program in 1946. Psychiatry in the first year consisted of three introductory lectures. The second and third years covered a comprehensive survey of the entire field, while the fourth year consisted of individual work with patients in small groups.[177]

Despite the money provided to expand the staff and fund students, there was still difficulty in attracting graduate physicians to the service. A committee established in 1950 by Richard Montgomery, director of the Hospitals Division, concluded that there was an urgent need to improve buildings and clinical facilities available to the students.[178] Although TPH was considered by students to be the only existing centre offering quality training, it too was lacking in both facilities and diversity,[179] especially important if TPH wanted to meet the requirements of the Royal College. Thus, as Stokes explained in 1950, he needed to expand the facilities for teaching.

> The TPH itself has gravely limiting facilities both in-patient and out-patient work, for dealing with the wide sweep of psychiatric disorders. The university Department of Psychiatry has therefore continued in the policy of fostering other associations to broaden the field of experience for psychiatric training.[180]

The chairman of medicine, Ray F. Farquharson, was also reorganizing his department. He integrated the three medical wards, resulting in the loss of the neuropsychiatric ward at TGH, in operation since 1911.[181] This was replaced in 1949 by a psychiatric unit in the Wellesley Hospital (from 1949–60 the hospital together with the psychiatric unit was administratively part of TGH),[182] where Stokes was given admitting privileges. This move effectively expanded the facilities of the TPH and provided the first bridge between the Department of Medicine (neurology) and the Department of Psychiatry. This, explained Stokes:

> will play an outstanding role in the integration of medical and psychiatric concepts, in the development of psychosomatic problems, and in offering an experience to postgraduate students of those less florid forms of psychiatric illness.[183]

The Wellesley arrangement was indeed "the first major inroad of psychiatry into the teaching general hospitals," and part of the larger move towards the integration of psychiatry with mainstream medicine.[184] The model was soon extended to other teaching hospitals: Toronto Western Hospital in 1953, St. Michael's Hospital in 1954, and Women's College Hospital in 1956. During the fifties, the slow and difficult integration of psychiatric services into the general hospitals proceeded.[185] By 1953, Stokes felt confident that, with nine centres for teaching, all aspects of his "liberal psychiatric education" were covered.[186] By the end of the decade, 11 hospitals and institutes were affiliated with the Department of Psychiatry for clinical teaching, while centralized courses were given at TPH.[187] Abe Miller remembers that Stokes "promoted psychiatric units in general hospitals to bring psychiatry into the mainstream of medicine."[188]

A growing emphasis on psychoanalysis was particularly apparent in the curriculum at TPH. For instance, in 1957 postgraduates at the outpatient department (OPD) spent a full month on inter-psychic functions and covered such topics as "libido (mental energy) and its instincts and their perversions, self and its divisions, and Ego self." Other essential subjects included "birth trauma and the first five years of life, and the triangle of mother, father and child."[189] The influence of depth psychology and Freudian language are obvious, so is the emphasis on sociology and psychology. Stokes himself felt that psychoanalysis was not practical, but that it was helpful as a therapeutic approach.[190] He did, however, appoint a number of psychoanalysts to the staff.[191] Psychotherapy, too, was a part of Stokes' broader vision of mental illness, encompassing many new fields, particularly in the social sciences. He said, "The widening of psychiatric horizons to a greater vision than the necessities of custodial care has attracted men of better quality and in greater numbers."[192]

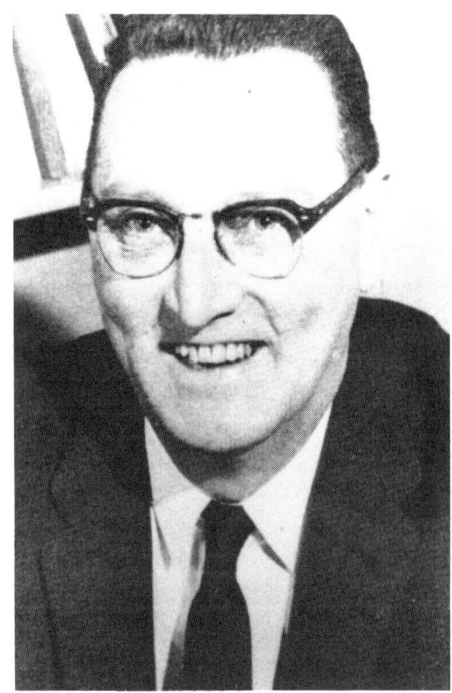

John Dewan (1909-1986), director of the Outpatient Department at TPH, 1946–60; director of TPH, 1960–64.

SERVICES

Government funding helped expand facilities and services at TPH in the postwar era. Many of these new services reflected the shifting emphasis within psychiatry, for example, the establishment in 1946 of a modern outpatient department organized under John Dewan. Additional money provided a new lecture room, an expansion of the library, and an increase of clinical facilities.[193] In particular, senior appointments were made in sociology (John Seeley), social work (Morton Teicher), and clinical psychology (G. Elliot and C. Pivnick). Ken Gray was appointed assistant professor for forensic psychiatry and began developing the field in Toronto in cooperation with the court.[194]

Thus TPH was moving with the times. A children's clinic was established in 1947, but not until 1959 was a separate children's service established under Edward Rosen, as part of a two-year graduate course in child psychiatry.) Research was also being done on intra-uterine causes of mental retardation.[195]

Many of the new services were integrated with community agencies and programs. The Outpatient Department, for example, worked frequently with family physicians.[196] This new outreach reflected psychiatry's improved public image, a consequence of the discipline's recent inclusion in general hospitals.[197]

The expansion of services placed greater demands on the time of the staff. Stokes remarked ironically, "It is a curious matter of reflection that whereas the hindrances to the development of psychiatry in the past were those of disclaim now they include demand."[198] Many of these clinical services depended heavily upon graduate physicians-in-training for staff. Some 30 to 40 graduates supported by educational bursaries staffed many of the clinics of TPH. This cost the Ontario Hospital Service nothing, but restricted the effectiveness of teaching in the Department of Psychiatry. As Stokes said,

> Without the educational relationship the clinical services educational development is impeded....In the long run the university requirement is a modern psychiatric institute where teaching and research, adequately financed, are based on exemplary but unharassed clinical investigation and treatment.[199]

TREATMENT

In the postwar era, with the exception of the shock therapies, very little could be done for patients with psychotic illness. Thus, psychology and psychotherapy became the cornerstones of psychiatric care.[200] Great strides were made in developmental psychology, sociology, and psychoanalysis. In keeping with this burgeoning of psychological therapies, a committee was appointed in 1953 to consider the methods of treatment in the department of psychiatry. The committee apparently arose out of concern of some members of the department that psychotherapy was receiving too little attention.[201] The committee stressed the need for integrating disciplines and for proper follow-up. "It is agreed that psychotherapy is a fundamental requirement in the treatment of psychiatric disorders."[202]

As a place, TPH was changing. In keeping with the then fashionable ideas of community psychiatry, the hospital had adopted a "community living" approach to care, with the ward as a miniature community. Rather than the traditional custodial-inmate relationship of a mental hospital, TPH was stressing an informal, open-door policy.[203] Mental illness was now regarded as a breakdown in living, and treatment centred on readjusting people to society. These principles, also known as milieu therapy, represented all that was new and progressive in psychiatric care in the 1950s and 1960s. The essence of the therapy was providing a normal, healthy environment for the patients. This was a natural reaction to the traditional mental hospital. Philip Melville explained:

> The traditional mental hospital leaves it up to the patient to decide how he will behave. People who have emotional disturbances are inclined to withdraw when their problems become too hard to deal with... We can't take out a patient's problem but we can help him deal with them in an acceptable and positive way... We try to construct an atmosphere where behaving in a sick way is not very acceptable.[204]

The onrush of milieu therapy did not imply that physical therapies were completely discarded. In fact, insulin and electroshock continued to be important methods of treating mental illness. But the postwar period is more often remembered for the use of psychosurgery.

Lobotomy

It is easy to look back on this era and condemn the drastic measures that were taken as quackery or a sinister program of social control. But it is more useful to attempt to understand the contemporary climate that produced such "Great and Desperate Cures."[205] While the new, psychologically oriented psychiatry and psychoanalysis were dealing with breakdowns in living and neurotic illness, the problem of severe psychotic illness was still largely unaddressed. The leucotomy operation or incision into the brain itself was developed in 1935 by Egas Moniz of Portugal. It was brought to the United States and championed by neurologist Walter Freeman and his partner James Watts, a neurosurgeon, in 1937. As with insulin, metrazol, and electroshock, leucotomy was rapidly accepted despite the tenuousness of the theory and inadequacy of evidence supporting it.[206] Moniz's theory was based on the assumption that all serious mental disorders were the result of fixed thoughts maintained by nerve pathways in the frontal lobes of the brain. Destruction of these abnormal pathways was the only effective cure.[207]

Although the early 1950s became the heyday of psychosurgery, lobotomies began at TPH during the war. In January 1938, the Ontario Department of Health sent Farrar, neurosurgeon Kenneth McKenzie, and a Dr. Van Wagenen, to Washington to visit Freeman and Watts and learn about lobotomies.[208] In their report to Deputy Minister of Health Bernard

McGhie, McKenzie and Farrar expressed some reservations about the selection of patients, but felt that the procedure had promise. They concluded that: "... We saw enough to make us feel that we would be justified in doing at least three or four carefully selected cases here."[209] The favourable impression the famous neurosurgeon Harvey Cushing had of the procedure was also an important factor in their assessment. On their way home from Washington, Farrar and McKenzie visited Cushing in Boston. McKenzie, who had studied under Cushing, reported that Cushing was interested and felt there was something in it.[210] Staff physician Mary Jackson also remembers that Cushing had been reported as saying that it was a "weird" procedure, but adding: "I can't help but feel there is something in it."[211]

As it turned out, the first lobotomy (more accurately a bilateral frontal leucotomy) was not done until July 1941. The patient was diagnosed as an involutional melancholic with pronounced psychotic symptoms. For two years she had failed to respond to shock therapy and symptomatic treatment. After surgery her condition improved sufficiently that in two weeks she was discharged to a boarding-out home and was considered to be in social remission.[212] A study of the procedure became incorporated into the research unit at TPH. By the following year, nine operations had been performed by McKenzie at TGH. The patients were selected from various Ontario hospitals, and transferred to TPH where they were examined and tested for suitability. Those chosen were chronic psychotics on whom insulin and electroshock had failed. The hospitals 1942 report to the Rockefeller Foundation noted:

> This neurosurgical procedure resulted in the discharge or the improvement of all cases in this group of patients, who previous to this treatment were considered to be chronically mentally ill with little hope of improving under routine hospital care.[213]

By summer 1944, 19 operations had been completed and the group was anxious to expand the series to 100 cases to make the results statistically significant. Ten of these first nineteen cases were considered to have recovered, six had improved, and only three had failed.[214] Nevertheless, the leucotomy program was one of the casualties of the end of Rockefeller funding. The operations ended in 1944 due to lack of nursing staff and available beds at TPH. Lionel Penrose's report in December 1944 concluded that:

> It is apparent that the results from this treatment are much more satisfactory than the results from the shock therapies, and this is also more striking on account of the fact that the patients who

are selected for this form of treatment are usually hopeless from the standpoint of ordinary forms of treatment.[215]

By 1947 interest again grew in reestablishing the leucotomy program at TPH,[216] partly as a result of pressure from patients' relatives, who were aware that the operation was being done in the United States: "They are rather critical of the fact that no provision is made for it in Ontario Hospitals."[217] Public pressure was evidently quite intense. Charles Hanna, superintendent at Brockville, remarked in a letter to Stokes on the effect that the press was having on the public:

> The publicity in the press and magazine articles is rendering the general public acutely aware—perhaps to an exaggerated degree—of the results obtained through surgery. [They] are quite aggressive in their attitude that something be done, even if it is as a last resort.[218]

Reacting to public pressure and desperate to do something about overcrowding, the superintendents pushed to have a large-scale leucotomy program. Montgomery indicated that the department was purposely going slow on the proposition.[219] The Department of Health sent an outline to all superintendents detailing how patients should be selected for leucotomies. Stokes, who prepared the memo, warned:

> It is clear, on account of widespread and uncritical lay publications, that great pressure is being exerted by relatives and interested persons to have this operation performed indiscriminately without regard to a proper medical judgement. Unless the tendency to an indiscriminate application for supposed automatic benefit is resisted both the project and the method are likely to fall into disrepute.[220]

The leucotomy program began again at the end of April 1948. The cost was $150 per patient per week.[221] One patient a week was transferred to TPH for a week of pre-operative testing. The surgery was performed by McKenzie at TGH, after which the patients spent a further five to six weeks at TPH before returning to their home hospital. This small-scale program did not satisfy the demand. By the next summer, the Department of Health was inundated with requests from relatives and hospital superintendents. Stokes objected to the expansion of the leucotomy program on the grounds that the operation was not yet accepted as a standard procedure, and that careful control was needed to prevent things getting out of hand.[222] In September 1949, Eric Clarke (son of C.K. Clarke) submitted a review of the literature on leucotomy to the superintendents' conference, concluding that: "... A majority of the articles are so devoid of any critical appraisal as to make it impossible to arrive at any conclusion." While the operation had been done around the world for 12 years (10,000 to 12,000 cases), Clarke noted that no long-term critical study had been undertaken. In particular, there was no standard for measuring improvement, and many of those listed as recovered were designated as such because they were out of hospital, which Clarke felt was a meaningless term.[223]

Despite these objections, in the fall of 1949, funding was secured from the federal government and arrangements were made to have patients transferred to the New Toronto Hospital instead of TPH (which could not accommodate them).[224] As the program increased, so did the demand. In June, Stokes had a circular sent around to the Ontario Hospitals informing them that the program was suspended until the waiting list of 30 patients was cleared.[225] The response was immediate. John Senn in Hamilton asked if McKenzie could do a number of operations there. The psychiatric hospital in London, Ontario, requested to have its own leucotomy unit.[226] Later that summer, at a meeting between Stokes, McKenzie, and the Department of Health, it was agreed to increase the leucotomy program by establishing a unit at Queen Street. TPH would continue only in the area of research and not service.[227] The program continued to expand with the Ontario Hospitals in London, Kingston, Whitby, Hamilton, St. Thomas, and New Toronto all eventually participating. These continued over the next decade and were deemed to be of great value: "We consider our results with lobotomy one of the most satisfactory achievements in therapy that we have ever participated in."[228] George H. Stevenson, superintendent of the Ontario Hospital, London, also stirred up media support for the program. On a number of occasions he released claims of "Amazing Results" to the newspapers, providing the very sort of uncritical press coverage that Stokes had cautioned against.[229]

Leucotomy has been criticized as an operation done to ease patient care at institutions. A program begun at the Ontario Hospital Hamilton was in fact designed for this purpose alone. According to a study done in 1958,

> Because of this problem [over-crowding], it was felt that there was need for a leucotomy program which concentrated on the disturbed patients who present a difficult nursing problem, not so much to get out of hospital as to relieve the overall nursing problem.[230]

The authors concluded enthusiastically that "most of the patients are more content and easily managed."[231] The most ardent proponents of an extensive leucotomy program were the superintendents of the biggest and the most overcrowded of the Ontario hospitals.[232]

Provincial officials realized that widespread leucotomies helped relieve overcrowding in the hospitals. In 1953, the minister of health affirmed his support in a letter to the director of the hospitals division: "I would like to give you my complete approval regarding the carrying on of leucotomy operations in as many of our Ontario Hospitals as possible."[233] In virtually all their reports to the Department of Health, superintendents stressed the positive effect that lobotomies were having on the staff and the management of the patients. In 1953, Martin Fischer of New Toronto summarized the results of their leucotomy program: "The nursing problem has certainly been reduced to a minimum in most cases."[234] Hanna in Brockville, commenting on a patient he felt would be a good candidate for a lobotomy, remarked: "There is a good possibility of making her a more manageable hospital patient."[235]

The role of TPH over this period became, as it did in most areas, one of research rather than service. When the leucotomy program resumed in 1948, TPH initiated a five-year study of the procedure, under the direction of Abe Miller.[236] The study, including various departments at TPH (nursing, psychology, neurophysiology, social services), and the biochemical laboratories of the Department of Health, involved the selection and follow-up of 150 leucotomized patients. Its general conclusion was that, although a small percentage of patients did not improve after the operation, 55 percent were out of hospital.[237] Even in 1967, when he again reviewed the patients from the study, Miller concluded that,

> Its value as a treatment method in psychiatry is clearly limited... [Nonetheless, in] certain chronic, intractable, distressing psychiatric conditions lobotomy can be a useful therapeutic technique.[238]

By the time Miller's initial report on the lobotomy program was published in 1954, interest in the treatment had begun to decline. Leucotomy would continue at many Ontario Hospitals into the next decade, until finally falling out of favour by the late sixties.[239] Burdett McNeel, chief of the mental health branch, summarized the feeling of the time in 1959: "There is a wide-spread feeling in psychiatric circles that lobotomy is a thing of the past. This has happened to all therapies. They are used intensely and then abandoned."[240]

The retirement of the principal neurosurgeon, Ken McKenzie, from TGH in 1952 probably contributed to the decline in the number of leucotomies performed.[241] But in the long term the introduction of psychoactive drugs, beginning with chlorpromazine in 1952, was a more important factor.[242] In many respects, leucotomy and the shock therapies can be considered as the results of the same therapeutic environment. Somatic views of mental illness still held sway. The rapid and virtually unquestioned acceptance of all these new therapies was largely the result of the absence of any other effective somatic treatments. As Abe Miller later observed,

> It is important to remember that the surge of enthusiasm for psychosurgical treatment during the 1940's was motivated by ineffectual psychiatric therapy, particularly that available for the treatment of patients with intractable and distressing mental disorders.[243]

The decline in the use of shock therapies at this time was also a direct result of the invention of the first antipsychotic drugs.

Drugs

The first neuroleptic drugs had a great impact. One remembers that as late as 1950 hydrotherapy was still an essential part of the physical therapy regime. Claire Muller, a student nurse at TPH in 1949, recalls that "the baths" were still in constant use. She also remarks, "In those days, with so few drugs, the physicians depended upon psychological analysis and positive thinking to help their patients."[244] Shock therapy and lobotomy had been only a limited success.

> I think perhaps those who didn't experience what it was like before don't realize just how helpful [drugs] have been in shortening the amount of time patients are in hospital, and the severity of their symptoms and the fact they can get back into the community.[245]

Investigations into these new antidepressant and tranquillizer drugs helped revive research at TPH during the 1950s and 1960s. A drug research unit with clinical facilities at TPH, St. Michael's Hospital, and the psychiatric hospitals at Whitby and Queen Street was established in the 1950s by the University-Provincial Drug Research Committee, chaired by John Lovett-Doust. A diverse group of experts at the various hospitals worked on antidepressants and tranquillizers.[246]

Expanding Horizons

Between 1945 (when the Rockefeller Foundation grant ended) and 1948 (when federal Mental Health Grants began), research at TPH was very limited. In fact, no research was published in 1946 or 1947. The Advisory Committee on Mental Health concluded in 1948 that the promotion of research was of paramount importance.[247] The province's need for the "production line" training of staff conflicted with Stokes' ideas about quality of training. The problem, Stokes continued, was that the demands of teaching and providing services gave the senior staff very little time for research.[248] Research did, however, continue to develop under the federal grants.[249] Stokes worked hard to place TPH at the forefront of modern psychiatry, recruiting a diverse group of people. Morton Teicher recalls: "Stokes' breadth of vision meant that many exciting types were about the Department of Psychiatry."[250] New sources of funding allowed for this infusion of new blood and energy at TPH.

The effect of this funding may be seen in a doubling of publications by staff members after 1951. Furthermore, the interests of the department became diversified. In 1949, the Forest Hill Project, a five-year study of the mental health of school children in a community, was begun. It was to apply the knowledge of psychiatrists and psychologists to improve the mental health of children. The study, the first major psychological research project undertaken in a Canadian community, focused on the emotional adjustment of school children by examining all aspects of their life in a community.[251] There was also a great deal of work done on group dynamics and group therapy. Although psychology at TPH had branched out, psychometrics still played a central role in psychological research. Speech pathology was another important research interest that saw Ernest Douglass and, later, John C. Richardson studying stuttering and aphasia.[252] Throughout the 1950s, "psychotherapy" was the catchword and numerous papers were devoted to this subject. Still others were distinctly Freudian in nature, such as Eric Boothroyd's "Occupation and the Ego"[253] and Alan Parkin's study of sleep during psychoanalysis.[254] The many fields that were studied at TPH in the 1950s and 1960s show how much psychiatry had expanded its horizons since the war. Stokes was anxious that the psychological aspects of psychiatry not be overlooked and were adequately supported:

> ...Disturbances may be described and understood in both physical and psychological terms. Unfortunately there is a disparity in precision both of description and understanding... Physical abstractions issue from a century of triumphant technology: psychological abstractions by comparison are naive and without equivalent technical support. Because of this disparity medical practice naturally favours the present strength of its physical techniques... But the problems of all ill people will be contained only when the physical and psychological abstractions are reunited in a unity of knowledge.[255]

Yet not all the work at TPH was in this vein. Especially towards the end of the 1950s, numerous papers appeared on drug therapy, physiology, and endocrine studies. While Stokes was keen to encourage research in all areas relating to mental illness, he continued the strong tradition of biological research at TPH, bringing Rolv Gjessing, the famous Norwegian psychiatrist, to Toronto. Stokes had studied under Gjessing in Norway while on a Rockefeller Travelling Fellowship in 1937–38.[256] Gjessing had been a general practitioner, later turning to psychiatry and becoming superintendent of the Dikemark Mental Hospital near Oslo. He quickly took an interest in schizophrenia. After visiting many leading American centres of psychiatry he felt, as a growing number of people did, that schizophrenia was too general a label for what he believed were a number of different disorders. Gjessing defined one group which he called periodic catatonia. He concentrated his work on these patients who went through periodic remissions, and followed each case meticulously. As a result of their remissions, these cases acted as their own "control." By studying metabolic differences between the symptomatic and nonsymptomatic phases of the disease, he could establish the key metabolic changes. Gjessing's work had become well-known, widely accepted[257] and made an impression on Stokes when he was in Norway.

In 1947, Stokes arranged with the help of federal grant money to bring Gjessing to Toronto, and to set up a metabolic clinic and laboratory at TPH. Gjessing's arrival brought instant international recognition to the hospital. John Dewan described the atmosphere of the time: "... It was a real live place. You felt things were happening. Reaching out. They weren't accepting everything simply because it was in front. When Dr. Gjessing came it was a great morale booster."[258] Biochemical and metabolic work in periodic catatonia became the flagship of research at

TPH. Gjessing's studies helped establish the relationship between metabolic function and mental states.[259] After Gjessing left, this work was continued by his collaborator, Allan Gornall of the Department of Pathological Chemistry.

In 1952, Stokes brought John Lovett-Doust, an expert in physiological psychiatry, from the Institute of Psychiatry at the University of London.[260] Lovett-Doust initiated a program of biochemical and physiological research, relating low oxyhaemoglobin levels to disturbances in schizophrenics.[261] He also headed the research laboratory at TPH. In 1959, the small facilities for metabolic study were expanded to include a clinical research unit of six beds, also in the charge of Lovett-Doust. Genetics, neuroanatomical studies, and mental retardation were other areas of research added to TPH.[262]

Despite the trend elsewhere in psychiatry away from organicity, organic psychiatry was strongly entrenched at TPH throughout this period, perhaps—according to Stokes—the most important aspect of research there in the 1950s. In 1958, John Dewan and William Spaulding, director of the OPD at TGH, published *The Organic Psychoses: A Guide to Diagnosis*. In the foreword, Stokes lamented the one-sided approach that psychiatry had assumed: "It is astonishing, particularly when cellular and chemical pathology are in rapid advance, that the field of the organic psychoses has been relatively neglected in practice."[263] Drawing on the wealth of biochemical studies done by TPH and other associated university departments over the years, Dewan and Spaulding tried to approach the diagnosis of organic causes of psychosis systematically. They noted:

> The frequency with which the physical factor is overlooked and the tendency to uncertainty (sometimes unavoidable) in understanding the causation of mental disorders have been an additional reason for writing the guide to the diagnosis of organic mental illness.[264]

It would be some time before the pendulum in psychiatry would swing back towards organicity, but the seeds had been sown and well preserved at TPH.

Planning the Clarke Institute of Psychiatry: the Borden Report

By the 1950s, both the population of Ontario and the services of the hospital had grown beyond all original estimates. From the end of 1948 to 1955, over 4,000 beds had been added in Ontario—well short of the 12,000 that were deemed necessary by the 1951 Health Survey Committee Report. A new psychiatric institute was one of the priorities of the report.[265] A brief on the state of planning stated:

> Following discussion between the Ministry of Health and the University in late 1951 it was agreed to develop plans for the expansion of the TPH, and for its reconstitution as an outstanding treatment, training and research centre in psychiatry, serving the whole province.[266]

In December, a ministerial committee of development of TPH was appointed, with forensic psychiatrist Kenneth Gray as chairman. The following spring, the *Toronto Star* announced that a new 200-bed psychiatric hospital was to be built in Toronto, a teaching and research centre to replace the overstrained TPH. Construction was to begin within two to three years.[267] The site recommended by the committee was the northwest corner of College and Elizabeth streets beside the Banting Institute.[268] The expropriation of this land was set as the number one priority and was soon purchased for $250,000. By the spring of 1954, 18 reports of various working groups on design were submitted, and the Ministry of Health and the architect had agreed on the site. The plan at this stage was to construct a new building at a cost of seven to eight and a half million dollars and connect it with the old TPH.[269] However, in October, the plan was shelved because no money was made available by the province.[270]

In the meantime the University of Toronto had appointed a committee to inquire into the running of the department of psychiatry. The report singled out the lack of adequate facilities: "... Without doubt the existing facilities at TPH for teaching and research and we believe, also in the clinical field, are completely inadequate to meet the demands made upon it and the urgent needs of the university."[271] No significant additions had been made to the hospital in the 30 years since it had opened. Research facilities were severely limited and although the reputation was high, "Development is continuously impeded and obstructed by lack of facilities."[272]

In addition to such physical limitations, the report pointed out that complex financing had fostered an ambiguous role for TPH and led to administrative confusion. Funds were drawn from five different budgets, and the relationship of TPH to the Ontario Hospital Service had never been clearly defined.[273] It was recommended that the professor of psychiatry be relieved of the burden of running the hospital. Stokes had in fact made this request before: "because he found the combined office an almost impossible burden in view of the complex financing patterns and the ill-defined relationship with the Ontario Hospital service."[274] (It was not until late 1960 that John Dewan assumed the responsibility of director of TPH, four years later moving on to become medical director of the Ontario Mental Health Foundation. Thereupon Charles Roberts became director of TPH (see his memoir at the end of this volume), with Mary Jackson acting as assistant medical director.) The Borden Committee concluded that plans should go ahead immediately for a new Ontario Psychiatric Institute on a site near the University of Toronto and other hospitals. The new hospital was to be run by a board of trustees and financed by the province. In the interim, they recommended that a director be appointed and that the complicated finances be immediately examined and simplified. The Borden Committee also felt that the site at College and Elizabeth was too small.[275]

When planning resumed in 1958 these recommendations effectively became the university's proposal for the new psychiatric institute. As a competitor, the Toronto General Hospital attempted to relocate psychiatric teaching and research within its own walls. According to Robert Pos, head of the department of psychiatry at TGH, this was the work of the Committee of the TGH on Psychological Medicine.[276] In the Ministry of Health correspondence, it is only noted that the proposal was submitted by "an interested citizen."[277] Why the Department of Medicine wanted to wrest control of psychiatry is unclear. In any event, the Ministry of Health was not interested in this proposal. Burdett McNeel, chief of the Mental Health Branch, felt the general hospital was the wrong place for psychiatry. The types of cases seen in a general hospital were narrow, and the medical staff were preoccupied with private practice; McNeel thought this would limit research. Additionally, to make the shift worthwhile, too many facilities would have to be added to TGH.

McNeel objected to the university's proposal because it would remove the new hospital from the Ontario Hospital Service, although the province would still be funding the hospital. Either proposal he felt would create two classes of patients and staff by relegating the less favourable cases to the Ontario hospitals. "If the universities and general hospitals are placed in the position of obtaining the Kudos and passing on the drudgery to the Mental hospitals, any incentive to continue the struggle will be lost."[278] This is effectively what had happened at TPH. Its very mandate was to send those patients who were diagnosed as insane to the mental hospitals, and keep those it could treat or needed for research. As far as the university and the Department of Psychiatry were concerned, the emphasis was on "the development of a centre for research, study and learning, rather than one for service."[279] This was how TPH had been operating since the late 1930s. The real point of the university proposal was to remove the administrative nightmare inherent in the three levels of government.

The original concept of TPH as a collaborative effort of government, university, and community was a laudable one. It is not possible to state briefly all the reasons for the breakdown in this collaboration. Yet it was the growing prominence of teaching and research that changed significantly TPH's original role as primarily that of a reception hospital.[280]

How the drama played out may be briefly stated. McNeel proposed that the new institute remain as part of the Ontario Hospital Service and be run by the province. The province, while recognizing the leadership of TPH, was unwilling to give up its control of TPH or sanction the establishment of any one hospital as the centre of psychiatry in the province. The university, represented by Dean MacFarlane, Stokes, and Arthur Kelly, was unprepared for the government's proposal, and was, of course, unequivocally opposed to the proposal of the Toronto General Hospital. The university suggested another committee to settle the issue.[281] In December 1959, McNeel and Stokes reached a compromise agreement. The government would operate the hospital and provide the staff, as before. The university was to look after research, teaching, and necessary staff. Instead of the board of trustees which the university had wanted, three committees were established: the Institute Committee, chaired by the professor of psychiatry, would look after education and research; a hospital committee, composed of the superintendent, the professor, the director of nursing, and the business administrator, would run the hospital; and an advisory committee to the minister of health, made up of representatives from the government, the university, and the community, would advise on matters of policy. This agreement did little to remove the administrative confusion surrounding TPH; it still remained within the Ontario Hospital Service, and although the city was removed from the administration, the position of the hospital was still somewhat ambiguous.[282]

On several occasions over the next couple of years, the special subcommittee for the psychiatric hospital and institute forwarded plans to establish the new hospital as a separate corporation, but the government would not move. The government was not interested in any new course for TPH; as far as it was concerned, the new hospital was first and foremost to provide more facilities for the care of the mentally ill in keeping with the Ontario Hospital tradition. Minister of Health Matthew Dymond reminded the vice-president of the university that the new hospital would remain as a unit of the Ontario Hospital Service under the direction of a superintendent appointed by the ministry. He noted, "The facilities of the hospital will at all times be made available for the teaching and research function of the institute, provided this is in keeping with good patient care, as decided by the director of the hospital."[283]

From early 1960, when the province agreed to spend $5 million on the new hospital, the project became bogged down in red tape—chiefly over the location of the building. Although the current site at the corner of College and Huron streets was chosen in 1960, zoning laws in the newly acquired west campus held up construction until summer 1963. In order to accommodate the building, a small street behind the site would have to be closed. The aptly named Division Street became the source of two years of delays until the way was finally cleared in spring 1963.[284] When tenders were called in July 1963, the cost had jumped to $6.6 million.[285]

As planning went ahead for its replacement in the 1950s and 1960s, TPH found a new role as the bridge between the old and the new — between asylum psychiatry and general hospital and community-based psychiatry. There seems also to have been a real sense of change: psychiatry was bursting out of its isolation and becoming a respectable branch of medicine. Between the opening of TPH in 1925 and the Clarke Institute of Psychiatry in 1966 lay 40 years of vast changes.

ENDNOTES

[1] An unknown number of documents from TPH were deposited at the Clarke Institute of Psychiatry, nearly all of which have since been lost or destroyed. Thus, there are many gaps in documentation. The material for this chapter was assembled from a number of sources. Many sources were found in the Archives of Ontario. The Rockefeller Archive Centre in Tarrytown, New York, was also of considerable use. In addition, material relating to the Department of Psychiatry (annual reports, appointments of the professor, etc.) is located in the University of Toronto Archives. Where possible I have drawn upon memoirs and interviews with those involved with TPH, but have avoided using these as the sole source of evidence for any particular point.

[2] Harvey G. Simmons, *Unbalanced: Mental Health Policy in Ontario 1930-1989* (Toronto: Wall & Emerson, 1990), p. 48.

[3] R.C. Montgomery (director Hospitals Division) to R.T. Kelley (Minister of Health) February 14, 1949. By March 1936, there were seven clinics including the TPH. From June 1930 through March 31, 1947, 56,344 new cases were seen in these clinics.

[4] D.G. McKerracher (for the Royal Commission on Health Services), *Trends in Psychiatric Care* (Ottawa: Queens Printer, 1966), p. 79.

[5] Simmons, p.37.

[6] Alex Richman (for the Royal Commission of Health Services), *Psychiatric Care in Canada: Extent and Results* (Ottawa: Queens Printer, 1966), p. 53.

[7] See J.S. Tyhurst et al., *More for the Mind: A Study of Psychiatric Services in Canada* (Toronto: CMHA, [c1963]).

[8] Simmons, pp. 42-43.

[9] McKerracher, p. 79.

[10] Commission for Survey of Hospital Needs in Metropolitan Toronto, "Mental Care in Metropolitan Toronto," March 1965, p. 17 [Metro Archives]. Six Toronto hospitals had psychiatric units with a total of 198 beds in 1963. A further 279 were to be added by 1970. In addition, there were outpatient departments attached to the Ontario hospitals.

[11] Farrar quoted in *Toronto Telegraph* May 8, 1925, p. 4. For reasons of public image Farrar was also anxious that the hospital be called the Toronto 'Psychiatric' and not 'Psychopathic' as the ministry had suggested. Psychopathic was a more commonly used term and thus had attendant connotations. Psychiatric was a newer and more scientific term. In addition, Farrar wished his title to be that of director rather than superintendent as was the practice in the Ontario hospitals. [H.M. Robbins (deputy provincial secretary) to Lincoln Goldie (provincial secretary) February 19, 1926, p. 4. Archives of Ontario RG 10 107-0-1009.]

[12] Department of Psychiatry, *Annual Report, 1956,* (hereafter cited as DPR) University of Toronto Archives.

[13] McKerracher, pp. 77-78.

[14] Robert Falconer (university president) quoted in *The Mail and Empire* October 13, 1923, pp. 4-5.

[15] Province of Ontario, Hospitals Division, Department of Health (HD). *Toronto Psychiatric Hospital Report Covering Period 1926-32,* (Toronto: Queens Printer, 1932), pp. 7 and 12. Report hereafter cited as HD 1926-32.

[16] Ibid., p. 10.

[17] Ibid., pp. 17-18.

[18] Most of the specific services of TPH are dealt with in detail in other chapters.

[19] S.W. Hamilton and G.A. Kempt for the Mental Health Survey Committee, "Survey of Ontario Hospitals," (1937), p. 3. Archives of Ontario RG 10 107-0-421.

[20] Archives of Ontario RG 10 107-0-1010.

[21] "Hospital for Mental Cases Would Have Wider Powers," *Toronto Star* February 13, 1926. See also Robbins to Goldie, January 14, 1926, and February 19, 1926. Archives of Ontario RG 10 107-0-1009.

[22] Robbins to Goldie, March 24, 1926, p. 3. Archives of Ontario RG 10 107-0-1009.

[23] Robbins to Goldie, March 26, 1926. Archives of Ontario RG 10 107-0-1008.

[24] Memorandum of the conference, January 6, 1926. Archives of Ontario RG 10 107-0-1009.

[25] HD 1926-32, p. 5.

[26] Robbins to Goldie, January 14, 1926. Archives of Ontario RG 10 107-0-1009.

[27] Statutes of Ontario. Chapter 71 "Psychiatric Hospitals," pp. 493-99. (Toronto: Clarkson W. James, 1926).

[28]Robbins to Goldie, March 24, 1926, p. 4. Archives of Ontario RG 10 107-0-1009.
[29] Robbins to Goldie, February 19, 1926, p. 3. Archives of Ontarion RG 10 107-0-1009.
[30]Ibid.
[31]*Toronto Star* February 1926.
[32]Statutes of Ontario. Chapter 71, "Psychiatric Hospitals," section 10, subsection 4 0. 495. (Toronto: Clarkson W. James, 1926).
[33]Ibid., section 12, p. 496.
[34]Robbins to Thomas F. Rooney (city relief officer), September 15, 1926. Archives of Ontario RG 10 107-0-1010.
[35]Robbins to Goldie, January 15, 1927. Archives of Ontario RG 10 107-0-1014.
[36]There was also a good deal of wrangling over the cost and extent of the city's responsibility for the equipping of the hospital. See also Cyril Greenland's chapter (Chapter 2).
[37]"City May Have to Pay For Outside Patients — Relief Officer Opposed to Amendment to Psychiatric Act," *The Globe* February 24, 1926, p. 1.
[38]Robbins to Goldie, November 21, 1928. Archives of Ontario RG 10 107-0-1009.
[39]W.G. Angus (city solicitor) to G.A. Brown (provincial auditor), December 20, 1929. Archives of Ontario RG 10 107-0-1009
[40]C.M. Colquhoun (city solicitor) to Bert S. Wemp (mayor) March 12, 1930 (Board of Control-Associated Documents 1930, March 18. #853, Box #222, City of Toronto Archives). Also city relief officer to Nathan Phillips March 23, 1931 (Board of Control-Associated Document 1931. March 26 #1023 Box #241).
[41]*Borden Committee Report of 1956,* January 12, 1956. (Hereafter cited as Borden) Clarke Institute of Psychiatry.
[42]See Edward Shorter's chapter on Farrar (Chapter 3).
[43]DPR April 30, 1926. Lectures included: psychopathology and the developmental process of psychiatric conditions, particularly hereditary and constitutional tendencies. In the 1920s and 1930s, the organic theory of mental illness was still very much in the forefront in Canada.
[44]These included: dementia praecox, manic depressive psychoses, epileptic states, senile and arteriosclerotic psychoses and neuro-syphilis.
[45]HD1926-32, p. 11.
[46]Archives of Ontario RG 10 107-0-336.
[47]HD 1926-32, p. 11.
[48]Farrar's education was solidly in the organic field of psychiatry, neuropathology in particular. See Shorter chapter on Farrar (Chapter 3).
[49]DPR 1932 and HD 1926-32, p. 11.
[50]HD 1926-32, p. 11.
[51]DPR 1933.
[52]Ruth MacLachlan Franks, "The Pathogenesis and Prevention of Suicide," (Ph.D. thesis, University of Toronto, 1936).
[53]DPR 1936.
[54]DPR 1932; DPR 1933; and HD 1926-32, pp. 8-9.
[55]HD 1933. For further discussion of the nursing program and education refer to the nursing chapter.
[56]This emphasis on psychiatry was recommended in a 1930 report for the Rockefeller Foundation prepared by Dean David Edsall. In "Mental Health Memo Regarding Possible Psychiatric Developments," Edsall stressed the huge economic losses due to mental illness and the backwardness of the field. By the early 1940s,

three-quarters of the Rockefeller Foundation's funding in the medical sciences was devoted to psychiatry and related fields. [Rockefeller Foundation Archives RG 3 series 906, box 2, folder 18, Program and Policy — Psychiatry, The Emphasis on Psychiatry, p. 12.]

[57] Rockefeller Foundation RG 1.1 series 427, box 1, folder 1. Clarence Hincks originally approached the Rockefeller Foundation in November 1923 for a grant.

[58] Rockefeller Foundation minutes 20106, 20107.

[59] Rockefeller Roundation RG 1.1 series 427, box 10, file 79. Minutes 20129, 20130, November 18, 1920. See also Cyril Greenland's chapter (Chapter 2).

[60] George E. Vincent (president of the Rockefeller Foundation 1917-29) to Robert Falconer, November 22, 1920. Rockefeller Foundation RG 1.1 series 427, box 10, file 79. (George Vincent was also a cousin of Vincent Massey.)

[61] Falconer to Richard M. Pearce (director of the Rockefeller Foundation Division of Medical Education 1920-30), June 20, 1923; and Edwin R. Embree (secretary of the Rockefeller Foundation) to Falconer, December 6, 1923. Rockefeller Foundation RG 1.1 series 427, box 10, file 79.

[62] Clarence Hincks to Farrar, March 16, 1931. Farrar private archive, Rockefeller Foundation file.

[63] Farrar to Spaulding, October 11, 1935. Farrar private archive, Rockefeller Foundation file.

[64] Memorandum Farrar to Dean Primrose on improvements with Rockefeller money via CNCMH. December 1930. Farrar private archive, Rockefeller Foundation file.

[65] Memorandum of October 5, 1936, interview Gregg with Farrar. Rockefeller Foundation RG 1.1 series 427, box 10, file 81, "Teaching has had concentrated attention during the past five years. An attempt to give better post-graduate instruction to the Ontario Hospital Service."

[66] Copy of an order-in-council approved by the lieutenant-governor, December 3, 1934, p. 2.

[67] H.J. Cody, university president, to J.G. FitzGerald, dean of medicine, University of Toronto, September 18, 1932. Farrar private archive.

[68] *AJP* 91: 944-45 (January 1935).

[69] See Cyril Greenland's chapter (Chapter 2).

[70] See Edward Shorter's and Cyril Greenland's chapters (Chapter 3 and Chapter 2). Farrar was briefly superintendent at Homewood before going to Toronto.

[71] Hobbs to Farrar, November 17, 1924. University of Toronto Archives.

[72] Farrar to Evelyn Farrar, a Wednesday, Christmastime late 1920s. Farrar private archive.

[73] Farrar to Hobbins, November 20, 1930. Farrar private archive.

[74] *Ontario Medical Registry* 1954.

[75] B.T. McGhie (deputy minister of health) to Farrar, April 13, 1934. Farrar private archive.

[76] Interestingly, Mitch Hepburn shows up later on in regard to Ontario Hospitals. St. Thomas Hospital was built on land that was right next to the premier's farm. A personal letter from its first superintendent, W.B. Smith, to Farrar (undated but presumably during his short tenure between April and October 1939 when the province gave the facility over to the air force) relates: "I hope the hospital will not become too much of a political football, but we are so close to Mitch's farm we can almost hear him 'listening to the grass grow.'" Smith to Farrar sometime in 1939 (page missing). Farrar private archive.

[77] Ontario Department of Health, Hospitals Division, staff records of Ditchburn, Eileen E.H., March 1, 1934, and Foley, Myrtle (Mrs.), January 20, 1934. Farrar private archive.

[78] Eileeen E.H. Ditchburn to C.B. Farrar, February 26, 1934. Farrar private archive.

[79] See Margaret Gorrie's chapter (Chapter 9).

[80] See also Cyril Greenland's chapter (Chapter 2).

[81] Hamilton and Kempt, p. 3.

[82] Robbins to Farrar, August 2, 1930. Archives of Ontario RG 10 107-0-1009.

[83] HD 1933, p. 116.

[84] Farrar to Robbins, August 16, 1926; Farrar to Robbins, March 18, 1926; and Farrar to Robbins, October 20, 1930.Farrar private archive, TPH personnel file.

[85] Archives of Ontario RG 10 163-0-421. S.W. Hamilton and G.A. Kempt for the Mental Health Survey Committee, "Survey of Ontario Hospitals" (1937), p. 61. The survey was commissioned in the wake of the Depression by Premier Mitch Hepburn and Dr. J.A. Faulkner, minister of health. In their introduction, the two American doctors explained that the study was motivated by "a series of unhappy occurrences that attracted unfavourable attention even outside the circle of officers responsible for the health of the patients." (p. 5) In addition, there was a severe shortage of physicians because many had left the service for financial reasons.

[86] Robbins to Goldie, March 24, 1926. Archives of Ontario RG 10 107-0-1009.

[87] John Dewan, "Psychiatry in Ontario 1930-70," (1978), pp. 11-12. QSMHC Archives.

[88] Elliot S. Valenstein, *Great and Desperate Cures: The Rise and Decline of Psychosurgery and Other Radical Treatments for Mental Illness* (New York: Basic Books, 1986), pp. 46-48.

[89] Hans Hoff, "History of the Organic Treatment of Schizophrenia" in Max Rinkel and Harold E. Himwich, *Insulin Treatment in Psychiatry* (New York: Philosophical Library, 1958), pp. 3-18.

[90] Valenstein, pp. 46-48, provides a complete narrative upon which most of this account is based. See also Rinkel and Himwich, pp. 3-18.

[91] See Valenstein, p. 52.

[92] Hoff, p. 11. Sakel's working theory held that under the influence of shock treatments, sick and defective cell connections in the brain would be separated. Sakel believed that such defective connections were caused by psychological influences in cells that were genetically vulnerable.

[93] See also F.E. James, "Insulin Treatment in Psychiatry," *History of Psychiatry 3*: 221-35 (1992).

[94] Bellevue was the hospital of Joseph Wortis, who had been in Vienna during Sakel's early experiments and was one of the major U.S. proponents of the treatment.

[95] *Toronto Telegram* May 19, 1937, p. 18.

[96] Farrar in *Toronto Star* May 20, 1937, p. 14. Dr. L.S. Penrose mentioned in his 1941 report to the superintendents on therapies in the Ontario hospitals that one of the most important results of the adoption of shock therapies was families' gratification at active treatment. Superintendents' Conference, April 25, 1941. Archives of Ontario RG 10 107-0-342.

[97] See *Toronto Star* May 20, 1937.

[98] DPR 1937 and 1938.

[99] James E. Shelley, comp., "A Survey of Manuscript Sources for the History of Psychiatry and Related Areas in the Rockefeller Archive Centre" (Tarrytown, NY: Rockefeller Archive Centre, 1985).

[100] Rockefeller Foundation policy, excerpt from Trustees Confidential Bulletin, "The Emphasis on Psychiatry," October 1943. Rockefeller Foundation RG 3 series 906, box 2, folder 18.

[101] Alan Gregg's Diary, Toronto, November 22, 1937. Rockefeller Foundation RG 1.1 series, Box 10, folder 81.

[102] Memorandum of October 5, 1936, interview of Gregg with Farrar. Rockefeller Foundation RG 1.1 series 427, box 10, folder 81.
[103] Farrar to Gregg, November 30, 1936. Farrar private archive, Rockefeller Foundation file.
[104] Memorandum of Gregg's interview with Hincks October 26, 1936. Rockefeller Foundation RGD 1.1 series 427, box 10, folder 81.
[105] Robert A. Lambert, memorandum on Farrar. Rockefeller Foundation RG 1.1 series 427, box 10, folder 81.
[106] University of Toronto Professor Michael Bliss, personal communication, October 14, 1992.
[107] Gregg to B.T. McGhie, January 12, 1938. Rockefeller Foundation RG 1.1 series 427, box 10, folder 82.
[108] Norma S. Thompson (secretary of Rockefeller Foundation) to Cody, January 24, 1939. Rockefeller Foundation RG 1.1 series 427, box 10, folder 83. See also minutes 39001, January 20, 1939. Rockefeller Foundation RG 1.1 series 427, box 10, folder 81.
[109] DPR 1939. Lorne D. Proctor succeeded McNeel in 1941.
[110] DPR 1940. See also Farrar to Gregg, August 13, 1940. Rockefeller Foundation RG 1.1 series 427, box 10, folder 83.
[111] Dr. G.E. Hall to Farrar, August 10, 1940. Rockefeller Foundation RG 1.1 series 427, box 10, folder 83.
[112] B.H. McNeel, J.G. Dewan, C.R. Myers, L.D. Proctor, J. E. Goodwin, "Parallel Psychological, Psychiatric and Physiological Findings in Schizophrenia Patients Under Insulin Shock Treatment," *AJP* 98: 422-29 (November 1941).
[113] "Report of the Research Unit of the Toronto Psychiatric Hospital During the Past Five Years," August 1943. Rockefeller Foundation RG 1.1 series 427, box 11, folder 85. See also L.D. Proctor, J.G. Dewan, and B.H. McNeel, "Variations in the Glucose Tolerance Observations in Schizophrenics Before and After Shock Treatment," *AJP* 100: 652-58 (March 1944).
[114] Farrar to Gregg, March 3, 1941. Rockefeller Foundation RG 1.1 series 427, box 10, folder 83. Certainly, Lucas's touching anecdote of Banting's last day in Toronto was reason for the inclusion of the letter. "It may interest you to know that the last thing Banting did before leaving the laboratory on the Saturday he left Toronto, was to read the reports of your part of the joint project being carried on under the Rockefeller grant. He expressed continued interest in the problem and growing satisfaction with the results. He was especially interested in the biochemical section and at one point interrupted his reading to exclaim, 'This gives me a new idea.' The following day he wrote to Miss Gairns and referred to the idea provoked by the report, saying he longed for the day when he could get back to working with his own hands and expressed regret that he would have to wait for this until the war was over." Dr. C.C. Lucas to Farrar, February 27, 1941. Rockefeller Foundation RG 1.1 series 427, box 10, folder 83.
[115] N.L Easton, "Metrazol As Used in the Treatment of Schizophrenia" (1938). Archives of Ontario RG 10-107-0-30.
[116] Valenstein, p. 50.
[117] D.R. Fletcher to R.C. Montgomery, January 6, 1938. Archives of Ontario RG 10-107-0-30.
[118] Valenstein, p. 50.
[119] N.L. Easton (1938).
[120] "Discovery of Metrazol Helps Dementia Praecox Cases: Patients Treated at Ontario Hospitals in New Toronto and London: Cheap and Easy," *Toronto Star* May 27, 1938, pp. 1-2.
[121] Memorandum, Montgomery to McGhie, April 22, 1938. Archives of Ontario RG 10-107-0-30.

[122] Memorandum, Montgomery to McGhie, April 4, 1939. Archives of Ontario RG 10-107-0-31.

[123] "Metrazol Treatment in Ontario Hospitals" (1939). Archives of Ontario RG 10-107-0-31. The committee consisted of McGhie, deputy minister of health; R.C. Montgomery, director of Hospital services; Farrar; C.H. McCuaig, chief of staff at TPH; G.E. Hall, associate professor of medical research at the Banting Institute; and N.L. Easton, director of research for the Department of Health.

[124] Memorandum from Easton to the superintendents of Ontario Hospitals November 10, 1939. Archives of Ontario RG 10-107-0-31. See also N.L. Easton and Joseph Sommers, "The Significance of Vertebral Fractures as a Complication of Metrazol Therapy," *AJP* 98: 538-43 (January 1942).

[125] Ontario Hospitals memorandum, August 13, 1940. Archives of Ontario RG 10 107-0-32.

[126] Montgomery to L.P. Teevens, November 1, 1940. Archives of Ontario RG 10 107-0-32. In autumn 1940, metrazol became prohibitively expensive because it was imported from Germany and had a very high duty imposed upon it. This remained a problem for several months until an American supplier could be found.

[127] Valenstein, pp. 50-52.

[128] J.D.M. Griffin, *N.C.M.H. Bulletin* (February 1941). Archives of Ontario RG 10-107-0-44.

[129] Ibid., p. 2.

[130] Memorandum, Farrar to C.H. Lewis (director of the hospital division) September 8, 1942. Archives of Ontario RG 10-107-0-44. See also "TPH Research Unit Annual Report" (1941). Rockefeller Foundation RG 1.1 series 427, box 10, file 84.

[131] "Minutes of Committee on Shock Therapy," July 11, 1942. Archives of Ontario RG 10-107-0-44.

[132] Farrar private archive, Farrar's patient file.

[133] *McGraw-Hill Encyclopedia of Science and Medicine* (New York: McGraw-Hill, 1992), vol. 6, p. 142.

[134] "Report to the Rockefeller Foundation for Medical Research on Electroencephalographic Studies of Schizophrenics" (December 1941). Rockefeller Foundation RG 1.1 series 427, box 10, file 84.

[135] Gregg's diary, April 8, 1942. Rockefeller Foundation RG 1.1 series 427, box 10, file 84.

[136] Best to Gregg, Feb 5, 1943. Rockefeller Foundation RG 1.1 series 427, box 11, file 85.

[137] Farrar to Gregg, Jan 28, 1943. Rockefeller Foundation RG 1.1 series 427, box 11, file 85.

[138] E.V. Gifford and C.R. Myers, "Measuring Abnormal Pattern on the Revised Stanford Binet Scale. (Form L)," *Journal of Mental Science* 89: 92-101 (January 1943).

[139] Gregg to Farrar, Sep 8, 1943. Rockefeller Foundation RG 1.1 series 427, box 11, file 85.

[140] Lorne Proctor, "Synopsis of Research Activities Toronto Psychiatric Hospital Research Unit" (December 1944). Rockefeller Foundation RG 1.1 427, box 11, file 86.

[141] DPR 1945.

[142] DPR 1943.

[143] Dewan, p. 9.

[144] Robert Pos, "History of Psychiatry at Toronto General Hospital till 1975" (Unpublished, 1992), p. 23. QSMHC, Griffin-Greenland collection.

[145] Pos, p. 13. See also Cyril Greenland's chapter (Chapter 2).

[146] Pos, p. 22.
[147] Alan Parkin, *A History of Psychoanalysis in Canada* (Toronto: The Toronto Psychoanalytic Society, 1987).
[148] Pos, p. 23 and 29.
[149] Farrar to Gregg, December 15, 1944. Rockefeller Foundation RG 1.1 series 427, box 11, folder 86.
[150] Memorandum of Gregg's interview with Hincks, October 26, 1936. Rockefeller Foundation RG 1.1 series 427, box 10, file 81.
[151] Dewan, p. 4.
[152] See Shorter chapter on Farrar (Chapter 3).
[153] Farrar to MacFarlane, May 13, 1946. University of Toronto Archives, Department of Psychiatry file.
[154] Angus to Farrar, February, 11, 1946. University of Toronto Archives, Department of Psychiatry file.
[155] Farrar to MacFarlane, May 13, 1946. University of Toronto Archives, Department of Psychiatry file.
[156] Farrar to Angus, May 13, 1946. University of Toronto Archives, Department of Psychiatry file. MacFarlane consulted Professor D.K. Henderson of Edinburgh, Sir Charles Symonds of London, Sir Francis Fraser (British Postgraduate Medical Federation, London), Sir Allen Daley (London), and Dr. Aubrey Lewis (Maudsley Hospital, London). Besides Farrar, Gregg of the Rockefeller Foundation was the only non-Briton asked for recommendations.
[157] MacFarlane to Farrar, November 22, 1946. University of Toronto Archives, Department of Psychiatry file.
[158] The others were Dr. L.R. Angus and Dr. R.F. Barbour, a Scot working at the time in Bristol. (Barbour was also a surgeon and had trained at the Boston Psychopathic Hospital, Johns Hopkins and Maudsley Hospital. He was not highly recommended, but it is of note that he was particularly interested in psychoanalysis.) Another Scot, Thomas Arthur Munro, was also considered. Although Barbour and Munro had similar backgrounds and had worked in the same American hospitals, Munro was inclined towards research, with an interest in heredity. A rather inexperienced J. Allan Walters of Toronto was also on the list. According to MacFarlane's letter to Farrar on November 22, 1946, Dewan was also considered. University of Toronto Archives, Department of Psychiatry file, 1949.
[159] A.B. Stokes, "Somatic Research in Periodic Catatonia," *Journal of Neurology and Psychiatry* (New series) 2 (3): 243-58 (July 1939); A.B. Stokes, "Psychological Aspects of Deafness," *Proceedings of the Royal Society of Medicine* 34: 309-20 (February 7, 1941); A.B. Stokes, "Effects of Drugs in Myotonia," *Lancet* 11: 979 (1939); A.B. Stokes, "Social Skill in Industry," *Industrial Welfare* 28: 128 (1946).
[160] L.S. Maclay to Hyland. University of Toronto Archives, Department of Psychiatry file: "Candidates for the Chair of Psychiatry". In his reference, Aubrey Lewis, an opponent of psychoanalysis, lists Stokes' shortcomings and comments: "On the clinical side, I suppose it could be reckoned as a failing that he is more interested in direct clinical observations than in their interpretation by psychoanalytical and kindred methods." See also Shorter chapter on Farrar (Chapter 3).
[161] Dewan, p. 9.
[162] Abe Miller, transcript of "Round-table Discussion of history of TPH at Queen Street Mental Health Centre," May 1, 1992, p. 5. Available at the QSMHC Archives, Griffin-Greenland Collection.
[163] DPR 1947-48.
[164] DPR 1947-48, p. 3.

[165]"Minutes of Advisory Committee on Mental Health" October 1-3, 1947. Archives of Ontario RG 10 107-0-505.

[166]Montgomery to Russell T. Kelly (minister of health), August 12, 1949. Archives of Ontario RG 10 107-0-497.

[167]*Globe and Mail* March 19, 1949, p. 5.

[168]Borden, p. 4.

[169]Memorandum, Mackinnon Phillips to L.M. Frost, September 16, 1953. Archives of Ontario RG 10 107-0-980.

[170]"Review of Community Mental Health Services 1955." Archives of Ontario RG 10 107-0-624.

[171]Ibid.

[172]McNeel, in "Superintendent's Conference Minutes," November 18, 1960, p. 26. Archives of Ontario RG 10 107-0-1026.

[173]Montgomery to Russell T. Kelly, February 14, 1949. Archives of Ontario RG 10 107-0-497.

[174]*Globe and Mail* February 2, 1948, p. 8.

[175]Montgomery to Kelley, February 14, 1949. Archives of Ontario RG 10 107-0-497.

[176]DPR 1949.

[177]DPR 1946.

[178]C.H. McCuaig, "Report of the Committee on Attracting Graduate Physicians to the Ontario Hospital Service," April 1950. Archives of Ontario RG 10 107-0-348.

[179]C.H. McCuaig, "Minutes of Superintendent's Conference," January 13, 1950, p. 3. Archives of Ontario RG 10 107-0-348.

[180]DPR 1950.

[181]Pos, p. 29-30.

[182]DPR 1950-51 and Pos, p. 30.

[183]DPR 1949.

[184]Pos, p. 31.

[185]Ibid., p. 30-38. It was not until 1958 that Farquharson and Stokes agreed on an arrangement for psychiatry at TGH. Under this agreement, appointments would be joint to the departments of medicine and psychiatry. Graduate teaching, training, and research would fall under the professor of psychiatry, while administrative and patient care would fall under the jurisdiction of the professor of medicine.

[186]DPR 1952-53.

[187]DPR 1957-58.

[188]Abe Miller, transcript of "Round-table Discussion of History of TPH at Queen Street mental Health Centre," May 1, 1992, p. 5.

[189]"Curriculum for Post Graduate Teaching, O.P.D." July 1957. Clarke Institute of Psychiatry, TPH file.

[190]Jack Griffin personal communication.

[191]DPR 1953-54.

[192]DPR 1950-51.

[193]Ibid., 1950-51.

[194]DPR 1948-49. See also Turner chapter (Chapter 16).

[195]"Superintendents' & Directors of Mental Health Clinics Meeting Minutes," November 19, 1959. Archives of Ontario RG 10 107-0-1025 and DPR 1959-60.

[196]DPR 1950-51.

[197]Simmons, p. 60.

[198] DPR 1957-58.
[199] DPR 1956-56.
[200] "Open House summary of services at TPH," May 1961, p. 3. Clarke Institute of Psychiatry, TPH files.
[201] Apparently, Davis and Cappon had been concerned about this for some time and had submitted a memorandum to this effect to Stokes in 1950. See preamble to the Report.
[202] "Report of the Board of Teachers Subcommittee for Treatment in the Department of Psychiatry," January 1953. Clarke Institue of Psychiatry, TPH files.
[203] *Toronto Star* May 2, 1960. In 1960, the *Mental Hospital Act* was amended to provide for open wards for patients not requiring restraint. The object was to adopt provisions similar to those of public hospitals. McNeel explained that this was now possible: "because significant advances have taken place in the field of medicine within the past twenty-five years." Memorandum, B.H. McNeel to C. Walker, solicitor, Department of Health, December 9, 1960. Archives of Ontario RG 10 107-0-1026.
[204] *Globe and Mail* August 6, 1965.
[205] Valenstein, *Great and Desperate Cures*. This book provides an excellent account of the introduction of lobotomy to North America. The history of lobotomy is a detailed and controversial topic. While a study of lobotomy in Ontario merits a separate chapter or book, a separate chapter in this work would give it undue emphasis in the overall history of TPH. Thus, I have attempted to highlight the main points of the story as they relate to developments in Ontario and TPH.
[206] Valenstein, p. 141 and 62.
[207] Valenstein, p. 84.
[208] Farrar to Eric K. Clarke, January 31, 1938. Farrar private archive, Freeman corr. file.
[209] K.G. McKenzie to B.T. McGhie, February 17, 1938. Farrar private archive, Freeman corr. file.
[210] Ibid.
[211] Abe Miller, transcript of "Round-table Discussion of History of TPH at Queen Street Mental Health Centre," May 1, 1992, p. 8.
[212] "TPH Research Unit Annual Report 1941." Rockefeller Foundation RG 1.1 series 427, box 10, file 84.
[213] "Report to Rockefeller Foundation for Psychiatric Research on Schizophrenia," December 1942, p. 4. Rockefeller Foundation RG 1.1 series 427, box 11, file 85.
[214] "TPH Research Unit: Results of Bilateral Frontal Leucotomies, July 23, 1941 — July 31, 1944." Farrar private archive, lobotomy file.
[215] Abstracted in memorandum to J.T. Phair from R.C. Montgomery, June 11, 1945. Archives of Ontario RG 10 107-0-48.
[216] Montgomery to Sharpe, June 23, 1947. Archives of Ontario RG 10 107-0-48.
[217] Superintendent of New Toronto to Montgomery, May 27, 1948. Archives of Ontario RG 10 107-0-48.
[218] C.E. Hanna to A.B. Stokes, July 14, 1948. Archives of Ontario RG 10 107-0-048.
[219] Montgomery to W.H. Weber (superintendent of Whitby), January 14, 1948. Archives of Ontario RG 10 107-0-48.
[220] A.B. Stokes, "Prefrontal Leucotomy," August 13, 1948. Archives of Ontario RG 10 107-0-48.
[221] Memorandum, Montgomery to G. Firby, accountant, May 18, 1948. Archives of Ontario RG 10 107-0-48.
[222] A.B. Stokes, "Minutes of Superintendents' Conference," May 6, 1949, p. 8. Archives of Ontario RG 10 107-0-347.

[223] E.A. Clark, "Prefrontal Lobotomy: A Brief Review of Selected Literature," given at the Superintendents' Conference September 1949, Appendix B. Archives of Ontario RG 10 107-0-688.

[224] "Minutes of Superintendent Conference," October 14, 1949. Archives of Ontario RG 10 107-0-347.

[225] Stokes to Montgomery, June 2, 1950. Archives of Ontario RG 10 107-0-688.

[226] Stevenson (superintendent Ontario Hospital London) to Montgomery, June 7 and August 30, 1950; and J.N. Senn (superintendent Ontario Hospital Hamilton) to Montgomery, June 7, 1950. Archives of Ontario RG 10 107-0-688.

[227] "Minutes," July 12, 1950. Archives of Ontario RG 10 107-0-688.

[228] Stevenson to Montgomery, August 12, 1952. Archives of Ontario RG 10 107-0-688.

[229] "26 Mentally Ill Patients Recover After Operation," *Toronto Star* March 7, 1951, p. 3; "Amazing Results of Brain Surgery Seen at London" *Globe and Mail* August 26, 1952, p. 3; and "119 Lobotomies Done 50 Patients Released 25 To Go, None Worse," *Toronto Star* August 26, 1952, p. 1.

[230] B.A. Boyd, W.H. Weber, K.G. McKenzie, "Leucotomy — Its Therapeutic Value on the Disturbed Wards of a Mental Hospital," *Canadian Psychiatric Association Journal* 3 (4): 170-79 (1958). J.N. Senn, superintendent at Hamilton, was an early and staunch supporter of leucotomies.

[231] Ibid., p. 178.

[232] These included J.N. Senn and Stevenson.

[233] MacKinnon Phillips (minister of health) to Montgomery, April 27, 1953. Archives of Ontario RG 10 107-0-688.

[234] Fischer to Montgomery, April, 27, 1953. Archives of Ontario RG 10 107-0-688.

[235] Hanna to Montgomery, July 9, 1952. Archives of Ontario RG 10 107-0-688.

[236] DPR 1948-49.

[237] Abe Miller, "Presentation of Postoperative Data," in A. Miller, ed., *Lobotomy a Clinical Study* (Toronto: Ontario Department of Health, 1954), p. 15.

[238] Abe Miller, "The Lobotomy Patient — A Decade Later: A Follow-up Study of a Research Project started in 1948," *Canadian Medical Association Journal* 96 (15) 1095-1103 (April 15, 1967).

[239] See Geoffrey Reaume, "The Rise and Decline of Psychosurgery in Ontario," April 16, 1989, p. 9-10 (Unpublished. Kindly provided by the author, but also available at the QSMHC archives). As late as 1959, despite growing opposition to the procedure, a number of hospitals were still very keen to continue and very pleased with their results. See "Minutes of Superintendents' Conference," November 19, 1959. Archives of Ontario RG 10 107-0-1025. In 1961, fifty-eight leucotomies were performed in Ontario hospitals, including twenty-five at the hospital for the criminally insane at Penetanguishene, two at St. Thomas, three at TPH, ten in London, two in Kingston, and sixteen at Hamilton. This was a significant reduction from the 157 done in 1953. See memorandum from W.H. Weber (superintendent at Whitby) to C.A. Buck (director of Ontario Hospitals), December 8, 1961. Archives of Ontario RG 10 107-0-689. See also C.S. Tennant to Montgomery, February 9, 1954. Archives of Ontario RG 10 107-0-688.

[240] B.H. McNeel, "Joint Conference of Superintendents and Directors of Mental Health Clinics," November 19-20, 1959. Archives of Ontario RG 10 107-0-1025.

[241] Reaume, p. 12.

[242] Valenstein, p. 254.

[243] Abe Miller, "The Lobotomy Patient."

[244] See Muller chapter.

[245] Dewan, p. 12.

[246]DPR 1959-60.
[247]"Minutes of the Advisory Committee on Mental Health," June 26, 1948. Archives of Ontario RG 10 107-0-505.
[248]DPR 1950.
[249]DPR 1948-9. Report on Activities Under Grants, p. 4.
[250]"Round-table Discussion At Queen Street Mental Health Centre," May 1, 1992, p. 9.
[251]J.R. Seeley, R.A. Sim, E. Loosely, *Crestwood Heights* (Toronto: University of Toronto Press, 1956).
[252]E. Douglass, "Diagnostic Classification and Re-education in Aphasia" *Canadian Medical Association Journal* 69 (4): 376-81 (October 1953) and R.G. Arthurs, D. Cappon, E. Douglass, B. Quarrington, "Carbon Dioxide Therapy with Stutterers," in S.B. Wortis, *Year Book of Neurology, Psychiatry, and Neurosurgery* (Chicago: Year Book Medical Publishers, 1953), p. 390.
[253]W.E. Boothroyd, "Occupation and the Ego," *Canadian Journal of Occupational Therapy* 22 (4): 131-36 (December 1955).
[254]A. Parkin, "Emergence of Sleep During Psychoanalysis," *International Journal of Psychoanalysis* 36 (3): 174-76 (May-June 1955).
[255]DPR 1952-53.
[256]Stokes' curriculum vitae, University of Toronto Archives, Department of Psychiatry file.
[257]Dewan, P. 10.
[258]Ibid., p. 11.
[259]DPR 1950.
[260]Stokes to MacKinnon Phillips, November 22, 1951. Archives of Ontario RG 10 107-0-515.
[261]DPR 1952-53.
[262]DPR 1954-55.
[263]J. Dewan and W.B. Spaulding, *The Organic Psychoses: A Guide to Diagnosis* (Toronto: University of Toronto Press, 1958), p. v.
[264]Ibid., p. vii.
[265]C.A. Buck (inspector, mental health division) to J.T. Phair (deputy minister of health), August 28, 1956. Archives of Ontario RG 10 107-0-980.
[266]"Brief On the Present State of Planning of an Ontario Psychiatric Institute," February 22, 1955. Archives of Ontario RG 10 107-0-980.
[267]*Toronto Star* April 5, 1952, p. 29.
[268]Memorandum, G.E. Williams (deputy minister and chief architect) to S.J. Vame (assistant chief architect), January 22, 1952. Archives of Ontario RG 10 107-0-980.
[269]"Brief on the Present State of Planning of an Ontario Psychiatric Institute," February 22, 1955. Archives of Ontario RG 10 107-0-980.
[270]Borden, p. 11. See also "Ontario Psychiatric Institute," June 23, 1958. Archives of Ontario RG 10 107-0-900.
[271]Borden, p. 11.
[272]Ibid., p. 6.
[273]Ibid., p. 7-8 and Pos, p. 35.
[274]Pos, p. 35.
[275]Borden, p. 12-15.
[276]Pos, p. 35—6.
[277]F.R. Stone (vice-president administration, University of Toronto) to Matthew Dymond (minister of health), January 14, 1959. Archives of Ontario RG 10 6-0-900.

[278] Memorandum, B.H. McNeel to Mackinnon Phillips, October 15, 1958. Archives of Ontario RG 10 6-0-900.
[279] "Ontario Institute of Psychiatry," June 23, 1958. Archives of Ontario RG 10 6-0-900.
[280] Ibid.
[281] McNeel to R.A. Farrell (executive officer, premier's office), October 21, 1958. Archives of Ontario RG 10 6-0-900.
[282] McNeel to Stokes, December 17, 1958. Archives of Ontario RG 10 6-0-900.
[283] Matthew Dymond to F.R. Stone, June 19, 1961. Archives of Ontario RG 10 6-0-900.
[284] "All Star," *Toronto Star* supplement, Spring 1963. Clarke Institute of Psychiatry.
[285] *Toronto Star* July 8, 1963.

5

Farrar and the American Journal of Psychiatry

Peter Faux[*]

"The care of the human mind is the most noble branch of medicine."[1]

Clarence B. Farrar became the eighth editor of the *American Journal of Psychiatry* (*AJP*) in July 1931. Farrar's association with the *AJP* had begun in 1927, when he was appointed assistant editor of the *AJP*. Canada's initial involvement with this journal commenced, however, in 1904, when Edward Brush nominated C.K. Clarke as assistant editor to the editorial board. Farrar, during his own editorship, would nominate the following Canadians to the board: Alvin Mathers, professor of psychiatry at the University of Manitoba; Lorne Proctor, a graduate from the postgraduate psychiatric program at TPH; and Kenneth G. Gray, a lawyer-psychiatrist, who was professor of psychiatry at the University of Toronto.

Farrar's predecessors

The *AJP* was Farrar's life's work. As its eighth editor, Farrar represented a kind of fulfillment of the journal's long history. In 1844, 13 superintendents drew up the charter of the Association of Medical Superintendents of American Institutions for the Insane. Primarily from New England and the Eastern Seaboard, in number and ambition they resembled the signers of the Declaration of Independence. Five years

---

[*]Peter Faux, M.D., F.R.C.P. (C) has been chief of psychiatry at St. Joseph's Health Centre since 1990. He chairs the history of psychiatry section of the Canadian Psychiatric Association and is a book reviewer for the *Canadian Journal of Psychiatry*. In 1985, he authored *The House that Grew*, published by Boston Mills Publishing.

later, in 1849, Canada was also represented at the association's annual meeting in Utica, New York.

In July 1844, the first issue of the *American Journal of Insanity (AJI)* was published. The founding editor was Amariah Brigham, who, since 1842, had been the superintendent of the New York State Lunatic Asylum at Utica. He had the distinction of editing the first English language journal of psychiatry. An anonymous observer with an insider's knowledge noted,

> For C.B.F. it was a matter of pride that the *American Journal of Insanity* was the oldest psychiatric journal in the English speaking world, and that it, the French and the German were all founded within the same twelve months.[2]

Brigham published a quarterly of 96 pages in 1844. To attract readers, he set the subscription at $1.00 per annum. Farrar later recorded,

> But even before the second number had come from the press Brigham was able to report "a good, though not large, subscription list." He remarked that although "the establishment of the Journal was a rather hazardous undertaking," he was encouraged by the increasing number of subscribers. Indeed only two years later in the autumn of 1846, he could write to [Pliny] Earle: "There are now subscribers enough to pay." He did not say how many subscribers or exactly what he meant by "pay."[3]

Brigham balanced the books from his own pocket and for the first volume wrote all the articles. Soon, other psychiatrists were contributing and subscribers were supporting the *AJI*. Alfred P. Noyes noted,

> Amariah Brigham's place in the history of American Psychiatry is a secure one. Not only did he help found an organization, a journal, and a hospital each of which is still functioning well today, but, also, he approached the problem of insanity from a broad scientific and humanistic point of view and developed methods of psychiatric treatment that were second to none in his time.[4]

Farrar was dedicated to following in the tradition of Brigham, and his life as editor never deviated from the historical mold that was set by the *AJI*'s creator. Much that was said about Brigham became Farrar's story too. Both were superintendents of renowned institutions: Brigham at Utica State Hospital and Farrar at TPH.

From the beginning of his career, Farrar had shown a keen interest in the history of psychiatry. One of his first articles to appear in the

American Journal of Insanity was titled "Some Origins in Psychiatry."[5] Perhaps it was his interest in history that prompted Farrar to discontinue the numbering of the 13-year-old *AJP* (which succeeded the *AJI*) at volume 13 and, in July 1934, return the numbering system to the one begun by the *AJI* in 1844. He issued volume 91 and returned the journal to its origins.

Perhaps it was Farrar's sense of history as well that led him to increase the number of associate editors from six in 1931 (among whom were Charles Macfie Campbell and Harry Stack Sullivan) to twelve, which, with Farrar himself, returned the total number of *AJP* editors to the original number of thirteen founding superintendents. During his many years of editorship, the number of associate editors did not change. He was committed to upholding the principles of the journal which anchored the mutations of the organization in the declaration of their forefathers.

In 1851, Nathan D. Benedict, then superintendent of the Utica State Hospital, assumed editorship of the *AJI* until his retirement in 1854. He was followed by John P. Gray who became both editor of the journal and superintendent of the Utica State Hospital from 1854 to 1886. In the history of the journal, only Farrar would surpass his 33 years of editorship.

As Alfred Noyes described in his *History of Psychiatry*,

> The life of Dr. Gray presented an interesting contrast to that of Dr. Amariah Brigham. Brigham was a quiet research worker, a therapist, a student, a devotee of literature and art, and a writer. Gray was a man of action and activity who inspired and directed rather than gave his strength personally to research and therapy... In contrast to Brigham, who wrote almost constantly, Gray wrote little or nothing except the thirty-three routine annual reports required by his superintendency and such writing as was unavoidable in his capacity as chief editor of the *AJI*.[6]

In 1886, G. Alder Blumer was promoted to superintendent of the Utica State Hospital and assumed editorship of the *AJI*. During Blumer's tenure in 1892, the Association of Medical Superintendents of American Institutions for the Insane became the American Medico-Psychological Association, which then purchased the journal.

Richard S. Dewey became the fifth editor of the *AJP* from 1894 to 1897, and transferred it from Utica to Chicago. In 1895, Dewey became president of the newly formed American Medico-Psychological Association. In 1892 as well, membership was opened beyond superintendents of asylums and mental hospitals to include all practising psychiatrists. Shortly after Farrar assumed editorship in September 1931, he honoured Richard Dewey by publishing his picture in the journal. According to Farrar, Dewey's "innate modesty" kept him from publishing his own picture.[7] Farrar would later note of Dewey that, "the guiding motive of his life work [was]...the scrupulous, thoughtful consideration from first to last of the individual patient, in an endeavour to feel oneself in his place."[8]

Henry M. Hurd edited the *AJP* from 1897 to 1904. Prior to his years as editor, in 1889 he became superintendent of the Johns Hopkins Hospital where he was professor of psychiatry (and, as we have seen, known to Farrar) until 1906. Once Hurd assumed editorship, the journal left Chicago and came to Baltimore. (In 1899 Hurd was also president of the American Medico-Psychological Association.) His four-volume *History of the Institutional Care of the Insane in the United States and Canada*, published in 1917, became a landmark study for asylum psychiatric history of the twentieth century.[9]

Edward N. Brush, the sixth editor, began his term in 1904 and served until his retirement in 1931, a period of 27 years. In total, he completed 41 years of editorial service to the journal since, prior to becoming editor, he had served on its editorial board. (Not to be outdone, Farrar would serve for 43 years in editorial service to the journal: 4 years on the editorial board, 34 years as editor, and 5 years as editor emeritus.)

During Brush's editorship, in 1921 the American Medico-Psychological Association became the American Psychiatric Association and the *AJI* became the *AJP*. About his predecessor, Farrar said:

> The length and richness of his own experience, his long career as editor of the Journal, and his phenomenal memory, gave to Dr. Brush a grasp of the development of American psychiatry such as few men have had. His outlook was always conservative but catholic and tolerant, his patience untiring, his interest in the careers and advancements of the younger men unfailing.[10]

For Farrar, the mold of editorship which began with Brigham was completed by Brush. In those two editors, he had a guiding force that would direct him through his many years.

At the eighty-seventh annual meeting of the American Psychiatric Association in Toronto in 1931, Farrar presented Brush with an illuminated vellum scroll. At the top was a picture of the Utica State Hospital, where Brush began his career in 1878, and at the bottom was a picture of the Sheppard and Enoch Pratt Hospital, where Brush had been superintendent and where he edited the journal. Farrar became eighth editor of the *AJP* at the same 1931 annual meeting held in Toronto.[11]

ADMINISTERING THE AJP

Following the pattern of peregrination—50 years of editorship at Utica, 3 in Chicago and 34 in Baltimore—Farrar moved the journal's office from the Sheppard and Enoch Pratt Hospital in Baltimore to the TPH. From 1931 to 1938, he would thus conduct his editorial duties at the only hospital in Canada ever to house the *AJP*.

During his years as editor, Farrar moved his office four times within the city of Toronto: in 1938, from 2 Surrey Place in the TPH to 111 St. George Street where Clarence M. Hincks, a pioneer in mental hygiene in Canada (who also had served as director of the New York mental hygiene office), gave Farrar an extra room in his office. Almost a decade passed before Farrar retired in 1947, moving his office to a converted house at 113 St. Clair Avenue West. When the house was acquired by Imperial Oil in 1952, he moved down the street to another home at 216 St. Clair West, owned by Robert Noble, registrar of the College of Physicians and Surgeons for Ontario. When Noble died in 1960, Farrar shifted his office to nearby 200 St. Clair Avenue West.[12]

Farrar often worked seven days a week, walking daily to the St. Clair offices near his home. Never did he return home without manuscripts which he read before retiring. To keep up this pace, he increased the editorial assistants from one to two and was responsible for hiring, educating, and supervising them. Having been brought up before the age of the phone, he rarely used it except in case of emergency, and preferred to correspond in writing. Five boxes of this correspondence are housed in the archives of the American Psychiatric Association.

Working alongside Farrar throughout his 34 years as editor was Austin M. Davies, executive assistant, who operated from the American Psychiatric Association's headquarters in New York City. Polar opposites in temperament, Farrar's shy, retiring nature was balanced by Davies' outgoing and social character. Davies was in charge of advertising for the *AJP* and was also responsible for organizing the yearly meeting of the American Psychiatric Association. Davies, Farrar, and the Lord Baltimore Press (which published the bi-monthly journal) formed a trinity that managed the *AJP* until 1958 when Lord Baltimore Press was replaced by Hanover Press, owned by Ken Foley in Hanover, New Hampshire, the home town of Dartmouth College. Together, each working in his own city, they became a successful team that managed the *AJP* for 34 years.

Farrar was always treated as an American expatriate in Tory Toronto. It has been said that Farrar came to Canada in 1916 to enlist in the war effort, since the United States was not then at war. However, the real battle would take place with Canada Customs, who throughout his editorship questioned his foreign mail coming daily from across the United States and from around the world.[13] They often censored his incoming mail, and he would have to go to Canada Customs offices regularly to engage in yet another skirmish. Like the allies however, he won the war.

Farrar brought to the *AJP* his conviction that it was the organ of the American Psychiatric Association. To him, the journal was a reflection of the interests of all the members and an embodiment of the state of American psychiatry. His dream and mission was of a journal that represented a democratic and unified association. Always he decried the divisiveness that sectarianism fostered.

He fought at least three battles to uphold this vision. First, he withstood the efforts of William Menninger to reshape the editorship, then of Emile Blain to move both the American Psychiatric Association and the editorship to Washington, finally of Samuel Solomon to shift the publishing to the Grune and Stratton Publishing Company (where Grune would influence the editorial policy).[14] As the defender of the *AJP* as the democratic organ of American psychiatry, Farrar was undefeatable.

Farrar summed up his philosophy of American psychiatry by wondering,

> if in any other field of medicine or other science so many divisive trends develop as in psychiatry. Such division is of course in inverse proportion of the amount of solid knowledge on which the discipline is based. It is comforting to read the words of Sir Aubrey Lewis about the atmosphere in which for the most part British psychiatrists pursue their labours: 'although psychiatry in Great Britain is not homogenous, either in theory or practice, it is not sharply divided into recognizable schools, centred on prominent men with distinctive views.
>
> The climate of opinion is temperate; the intellectual winds are seldom sharp and nipping.'[15]

No matter what the winds were, nor even if they reached the intensity of gales, Farrar was unmoved in his Toronto citadel. The distance from Toronto to major American centres allowed him to go about his editorial work, politically speaking, in a temperate climate.

Farrar's influences

Farrar's own background influenced his work as editor. First, there was Osler. Years later, in 1965, Farrar remembered,

> at the head of a table sat Dr. Osler. He would ask us about the cases we had studied during the week and would bring out points we had missed or had not given sufficient emphasis. He would enliven the discussion by bringing out from his library in an adjoining room—the famous Bibliotheca Osleriana, which he later presented to McGill University—ancient books containing the original descriptions of the diseases we were talking about, written in many instances by the men whose names they bore.[16]

The resemblances between Farrar and Osler are interesting.[17] Both men had an intense love for their profession and its books, and Farrar amassed a library whose size rivaled Osler's. One of Farrar's earliest childhood memories was desiring for Christmas the works of Dante.[18] While his library was not as "rich" as Osler's, it remained a significant collection nonetheless and contained one of the few series of the *AJP* dating back to 1844.

Like Osler, Farrar maintained that psychiatry belonged in the mainstream of medicine and was against anything that would separate the two. In a book review of "Emotions and Bodily Changes" by Flanders Dunbar, Farrar wrote:

> The reviewer would be inclined to agree with the author's earlier opinion and that the term (psychosomatic) should become obsolete not so much because it suggests a dichotomy between soma and psyche but because it suggests a dichotomy between psychosomatic medicine and medicine.[19]

Two of Farrar's undergraduate years had been spent at Harvard, where one of his professors was psychologist William James. Of James, Farrar would say:

> partly it was James' style and partly it was the kind of man behind the style—which is of course only two ways of saying the same thing. "He was beautifully at home with the genius of our English

language." His sentences were models of clear and concise expression and there was the throb of life in them. They were set down with the true instinct of the artist who knew how to economize with words and to infuse into them the warmth of his own spirit.[20]

Farrar as writer was molded by James. For both men language provided the foundation of knowledge.

As an editor, Farrar brought to the task not only his education but also great erudition. He was able to give an expert opinion in clear and eloquent prose on many topics. Grammar was his love. Words were his inspiration. He said that he read each and every manuscript which crossed his desk. Having studied at school German, French, Spanish, Italian, Latin, and Greek he was able to peruse journals from around the world.

Farrar scorned loose usage. What he said about British psychiatrist John Conolly, could have just as appropriately been said about himself.

> The wisdom and insight and foresight of this great physician who was writing for the future as well as providing new prospects for his own times, and particularly his masterly use of the English language and his economy of expression, contrasting in that way with not a little of psychiatric writing of today, make the book a delight to read.[21]

For Farrar, as for his teacher William James, there was no royal road to the truth of the science of mind. Rather, it was the crossroads of many paths. Modern science had developed from a pluralistic background, and truth was not discovered but manufactured. Farrar would quote from James this insight:

> we have no basis for asserting the external world simply exists in its own right; the only world about which we can speak is that which is found in the collective consciousness of sentient creatures. The world therefore is not one but many...[22]

Germany too had formed Farrar. Later, he would say of his Heidelberg period:

> It was the reviewer's great privilege to be in Germany in the midst of that germinal season and to have worked under the guidance of Kraepelin, Nissl and Alzheimer... Appreciation of the value of that experience has grown with the passing years. There were giants in those days, and one cannot but think of how it might have seemed to have stood on the face of the planet in its earlier days when the mountains were thrusting up.[23]

It was Farrar's view that Kraepelin had taken psychiatry from its descriptive phase into its "heroic age." Never would Farrar lose his perspective of psychiatry as an international science. In 1954, he wrote in the *AJP* his personal memory of Kraepelin, whom he had described as the "greatest psychiatrist of his time."[24]

Interestingly, when he returned from Heidelberg, his attire was molded as well. In 1904, Farrar was wearing a plastron type vest which buttoned on the side, an attire he would retain for the rest or his life. Then, when he was in Ottawa as a psychiatrist and major in the Department of Soldiers' Civil Re-establishment, he made his own modification to the plastron vest. In his redesign there were two layers of warmth which then buttoned on both sides.

While Farrar always maintained a democratic approach towards science, he disliked what he considered religions that dared to pose as science. For Farrar, a religion was any body of metaphysics, blocking the truth of the human condition, which could only be achieved through the scientific method. In reviewing William Sargant's *Battle for the Mind*, Farrar said,

> He has described with great objectivity canine neurosis, voodoo orgies, Christian revivalist behavior disorders, hysterical snake-handling symptoms, mind changing by communist brainwashing—all as variations of pathophysiological-psychological phenomena. And yet, he seems to exempt in some manner or degree the morbid results of religious suggestion from the critical evaluation accorded to the brainwashing products as a whole.[25]

Needless to say, Farrar condemned the religion of Freudian analysis as a closed and non-scientific system. In 1943 he noted, "The world of science was democratic. Freud's world on the contrary represented a closed system, a 'block-universe' as James would call it; it is authoritarian and totalitarian, intellectual atavism."[26] Yet, when Freud arrived in London, Farrar wrote in the journal:

> In a peace loving country there is prospect that Sigmund Freud may abide in comfort to pursue the work which is his life, to bring to conclusion what may be his crowning work—the psychoanalysis of the Bible—and in these compensations perchance to forget the hardships he has undergone, the low estate to which his country has fallen, the perversion of science and the eclipse of scholarship which are now her lot.[27]

Farrar did not underestimate the role of sex in human behavior. At the Toronto Psychiatric Hospital, he pioneered forensic psychiatry and knew firsthand the intractability of sexual disorders. He ended his review of Havelock Ellis' book *Psychology of Sex* with the following quote from the author: "Sex lies at the root of life, and we can never learn to reverence life until we know how to understand sex."[28]

As a believer in science, Farrar spoke out in the journal against superstition, religion, faith healing, quackery, moralization, and any pseudo-scientific sect that claimed to have the answer to the human condition, agreeing with Carl Jung that:

> First of all it is needful for the physician practising psychotherapy to strive to free himself to the very utmost of preconceptions... Each patient must be accepted as a unique personality presenting unique problems; and just as important, each physician will evolve his own personal method... So true is this, the author comments, that "any physician who announces that he will give treatment according to this or that authority by such limitations compromises the very purposes of his treatment."[29]

Suspect of ideology in therapy, Farrar believed that a therapist must find his or her own path to mastery. He would agree with Pierre Janet: "What would one think of a physician who would presume to give digitalis to all his patients, or of another who might specialize in the giving of arsenic?"[30]

Prior to assuming editorship, Farrar met another individual who was also to have a profound influence on him for the rest of his life. His first book review that appeared in the *AJI* in 1908 was of *A Mind that Found Itself* by Clifford Beers.[31] Beers' influence upon Farrar is a reminder of Farrar's pluralism, an ex-psychiatric patient (as Beers was) among Osler, James, and Kraepelin. Beers became a lifelong friend. In a book review of the 25th anniversary edition of Beers' book in 1935, Farrar wrote:

> Mental hygiene is spread over the world almost like a religion... It may even safely be said that while a considerable number of people conduct their lives apparently quite satisfactorily without consciously practising any religion, those who habitually disregard the fundamental tenets of mental hygiene, which might equally well be classified among the so-called laws of nature, are headed for future punishment, not in the next world but in this... But mental hygiene as conceived by Clifford Beers is not a theory or body of doctrine merely, but a living agency and a powerful social force for human betterment. The book which launched this

movement, *A Mind that Found Itself,* has enjoyed a continuous and growing prestige and has come to occupy a place entirely its own among the great autobiographies of the world.[32]

Farrar's approach and the evolution of the AJP

When Farrar assumed editorship, he brought to the position his linguistic skills, his erudition, his knowledge of psychiatric and medical history, his clinical skills, and what one might call the American way. Farrar was the penultimate modern American psychiatrist—clinical, scientific, pragmatic, and imbued with a deep appreciation for the social. He had received the finest psychiatric training in America and Germany and never separated from his American roots. Throughout his years as editor, he would inform the members of the American Psychiatric Association of what was happening both nationally and worldwide. He promoted American scientific leadership, comparing it to earlier German advancements. Above all, he withstood inundation during the years of the rising tide of psychoanalysis. His ark was to carry all the species of American psychiatry.

In the end, Farrar lived out the prophecy of Edward Brush who said as Farrar became editor:

> There are many things in the present instance which the writer would gladly say about Dr. Farrar; but a long acquaintance with the Editor-elect has taught him that Dr. Farrar is a modest man, that though he has no inferiority complex he has on the other hand a woeful lack of comprehension of his peculiar fitness for the position to which he has been called...
>
> Let us therefore by force of circumstances be content with saying to the readers of the JOURNAL that in education, medical training and experience Dr. Farrar has laid a foundation upon which we predict will be built an editorial career which will enhance the reputation of the JOURNAL and of which his friends will have occasion to speak with gratification and pride.
>
> In turning over to Dr. Farrar the editorial conduct of the JOURNAL we do so with the most complete confidence in his ability to carry on the work and in a confident expectation of a progressive improvement in the character of the periodical.[33]

In 1944, the *AJP* celebrated its one hundredth anniversary. Farrar had achieved much since taking the job in 1931. The American Psychiatric Association had more than doubled its members (all of whom were subscribers) from 1,393 in 1931 to 3,050 in 1944. In addition, there were 1,589 other subscribers. When Farrar retired in 1965, the association had increased to over 9,000 members and the journal had 2,500 additional subscribers. The *AJP* was now delivered to every country in the world. While it had taken 77 years for the journal to reach an audience of 1,000, during Farrar's 34 years the number of recipients rose from 1,500 to 12,000.

In 1931, when he assumed editorship, he could take home from the annual meeting the articles required for the upcoming year of the journal in one suitcase. Later, his editorial assistant had to carry two suitcases. Even adding another assistant was eventually insufficient and after the Second World War, they had to ship a veritable carload of articles to Toronto by Canada Post. When Farrar began, all requests for reprints were sent directly to him. Later, the policy was changed to writing directly to the author.

In 1942, he changed the physical presentation of the journal, introducing a new layout and larger format which has remained to this day. It is a testimony of Farrar's perseverance that throughout the Second World War there was no break in continuity of the *AJP*. When he retired from the University of Toronto in 1947 at the age of 73, he devoted himself totally to the editorship of the journal, which in that year changed from a bi-monthly to a monthly publication.

Every year, Farrar journeyed south to the annual meeting of the American Psychiatric Association. There, the business meeting of the editorial board was conducted. Farrar was one of the few editors of the journal who never became president of the association. But he was without political ambition. All his energies were devoted to being editor. He held court with no party within the infrastructure of the association; instead, all his allegiance was to the association itself. On the merit of his record, he carried the annual meetings.

While Farrar's way to the meeting was paid, he only billed the association for the night of the meeting.[34] The annual meetings for Farrar were a highlight of the year, an occasion to mingle with old and new friends and exchange information. He loved to write letters and to meet and talk. The annual meeting also provided opportunities to indulge his taste in books and art by perusing local bookshops and visiting galleries.

A passion kindled during his years at the Sheppard and Enoch Pratt Hospital, he became so interested in art that he would lecture patients about its history. So well was he known in New York art circles that he acquired the distinction of being hailed as a "historian emeritus" of art. Throughout his editorship from 1931 to 1965, Farrar was never reimbursed. It was a labour of love. When he retired, he received an honorarium.[35]

The 1944 annual meeting of the American Psychiatric Association was held in Philadelphia. A century earlier, the 13 founders of the association had met in the same city. To commemorate its first hundred years, Farrar edited a centennial anniversary issue for the annual meeting. While Brigham had written the entire first issue himself, Farrar proposed the topics and selected the writers for the centennial issue.[36] From the four corners of the United States and Canada, the 27 authors summed up the state of American psychiatry: past, present, and future. This centennial issue stood apart, was not included in any volume, and became a beacon for historians of psychiatry. There was no disputing who its lightkeeper was. For Farrar, the special edition was a peak experience.

It has been said that one of Farrar's shortcomings was that, unlike Hurd, he never wrote a book. But for C.B. Farrar, the *AJP was* his book. Besides his editorship duties and his contributions to news and comments, Farrar wrote 77 articles: 29 appeared in the *AJI* and *AJP*; 48 were printed in other journals and periodicals.[37] He also penned 273 book reviews, beginning in 1908 and ending in 1965.[38] On a bi-monthly and then monthly basis, he reviewed the ever-changing world of books in psychiatry and kept his subscribers abreast of the latest developments.

In 1957, the *AJP*, under the aegis of the president of the American Psychiatric Association, Francis J. Braceland, celebrated a 25-year salute to Farrar. Braceland, who later would succeed Farrar, wrote this about his predecessor:

> The history of the Journal in the past twenty-five years is thoroughly intertwined with the history of the distinguished editor. Conservative, cautious, dignified and literate, it has been as sound and as careful in the minds of our colleagues as that famous institution on Threadneedle Street. Like the latter institution, its circumspection has not always been appreciated by some, but its solidity and its integrity have never been questioned.[39]

In 1961, at the third world congress of psychiatry in Montreal, Quebec, Farrar received an honourary doctorate for his life's work in psychiatry and his contributions to the *AJP*. The next year at the annual meeting of the American Psychiatric Association in Toronto, he was presented with an editorial chair and, in 1965, the *AJP* designated him editor emeritus. His last alma mater, the University of Toronto, conferred on him an honourary doctor of laws degree. In 1969 the Governor General of Canada granted him the medal of service of the Order of Canada, and he received the distinguished service award of the Thomas W. Salmon committee on psychiatry and mental hygiene. These awards tell a story in themselves.

In 1965, when Farrar ended his term of editorship in his ninety-first year, he quoted (using his favourite literary device of communicating through the words of others) William Hone on the need for sensitivity to the plight of editors. On another occasion, Farrar included, in his now classic article on psychotherapy, the vignette of how John Stuart Mill was cured of his mental disorder by reading from a Wordsworth poem and then concluded the article with a quote from *Anatomy of Melancholy*: "He doth the best cures, according to Hippocrates, in whom most trust."[40] The readers of the *AJP* for those 34 years had come to trust their editor and that was his greatest tribute. Over 25 years later, Lucy D. Ozarin conveyed their feelings when she wrote, "Clarence Farrar, in a sense, was the APA Journal."[41]

ENDNOTES

[1] Grotius, as quoted in the frontispiece of every *AJP* issue published under Farrar's editorship.
[2] An unsigned quotation on the reverse side of the photo of Brigham in the Farrar library in the Clarke Institute of Psychiatry.
[3] C.B. Farrar, "Forward," AJP Centennial Edition: v (April 1944).
[4] Alfred P. Noyes, *History of Psychiatry*, unpublished manuscript in the library of the American Psychiatric Association, p. 10-3.
[5] C.B. Farrar, "Some Origins in Psychiatry," *AJI* 64: 83-101 (January 1908); 66: 277-94 (October 1909).
[6] Noyes, pp. 10-9, 10.
[7] C.B. Farrar, "News and Comment," *AJP* 11: 26 (September 1931).
[8] C.B. Farrar, "News and Comment," *AJP* 13: 451 (September 1933).
[9] Henry M. Hurd, *The Institutional Care of the Insane in the United States and Canada* (Baltimore: Johns Hopkins Press, 1917), 4v.
[10] C.B. Farrar, "Edward Nathaniel Brush," *AJP* 12: 853 (January 1933).

[11] Previously, the only other annual meetings of the association to be held in Toronto were in 1871 and 1881.
[12] Personal communication with Joan Farrar.
[13] Personal communication with Joan Farrar.
[14] Personal communication from Joan Farrar's notes of her husband's conversations.
[15] C.B. Farrar, "Book Reviews," *AJP* 119: 701 (January 1963).
[16] C.B. Farrar, "I Remember Osler, Psychotherapist," *AJP* 121: 761-62 (February 1965).
[17] See Shorter chapter on Farrar (Chapter 3).
[18] Personal communication with Joan Farrar.
[19] C.B. Farrar, "Book Reviews," *AJP* 111: 799 (April 1955).
[20] C.B. Farrar, "Book Reviews," *AJP* 99: 631 (January 1943).
[21] C.B. Farrar, "Book Reviews," *AJP* 121: 620-21 (December 1964).
[22] C.B. Farrar, "Book Reviews," *AJP* 99: 772 (March 1943).
[23] C.B. Farrar, "Book Reviews," *AJP* 119: 190-91 (August 1962).
[24] C.B. Farrar, "I Remember Kraepelin," *AJP* 111: 379-81 (November 1954).
[25] C.B. Farrar, "Book Reviews," *AJP* 114: 1133 (June 1958).
[26] C.B. Farrar, "Book Reviews," *AJP* 99: 772 (March 1943).
[27] C.B. Farrar, "Book Reviews," *AJP* 95: 229 (July 1938).
[28] C.B. Farrar, "Book Reviews," *AJP* 91: 957 (January 1935).
[29] C.B. Farrar, "Book Reviews," *AJP* 111: 715 (March 1955).
[30] C.B. Farrar, "Book Reviews," *AJP* 4: 587 (January 1925).
[31] C.B. Farrar, "Book Reviews," *AJP* 64: 215-28 (July 1908).
[32] C.B. Farrar, "Book Reviews," *AJP* 92: 248-49 (July 1935).
[33] Edward M. Brush, "Notes and Comments," *AJP* 11: 188 (July 1931).
[34] Personal communication with Joan Farrar.
[35] Ibid.
[36] Farrar was also on the editorial board of J.K. Hall, ed., *American Psychiatry (1844-1944)* (New York: Columbia University Press, 1944), *Funk and Wagnall's New Encyclopedia* (New York: Funk and Wagnall, 1932) and the *Yearbook of Neurology and Psychiatry* (Chicago: Year Book Publishers, 1907).
[37] The following is a brief list of Farrar's articles appearing in the *AJI* and *AJP*:

1902	On the Typhoid Psychoses
1903	On the Motor Cortex
1905	Cytodiagnosis in Psychiatry
	Dementia Praecox in France...
1906	Dementia Praecox
	Depresso Affectur
	Depresso Psychomotoria
1907	Melancholia Vera
	Arteriosclerosis Cerebralis
1908	Some Origins in Psychiatry (3 papers)
1917	War and Neurosis
1919	Rehabilitation in Nervous and Mental Cases Among Ex-soldiers
1923	Neuropsychiatric Service of the Department of Soldiers' Civil Re-establishment
1931	Menopause and Psychosis
1933	Twenty-five Years of Mental Hygiene

1951 Suicide
1954 I Remember Kraepelin
      I Remember Nissl
1955 Psychotherapy
1957 I Remember C.K. Clarke
1960 I Remember Stewart Paton
1963 I Remember J.G. FitzGerald
1965 I Remember E.S. Southard
1965 I Remember Osler

[38] The following is a partial list of his book reviews that appeared in the *AJI* and *AJP* (some entries are reprints, or translations into English): Gregory Bateson (1943), Clifford Beers (1908), Hippolyte Bernheim (1949), Abraham Brill (1947), John Conolly (1964), Flanders Dunbar (1936), Emile Durkheim (1952), Albert Deutsch (1952), Havelock Ellis (1935), Sigmund Freud (1950), Ernst Feuchtersleben (1935), Aldous Huxley (1953), William James (1964), Pierre Janet (1924), Carl Jung (1954), Leo Kanner (1961), Moses Maimonides (1958), Margaret Mead (1943), Benjamin Rush (1950), and Kurt Schneider (1934).

[39] Francis J. Braceland, "President's Page," *AJP* 113 (10): 938 (April 1957).

[40] C.B. Farrar, "Psychotherapy," *AJP* 113: 865-70 (April 1957).

[41] Lucy D. Ozarin, "Clarence Farrar and the APA Journal," *Psychiatric News*: 19 (October 2, 1992).

6

Recollections of a Patient at TPH: Snakepit

Peter Keefe[*]

Away with her!
Poor soul, she speaks this in th'infirmity of sense.[1]
          The Duke of Vienna in Measure for Measure
          by William Shakespeare

My meeting with a former TPH patient for the purpose of obtaining a subjective account of a hospitalization was little different from most initial clinical psychiatric interviews. Much "clinical" information had already been conveyed over the telephone in the process of setting up our meeting; the patient's eagerness to volunteer her recollections, for example, had a pressured, compulsive quality. As some patients are, she was anxious to tell her story and, in that often telling moment of setting a time to meet, she had shown an immediate deference to the needs of my schedule. She, let's call her "E," was employed half-time as a clerical worker and had a demanding home life. Her deference reminded me of some downtrodden chronic psychiatric patients who assume that their time is not of the same currency as mine. Or, given that she was a former patient rather than a current one, had she for some reason felt a responsibility to tell her story? Perhaps this was a way of valorizing her experience by telling others. Realizing that first impressions can be misleading, I wasn't sure what to expect: a "chronic patient" of some sort

---

[*]Peter Keefe, M.D., F.R.C.P.(C) Int. Med., F.R.C.P. (C) Psychiatry, has been assistant professor of psychiatry at the University of Toronto since 1987 and staff psychiatrist at Mount Sinai Hospital since 1983. He is a participant in numerous professional associations and committees, including the Canadian Society for the History of Medicine and the History of Science Society in the United States.

or a kind of solid citizen, a volunteer even. As if "chronic patients" don't volunteer, one might ask.

I guessed which one E was in the waiting-room. Her manner of dress was somewhat downbeat set against Toronto's code of downtown female office garb: a denim skirt (or was it pants?), earth sandals, a fanny pack replacing a purse, and no noticeable make-up. Her face was a solid mask of anticipation, and her brow, furrowed vertically between her eyes, suggested a chronicity to her worriedness. Her eyes were of a light colour and alert.

I wondered if our meeting to talk about her past hospitalization had taken on the quality of a reckoning for her, as if her past was something for which she might be taken to task. As often occurs in an initial psychiatric interview, I, the psychiatrist, perhaps represented an authority figure who might sit in judgment on her past sins.[2] And yet, I was to hear that it was the hospital that was to be taken to task and that it was she who was to be reckoned with.

INTERVIEW

PK: How long ago was it?

E: I was about 20 so that would be about 40 years ago roughly. I was going to the outpatientt at Toronto General which at that time was in the old Sick Children's Hospital ground floor; and I was seeing a couple of psychiatrists there on a one-to-one basis; and I also had briefly some time with a group that was very short lived; then I had what was considered a crisis by the doctor there, a woman. At any rate, they decided I should go into Surrey Place [the TPH] because I was seeing things and I was in a very, very upset state, and I guess it was because of that they decided I should go into Surrey Place.

At the time, my sister who was about ten years older, was the one that signed me in. Because I was so distracted and upset, I really didn't think, "Well, why did she do the signing and where was my mother in all this?" Maybe my mother was just distraught with it all...I can't remember that. I was put in a public ward in Surrey Place and, well, it was like a snakepit. It was really really bad. It was frightening and it was...there was absolutely no privacy whatsoever; I don't even think there was toilet seats; no doors, no nothing, and I got a terrible case of constipation. I really refused to go their little handicraft workshops (what do they call them?)...occupational therapy rooms. I was very depressed and very unhappy in there.

Actually, my problems became secondary to what I was seeing around me. I mean, I was witnessing things that were just really terrible. One young woman was in there, she had wanted an abortion. She was told that she couldn't have an abortion. She made several attempts at suicide and she was swallowing pins in there. I was absolutely alarmed at was happening in this place. Nurses were pretty rough with her. You don't have to stay in bed. They would pull the blankets off her and just...it wasn't very, you know, it was upsetting. Now, maybe you better ask me some questions because I will just bubble over.

PK: When you say it was a public ward, how many beds would there be?

E: There were about four or five or maybe eight or ten beds in a room. It was quite a large room and it was one of several rooms. There were private and semi-private rooms there.

PK: What sort of treatment did you get?

E: When I got there, I forget the doctor's name, but he decided I was very sick... Because I wasn't combing my hair, because I was sleeping and because I wasn't participating in this occupational craft work or whatever, and I remember I would be upset, very upset. I would cry and whatnot, and they would come and give me a needle, you see, and calm me down and, I felt... I mean, in retrospect as I think back, I mean, this whole situation is actually feeding my upsetness. And, other people too, I noticed that they were reacting very much to this rather negative sort of thing that was happening, and, finally, I was set up for shock treatment and my sister had again signed the papers for this to happen... They had these rooms with baths where you would get in the bath and you were covered in canvas up to your neck and it was this dark, gloomy room; and this is for people who might get hysterical or whatever.

PK: Did you have those?

E: I think I was in there once... I did something that got me thinking I should have one of these baths... I just remember it was very dark in there, very...everything seemed dark and that's my memory of course.

But anyway I was signed for shock treatment. I was taken up to the room. It was a Sunday, I think,...and they had given me medication so that I wouldn't be upset,...and they had all these things clamped on my head and so forth, but they couldn't find the paper that was signed to give them permission. So, I could hear this all through this medication I was on and I never had it. They took all the equipment off and down I went.

Well, just after that, this Dr. [William] Mitchell turned up and he was a young man who had come from either England or Scotland and the whole place was just transformed. He became the head of that department and I had an interview with him shortly after he arrived and he said that there was absolutely no reason why I should have been put in there and he said I did have emotional problems and so forth, but nothing to, you know, end me up in this place... He immediately signed the release for me to go, and he said I was a bit eccentric, but that was about it and that,...through the years I probably would need a bit of help here and there. But he said,...that it has been a big mistake and the person who had signed me in, this person from Toronto General, had not really assessed the case properly according to him.

After that, I was finished with Surrey Place and doctors. I...once I was there, I was just...I just didn't want to go near any other of this kind of help...

PK: After you got out of the hospital how was your emotional state?

E: Shortly after, I met a man and eventually got married. I was pretty mixed up and that sort of was...another story. But as far as my experience in the hospital, as I say, it was a very negative experience with this doctor who was in charge and I remember the patients, they would be so frightened. I mean, if somebody said... "You know, you're going to have to go to Whitby..."

This was like a death sentence to them... There was one doctor, I remember...he came in one lunch hour and he was actually swinging this key chain like this [E demonstrates] with a pipe in his mouth and he came to this poor distraught girl who had been trying to kill herself, and he said, "Pack your bags you're going to Whitby." Just like something out of a horror movie...because really I think the people were very scared in there. They were very scared... Whatever was wrong with them was being fed, it wasn't being corrected. It was like this Mitchell, this Dr. Mitchell when he came, he would joke with people. He had them laughing. He had them not taking themselves seriously, you see, and this was a big, big difference.

PK: Had there been people in the Surrey Place [who were] there for a long time?

E: ... [Some] were certainly there sometime before I had arrived. It could have been two or three months. It seemed to me that people were there for months, not days or even weeks.

PK: Around that time some medications were being introduced to the field of psychiatry, antipsychotic drugs and so on, do you recall ever getting anything like that or having reactions to...

E: No. The only medication I was getting, as I recall, was if I was upset they would give me a hypodermic needle.

PK: But you don't know quite what it was?

E: Well, I guess to make me sleepy...to calm me down. But I don't recall taking except maybe for constipation...castor oil or something. But I don't remember taking pills...others were taking pills. Yes, I remember other people and maybe I was, but I remember definitely there was pill taking because this woman would drink the water first and then take the pill and I thought that was kind of strange, but, you know, that is something that I can't say for sure. Maybe I was on pills of some sort.

PK: What sense do you make of this whole episode of your life? When you think back of this hospitalization?

E: ... I'm grateful I did not have shock treatment. Absolutely... I thought when I was young...somehow there was an answer with psychiatry. Like I would find answers to my anxiousness and my problems. I was very, very mixed up as a young person and in a lot of pain mental...I mean emotional...and that sort of stuff. But I thought...that somehow something was going to be revealed to me. I was going to...like some people believe in God...well, I thought maybe, you know, something's going to happen. And I realized, "no, it's not going to happen this way in these places." I felt let down. I felt I had come for...well, I didn't go into the hospital for help, I was put there. But I had been going to psychiatrists for help, and I felt that this was no longer a way for me to get help.

PK: This as a result of the hospitalization?

E: Yes, yet I did go again...I did in later years go back to psychiatrists off and on.

PK: You went to psychiatrists in later years—what sort of treatment did you receive?

E: Really, I would go only in crisis...if I was having a crisis in my marriage. It was breaking up and,...being very upset, I went to an outpatient and Queen Street for, I think, it was marriage counselling. And then, I was referred to a psychiatrist... The benefit was that I could go and talk to someone who was objective and who wasn't part of this whole tangle that I was in. I think that was good. But as far as actually coming to grips with things in myself, I don't see that I got that from seeing doctors.

PK: How did you get it?

E: Or have I got it?... I feel basically I have an acceptance of what I am and who I am and at times this gets...kind of fragile, but it's there... I tried medication and I've thought, "oh, if I could just get that sense of well being...that sense of feeling good about myself." ...I think "well, I love being out in the nature." That's very good for me and so I look forward to my trips out into the country... I like studying...and I feel good about things. I feel that now I am on solid ground and when I had my daughter as a single parent (eventually it turned out that way), I felt good with her... This is good what I'm doing. ...In those ways,...I feel in touch with who I am, but, of course, there are other emotions that come along that sort of get me all turned around from the other time.

PK: What do you think precipitated your psychiatric problem?

E: I had a very devastating teenage life... I lost my virginity at 14 and part of the crisis...was because...I felt I identified with prostitution although I wasn't taking money from anyone, but I was having a lot of sexual affairs and they were very shallow and very physical. And I did get pregnant [at 20] and have an abortion and I nearly died from it because I got peritonitis.

PK: Was that a therapeutic abortion?

E: It was a backstreet. There was no way you could get an abortion in those days. It was strictly going into this dirty little apartment on Huron Street and I had to go back several times. It didn't work and, then, finally this woman gave me some quinine or whatever douche she was giving me and I started hemorrhaging. And my brother came in one day and he said, "What's wrong with her?" And my mother said, "Oh, she's just got the flu, she's alright...you know she'll be alright." And he said he didn't believe her and he took me to the hospital. And they said if I hadn't come that night I would have been dead because of this infection. So, I think that too was all escalating into this whole thing of getting into Surrey Place.

PK: When you had your treatment at Surrey Place did anyone talk with you about the abortion?

E: ...When I did see them,...they were taking brain scans or EEG and those kinds of things they were doing to me. I don't really remember any real therapy as like counselling or, you know, talking to the doctors about my problems in the hospital. I remember one of the nurses asking if I would like to go out one day. She would take me out, so I said, "Yes I would," but, you know, we just went out for the afternoon or something. But I can't really recall...going to a doctor's office and talking about my feelings at the hospital...

PK: The only interview that you seem to remember is the interview with Dr. Mitchell?

E: ...At one point they were going to get a room full of people and assess my case... That never came off because Dr. Mitchell came along...and instead I saw him and was released. But I don't remember any kind of therapeutic work in the hospital itself.

PK: Thinking back about Surrey Place again, was there a place for patients who were unruly?

E: Well, the ones that got hysterical started struggling with the...what do you call them? Not interns, but the men in white. They did have straight jackets, I think they put one woman in a straight jacket. They had these men who would come in, grab a patient, hold them and steady them and the baths were part of that... If somebody was getting out of hand, they would put them in the bath.

PK: Was the bath cool or warm?

E: ...It was warm. [They had] these big bath tubs and they were covered in canvas, so I guess you couldn't, you know, get your head under the water... Your head was sticking out of this canvas covered at the back...

PK: Did anyone harm themselves while you were there?

E: ...This one girl...who didn't want the baby. I mean, it was just grotesque. She was losing weight. She was about four months pregnant and she was losing weight... Then, she got a hold of a safety pin and swallowed it and she was having dreams of waking up in a coffin or all this kind of thing...and she is the one that they sent to Whitby... There was one woman in there with a lobotomy and she was just like a vegetable walking around. She just...she didn't respond to anything.

PK: Was that something that you were concerned about?

E: ...At the time I was in the situation, so I was part of that whole thing. Another woman had the shock treatment and something had happened to her jaw joint. And they sent her back. And I remember it was a weekend and she was suffering and they couldn't get a doctor to come to her. And all day...she was crying in pain and nobody would seem to do anything for her. It was a strange kind of experience. After I got out of there...that was all I could think about...was that place that I had been in.

PK: Did you have nightmares about it?

E: I can't remember that. I know it was quite an obsession with me though; it really stuck with me. Yes, again it was 40 years ago, it's hard to remember those feelings at the time... It was a real turning point for me because up to that point I had looked in this way for help. And after that, even though I did seek help, it wasn't quite in the same way.

COMMENTARY

E's vivid account of her hospitalization provides us with a picture of the TPH as "snakepit." This doesn't easily allow an exercise in what Andrew Scull calls "the liberal public relations theory of psychiatric history."[3] Yet, it does permit a number of readings.

From one vantage point this is an almost stereotypical story of involuntary hospitalization and dehumanization. From another it is a melodramatic rescue story wherein bad caregivers are vanquished by good. From a current diagnostic viewpoint it sounds like a case of post-traumatic stress disorder or brief psychotic disorder.[4] At the time of E's illness, stress reactions were largely associated with the war experiences of men. Brief or "benign" psychoses were seldom diagnosed and were scarcely referred to in official diagnostic nomenclatures.

Her story of hospitalization is also anecdotal social history. This is the account of a troubled young woman in Toronto in the 1950s for whom an unwanted pregnancy had grievous medical and psychological consequences. She did not conjure up her life-threatening peritonitis, an abdominal infection complicating her botched "back-street" abortion (a "criminal abortion" according to her medical record).[5] The plight of the psychotic pregnant patient on the ward tells us that this is indeed a story from another time. We hope. It also tells us, unsurprisingly, that TPH's practices reflected the social attitudes of the day.

TPH was no haven from society, much as E might have wished that. It is not clear what her mental state was at the time. A review of E's clinical record provides some objective corroboration, yet raises new questions. Her admission history on May 18, 1956, describes her symptomatology:

> One month prior to admission for a period of a week she was very upset, had visual hallucinations (1) of seeing a female shoulder on fire and (2) of seeing the players on a stage surrounded by fire. Over this period she heard laughing which was directed at her, and seemed to be in her head.

This episode suggests a psychosis and seems to have precipitated her admission. But there was no evidence of psychosis on examination of her mental state at the time of admission: "Speech: Logical, coherent, no evidence of thought disorder. Thought: Spends much of day in phantasy which makes up for what she misses in real life."

As is not unheard of in current clinical practice, there was disagreement over the meaning of her symptomatology. An extensive battery of psychological tests was carried out, including "projective" tests designed to elicit unconscious thoughts and feelings:

> The pseudo-hallucinatory perception of a burning shoulder...was hardly a real hallucination, but a not quite clear personality reaction towards a stress situation in the form of a very vivid day-dream. Hospitalization is not felt to be necessary.

The psychologist's view stands in contrast to the first medical progress note shortly after admission: "May 20, 1956. She is dishevelled, unkempt, neglectful of personal hygiene with long hair falling over her face. She resembles a patient one might see on the back wards of a mental hospital."

Ensuing progress notes over the following weeks suggest a picture of struggle with the assigned patient role: "May 23, 1956. Patient still withdrawn, seclusive, tearful, upset and unaccepting of the hospital. May 28, 1956. Patient has begun to tidy herself up... She accepts the hospital as a necessary evil."

There is little evidence of any psychotherapy, not that it would have been possible given the gulf between the patient and her caregivers. Occupational therapy notes shortly before her abortive ECT confirm her uninterest in personal therapeutic contact:

> June 5, 1956. She watches people who approach her rather suspiciously. It was suggested that she do some painting. The supplies are given her and are available for her all the time (they are left on the ward) but every time a staff member approaches her about it she says she does not feel like painting right now...

Medication consisted of Largactil (chlorpromazine) 50 milligrams by mouth three times daily and nightly sedation with sodium amytal "grains three," a common barbiturate sedative at the time. In Largactil she was taking a drug only recently introduced into the therapeutic armamentarium for psychosis.[6] It seems that she was seen as an incipient schizophrenic and her withdrawal from ward routines served to cast her even more in that light. The ensuing decision to embark on a course of ECT was probably seen as a way of breaking her out of a presumed schizophrenic withdrawal, a presumption reinforced by her initial presentation as a "back ward patient."

As is common throughout the practice of medicine, a diagnosis looked for is sometimes a diagnosis seen, even in the face of contradictory data. All the facts were poured into the diagnosis construct of her as schizophrenic. E's history, which might have supported another diagnosis, was available from her outpatient record. This told of the sudden death of her father when she was nine. Her allegations of physical or sexual abuse by an older relative when she was seven fell on deaf ears. In a constant financial crisis after the father's death, the family also fell into a state of chronic turmoil.

E's adolescent promiscuity and "criminal abortion" were not seen as relating to possible sexual abuse,[7] as they might be today. Perhaps her promiscuity and sordid abortion were seen as early signs of madness in themselves. Elaine Showalter has argued in *The Female Malady*[8] that there was a post-World War II shift in depictions of "female insanity" from hysteria to schizophrenia:

> Schizophrenia offers a remarkable example of the cultural conflation of femininity and insanity. First of all, unlike anorexia or

depression, schizophrenia is clinically and statistically not a predominantly female mental disorder... Nevertheless, schizophrenia does carry gender-specific meanings...the schizophrenic woman has become as central a cultural figure for the twentieth century as the hysteric was for the nineteenth.

Even so, some staff member used nineteenth-century literary allusions to insanity to describe her adolescent imbalance: "To her mother at this time she seemed like a Dr. Jekyll and Mr. Hyde, since her behaviour went to such extremes."

E's recollection of "identifying herself with prostitution" suggests her own equation at the time of female sexuality and madness. Sander Gilman has written of stereotypes of insanity, "The prostitute is the essential sexualized female in the perception of the nineteenth century. She is perceived as the embodiment of sexuality, disease as well as passion."[9]

E's longstanding outpatient diagnosis of psychoneurosis, including a sophisticated psychoanalytic understanding of her sexual guilt and an erotic transference in treatment, had little influence on her clinicians at TPH. Her outpatient record also indicated that her "burning shoulder" vision occurred on the anniversary of her abortion, thus linking her traumatic abortion directly to her mental illness—a link overlooked as schizophrenia came into the diagnostic foreground. The inpatient assessment incorrectly dated her abortion as having occurred two years previously, thereby attenuating that historical connection. Curiously, the earliest record of her hallucinations or pseudo-hallucinations[10] was actually that of a burning hand (the abortionist's?), later displaced to the shoulder in her painful recollection. These connections to the particulars of her suffering could have helped explain her symptoms as understandable post-traumatic reactions.

On June 1, 1956 a short clinical note indicated that the decision for ECT had been made: "Her two sisters were interviewed and they noticed a change in the past two months. They agreed to ECT as did the patient. Treatments to start next week."

Then came the unlikely twists, just as E had recalled them: the lost consent form, the deliverance from ECT and the arrival of the white knight, Dr. Mitchell:[11]

> June 11, 1956. This patient's clinical state is in no way schizophrenic at this time. In hospital she is inactive and seclusive but these are not unusual activities for her. She is not certifiable (I

would not certify her)...the sensible thing to do is to discharge her to the Out-Patient Department. In reviewing her history from the Out-Patient Department there is no reason to think that any thing but supportive occasional interviews are indicated.

June 26, 1956.

Discharge: Home

Condition: Unimproved

Diagnosis: Schizoid Personality 320.0

The question of historical truth (what the TPH was really like—the snakepit of E's recollections or the more humane institution recalled by its caregivers) is secondary to E's perception of a therapeutic gulf between her experience of being mentally ill and those attempting to make contact with her. This gulf remains a problem despite the advances of psychiatry.

Adolf Meyer, the foremost American psychiatrist of the first half of this century, commented on a similar contradictory account of subjective and objective reports of a mental illness:

> Unfortunately there is a tremendous tendency to pick out from reports and reminiscences the things that satisfy the sadistic attitude of those who are spreading the gospel of knowledge on the ground of ignorance. It is so easy in an account of this sort to see elements concerning which the host may be sensitive, concerning which the eager public will be very greedy because it tells them what things happen behind that veil which ought not to continue to be a veil... We know that the principal work and progress of the psychiatrist in this century—and the greatest gift that psychiatry can give in return for all it gets from the rest of medicine—is the fact of guidance in the sense of a collaboration between physician and patient as persons. That, I think, is the great gain of this century, the greatest and more important contribution that psychiatry is capable of making, that of understanding the active as well as the passive role of the patient in the sickness and in the treatment.[12]

E experienced a sense of failure and of being failed while in the throes of her personal crisis. She and Meyer, both observers and actors on the therapeutic stage, help us reflect on the challenge in human relations that mental illness can pose.

Endnotes

[1] William Shakespeare, *Measure for Measure*, Act V, Scene I (Toronto: Bantam Books, 1988). Isabella's story of sexual harassment wasn't believed either.

[2] Roger A. MacKinnon and Robert Michels, eds. *The Psychiatric Interview in Clinical Practice* (Philadephia: W.B. Saunders, 1971), p. 6.

[3] Andrew Scull, *Social Order/Mental Disorder: Anglo-American Psychiatry in Historical Perspective* (Berkeley: Los Angeles: University of California Press, 1989), p. 31.

[4] See "Brief Psychotic Disorder" in Harold I. Kaplan and Benjamin J. Sadock, eds. *Comprehensive Textbook of Psychiatry* Sixth edition. (Baltimore: Williams & Wilkins, 1995), pp. 1028-30.

[5] For a history of abortion, its methods and its complications see: Edward Shorter, *Women's Bodies: A Social History of Women's Encounters with Health, Ill-Health and Medicine* (New Brunswick, NJ: Transaction Publishers, 1991), pp. 177-224.

[6] Leo E. Hollister, "Antipsychotic Medication and the Treatment of Schizophrenia," in Jack D. Barchas, Philip A. Berger, Roland Clarenello and Glen R. Elliott, eds. *Psychopharmacology: From Theory to Practice* (New York: Oxford University Press, 1977), pp. 122-25.

[7] P. Susan Penfold and Gillian A. Walker, *Women and the Psychiatric Paradox* (Montreal: Eden Press, 1983), p. 157.

[8] Elaine Showalter, *The Female Malady: Women, Madness and English Culture, 1930-1980* (NY, Penguin Books, 1985), p. 204.

[9] Sander I. Gilman, *Difference and Pathology: Stereotypes of Sexuality, Race and Madness* (Ithaca: Cornell University Press, 1985), p. 94.

[10] Pseudo-hallucinations generally refer to hallucinatory experiences which the person recognizes as arising in the mind rather than "out in space."

[11] Mitchell's suicide at the beginning of a promising career sent shockwaves through the psychiatric community.

[12] See "The Discussion of Adolf Meyer" in Joseph A. Kindwall and Elaine F. Kinder, "Postscript on a Benign Psychosis," *Psychiatry* 3: 527-34 (1940).

7

Experiences of a Student Intern at TPH

W. Clifford M. Scott[*]

I remember how TPH got its name. In January 1925, the *Toronto Star* wrote: "it is within six weeks that the Psychopathic Hospital should be opened." C.B. Farrar was appointed professor and the name Toronto Psychopathic was changed to Toronto Psychiatric. Farrar felt that a hospital shouldn't be psychopathic. He hoped it wouldn't!

Farrar became to me an erudite professor, a kind man, a good teacher, an interesting writer, a helpful editor and a humanist, but a man not easy to know as a whole man. In 1925 he offered me a student internship at TPH in the middle of my fifth year of medicine. I was to live in the male nurses' quarters; eat with the staff; do physical examinations, blood counts and urine analyses; take blood samples, etc., and be of some use to B.T. McGhie, the one resident psychiatrist, who (with his wife) had an apartment across the hall from Farrar's and Clarence Crawford's offices. I was, of course, glad to accept.

Before I moved in, Farrar told me that the appointment of the two[1] student interns had been taken out of his hands (appointments were a political matter) and he wished me good luck. I appealed to my father, a Presbyterian minister in Omemee, who arranged for me to have an interview with the Minister of Health. The interview was short, but I got the internship. I later found that my father voted for the party not in

---

[*]W. Clifford M. Scott, B.Sc., Medicine, M.B., University of Toronto, 1927, has devoted a lengthy career to psychiatry in Canadian, U.S., and British hospitals and schools. After his internship at TPH and a fellowship in the Harvard Medical School Department of Psychiatry (where he taught at Harvard and the Boston Psychopathic), he spent the next twenty years in England primarily with London's Maudsley Hospital. He returned to Canada to teach at McGill University. Since his retirement he has been consultant psychiatrist to several Montreal hospitals and a practising psychoanalyst.

power! Thus, I learned that sometimes religion is more important than politics. It is ironic that what was most important in my case was the interaction between politics and religion since there was no chapel, denominational or otherwise!

When I attended Farrar's first lecture, given in the Anatomy Building, he surveyed the field and wrote the titles of three texts on the blackboard: Eugen Bleuler's[2] book on psychiatry had been translated into English, another text was in German, and one was in French. At least Farrar was very different from our other professors! During the eighteen months I was at TPH, Farrar's lectures were given there, and I skipped some of my other classes in order to hear him lecture again.

We had learned that he was a Kraepelinian; but I soon discovered he might be called a neo-Kraepelinian because he was much more a humanist than Kraepelin was reported to be. There was no library at TPH, only a bookcase in Farrar's office. When I moved in and saw him for the first time in his office as a very junior member of his staff, he loaned me two books. The first was *The Common Neuroses* by T.A. Ross,[3] and the second was a criticism of Freud, which, as I remember, was written by a psychiatrist more interested in legislation than in patients. I had already bought Bleuler's text months before and had devoured it.

Later, when Donald Campbell Meyers was dying of cancer of the pancreas, he asked me to take as many psychiatric books from his library as I wished. His wife and daughter went into the library with me and I left with about 30 to 40 books. I took them back to the TPH and put them in the bookcase in the male nurses' lounge. Most remained there when I left as it would have been quite a job to take them around with me. However, I took some to New York, left some with friends, and gave some away. These have nearly all disappeared. I have only two or three left.

Farrar's concern for facts, his poise, his dignity and his human interest certainly had a very good effect on all those who worked with him. We were a small group at the beginning and life in the TPH was quite enjoyable, especially on weekends and during holidays. His high standards may have had something to do with the fact that he published so little of his actual clinical work. In that way, he was like Adolf Meyer, the professor of psychiatry at Johns Hopkins University. A great writer and man of national repute, Meyer was always asked to write papers for congresses and societies that (because they were for formal occasions) were often rapidly published. Unfortunately, however, when Meyer's collected papers were published, the unpublished clinical reports and manuscripts (which I think would have been as numerous as the formal presentations) were not edited and published. I'm sure it must be the same with Farrar.

These two men were the best psychiatric interviewers I have seen at work. Farrar had great respect for patients (as he had for many other people), but he didn't have great respect for everybody. He talked about various types of reactions, several of which may be combined in one patient, without necessarily dignifying any of these reactions with the name of a "disease." In other words, he avoided the diagnostic problems associated with the idea of a disease concept in psychiatry.

I gradually was given more and more responsibility in examining patients. In time, I saw quite a number of male and female adult patients. I also saw quite a few people charged with criminal offenses because many police cases were brought in, as well as delinquent children. As a matter of fact, the only juveniles sent there at that time were young people charged by the police.

While at the TPH I wrote my first paper[4] which was published in the students' new journal. It was on the reciprocal relation between the populations of prisons and mental hospitals—when one goes up the other goes down. We have all watched a radical shift in a tragic direction during recent decades.

When I discussed applications for my first internship in psychiatry after graduating, Farrar gave me recommendations to Adolf Meyer at Hopkins, Thomas Heldt at the Ford Hospital in Detroit, and Albert Moore Barrett at Ann Arbor. During the Christmas holidays of 1926, I visited Heldt and Barrett and wrote to Meyer and the superintendent of the Manhattan State Hospital, Wards Island, New York. Heldt did not offer me a post. Although Barrett offered me a post, Farrar advised me not to go to Ann Arbor. He felt I should travel about, and if I started working with Barrett, I would fall in love with the place and stay. His advice was good, as I might have fallen deeply in love with it as I began to do at first sight. I have never visited Ann Arbor since.

As I could not afford the post Meyer offered, I accepted a junior post with Manhattan State Hospital. Its $1,500 a year salary with board and lodging allowed me to save for 14 months before taking up Meyer's offer in 1928.

After leaving Toronto I kept in touch with Farrar by letters, and his answers were always interesting. When I last visited him at his home, during our discussion he went to his bookcase, brought down a volume of Ezra Pound's Cantos, pointed to two (which illustrated our discussion) and hoped I would continue my interest in poetry.

Endnotes

[1] The second intern was interested in surgery, his saxophone, his external life and, minimally, in psychiatry.

[2] Eugen Bleuler, *Textbook of Psychiatry* (New York: Macmillan, 1924).

[3] T.A. Ross, *The Common Neuroses* (London: E. Arnold; New York: Longmans, 1923).

[4] W.C.M. Scott, "A Comparative Analysis of the Size of Certain Public Institutes in Canada with special reference to Mental Hospitals, "*University of Toronto Medical Journal* 3 (1): 27-28 (1925).

8

Memories of a Nurse

Claire A.(MacKid) Muller*

My recollections of Toronto Psychiatric Hospital are those of my student nursing days. In 1949, most big hospitals had nursing schools and the courses were three years long. Residence living was compulsory. For each school, there was a distinctive nursing cap, if not a uniform, and since many hospitals did not offer complete patient services, we nurses were farmed around to take training unavailable in our own bailiwicks. My home base was the Women's College Hospital and when I read on the posting list that I was to take my psychiatric training across the road, instead of having to go to St. Thomas, Ontario, I was thrilled. I soon discovered another thrill too. Our hospital was still on the "twelve hour" day, whereas TPH had modernized to the eight-hour day. Since no students were required to work the graveyard shift, I looked forward to a very agreeable two months.

On our first day, we trooped into the front hall at 8:00 a.m. sharp and were shepherded into a small lecture room. I can't recall how many of us there were, but since the hospital was small to begin with, there may have been as few as 16 of us. That first week, I think we all had lectures together, because I know we were split up into day and evening shifts at the end of a week or two. There were about three of us from the "WC" (as we called it) and the rest were from St. Mike's, Toronto East General, and Toronto General hospitals.

I think the first week we had lectures and visited the different sections of the hospital, and were assigned to accompany one graduate nurse for the day. Lectures were held almost daily after that, and slowly we assumed more responsibilities, but never gave drugs. The textbooks were

---

***Claire A. Muller, B.Sc.N., Women's College Hospital and the University of Toronto, is a teacher, amateur naturalist, feature writer and a strong supporter of environmental causes.

small, few in number, and limited in scope. Our first day on the wards, nearly all the patients were aware that we were new students, the men showing more interest that the women. A few patients asked us a little about ourselves, but our roles were to learn about them, so we were generally circumspect in our replies other than divulging names and hospitals. We were expected to be impersonal professionals. (This got the St. Mike's girls into trouble once. One of their classmates from "home base" was admitted as a possible schizophrenic and her classmates on duty at TPH fell over backwards trying to be helpful. The psychiatrist in charge of the case called us all into the lecture room and gave us a stern lecture making it very clear to us all that, "You must remain objective at all times and also must NEVER become personally involved and carry the case home with you at night.")

The thing which struck me most about TPH was the sterile drabness of the place. It certainly had all the earmarks of a hospital sickroom environment with sparsely furnished rooms, bare cream walls, and (except for little mats) bare floors sporting battleship linoleum. The dust mops were in evidence every day, and once a week the floors were washed and then the big polishers hummed over the Johnson's Brightest, and little wooden horses appeared which announced "FRESH WAX" from their dangling signs.

This "FRESH WAX" business reminds me of one woman patient who used to march very slowly down to the end of the hall, salute the little horse and march back around the horse and back down the hall again. Then she might stand rigid, staring ahead for a long time before saluting and repeating her performance.

Our first duties were to get to know one patient and her history (I say "her" because I was assigned to the women's floor first). We were free to ask questions and encourage any positive behavior. Our real job, though, was TO LISTEN. In those days with so few drugs, the physicians depended upon psychological analysis and positive thinking to help their patients. We helped bathe, dress, feed, and offer such solicitous service as seemed appropriate. Trips out to the garden or to the "OT" (occupational therapy department) were part of the routine. It was imperative to have a good memory, because anything of significance was to be written down, and I'd find myself rushing back to the nursing station to record whole conversations.

One floor was for women, one for men, and the top (third) floor, I barely recall, as we were only taken up there once. Violent patients were housed there in individual rooms and I believe each patient was locked in. It was a barren and strange place, and I felt uneasy in the eerie atmosphere of silence or mutterings or occasional shoutings, even with male attendants constantly on duty. I recall one schizophrenic man on a special diet which included prunes, and I thought his woman physician very courageous to try to treat him when he could have killed her (had he known any martial arts) before any attendant could have reached her.

There were also "the baths": one unit on the women's floor and one on the men's. I believe each had three large deep tubs in the high-ceilinged, echoing, tiled room. Usually, a patient would come in for a tub session either indifferent to the procedure or with smiling consent, but occasionally a violent patient would writhe, shout, bite, and flail as up to six people would steer, undress, and get the patient into place in the warm water with only the head showing above a canvas which covered the whole tub and fitted snugly around the patient's neck, reminiscent of the "living-head-without-a-body" which I used to ogle with awe at the Canadian National Exhibition as a little child.

As I said, the tubs had canvas covers, and these were hooked at intervals all around the edges. One could lift any section and check on a patient's well-being, but normally this was not necessary unless the patient's skin was becoming too wrinkled and needed more oil. As attendants in the room, we students would often be alone for our whole stint of duty there (I think we were relieved every two hours), and our duties involved taking and recording the water temperatures every fifteen minutes for a constant 98 degrees and recording any changes in patient behavior or physical state.

I recall one male patient particularly. He was a big farmer from western Canada, who had just had a prefrontal lobotomy, and his language would have done any sailor proud. I had come from a very narrow background of "Victorian gentility," and I thought it totally inappropriate for *any* young ladies to have to listen to such foul language with all the explicit sexual invitations. It horrified me. I didn't blame the patient. I thought the hospital authorities insensitive to the needs of women in general and female students in particular.

Generally, treatments of the times were limited. Electroshock treatments were common and insulin coma therapy was also used. I remember sodium amytal (7g injections, I believe) being used to encourage patients to voice deeper thoughts and emotions, and a solicitous physician would sit beside the patient, clipboard on knee, asking questions and recording answers in some quiet setting, often over long periods of time (i.e., as long as the drug seemed effective). The drugs of choice were very limited in those days too; chloral hydrate, phenobarbital, and paraldehyde being the ones I most readily recall.

Women physicians were just breaking into the medical field in those days, and women psychiatrists (a rare breed indeed) fought a constant battle to be accepted. It was amusing to me to see that the men in such a setting were expected to be particularly tolerant of their female counterparts, but the resentment still hung in the air like thin smoke. Male nurses also fought to create an attitude of acceptance and, individually encountered, most of them were well received, but, in general, patients, physicians, and nurses alike had trouble envisioning the male nurse role in the female bastion, so most of these men gravitated to urology, O.R., or psychiatry.

There was a male nurse at TPH (usually in charge of the men's floor). One evening, he, a male orderly, and I were on duty there. The male nurse was away, down at the end of the ward, giving the last of the evening medications, and most of the patients had settled down or were asleep. The orderly was off the floor for some reason or other, and I walked into the male wing. The big farmer with the lobotomy spied me and with a glint of sexual glee in his eyes, he leapt from his bed and headed in my direction. I didn't run—I flew—but I was only five feet tall and he was six feet four. I was terrified. As I ran, I pulled out the office door keys, reaching the door seconds ahead of him. I got the door open, slid inside and slammed the portal on his very breath. I sat on a chair in this nursing station and willed myself not to cry. Once I thought my voice was under control, I phoned for help while the big farmer shouted and pounded from without. In due course, people arrived, the patient was sedated, and the male nurse was very protective of my welfare for the rest of our evenings of duty together.

In those days, Huntington's chorea, carbon monoxide poisoning, dementia paralytica (neurosyphilis), degenerative psychoses, manic depressive psychosis, and schizophrenia (divided into simple, hebephrenic, and catatonic) were all diagnosed and treated under the same roof. Today, due to vast changes in prevention, proper classification (Huntington's), treatment, and the attitude of the informed public, professionals handle these cases in vastly different ways: more enlightened, more diverse (for chronic care especially), and with increasing breakthroughs in effective treatments. Of the neuroses, earlier treatment, new drugs, and counselling services within the community have broadened the focus for these victims of circumstance, attitude, and behavior.

As student nurses, most of us looked upon the whole field with misgivings and we'd spend long evenings talking among ourselves about how we felt emotionally and intellectually about this complex world of mental illness. I think I was not atypical of the majority of the student body at that time, for most of us shied away from this field where we considered so many cases hopeless (as indeed they were). I recall being offered a scholarship at TPH which I turned down with a polite smile.

Unlike medical illnesses (with exceptions like cancer clinics and intensive care units), psychiatric nursing gave many of us a feeling of being drawn into the vortex of the sick mind and I, for one, had just successfully escaped from a very unhealthy childhood environment and didn't want to be ensnared again. We students had high regard for the TPH staff in general, but we could see that some of the physicians had, themselves, been drawn into this vortex a little too far for their own good, and we were, thus, doubly suspicious of any constant participation in this field on our parts and fearful of warping of general outlooks on life.

Of the patients themselves, those who were able to be helped were very grateful. Alas, in those days there were so many unknowns and many many sick minds slipped beyond recovery. Of the neurotic patients, I can still see parallels today which seem all too familiar: There are still too many neurotic people out there who cannot function without the hospital crutch. When, in the 1980s, I had occasion to nurse in the psychiatric department of Sunnybrook Hospital, there they were again, as large as life, and just as dependent. The revolving door syndrome was alive and well—be it the eternal repeat visits to the couch or to the institution. They *still* appear to manifest a clear inability to "stand alone."

I have many vivid recollections of individual case histories: Thelma, who wept and wrung her hands and cried to Jesus, believing she had murdered her parents (except when fresh from a shock treatment, when her thinking was rational); Frank, who was always jumping into bed with the other men on the ward; the two fourteen-year-olds, who were incorrigibles and difficult to place in any treatment home; the sane young secretary, who had tried to kill herself because her parents had taught her that sexual feelings were evil; the spontaneous abortions in a bed or on a floor; catatonic Louise, who wedged her right hand in the hinged side of her door and pulled the handle with the other hand until the right hand fingers broke; Immogene, who thought she was Queen Hatshepsut of

Egypt and who sat bolt upright in bed with a turban on her head and demanded that we bow to her; the Huntington's chorea chap, who would go into a rage, and then, ashamed of his behavior, would crawl under his bedcovers and sob in humiliation; the compulsive hand washer, who wouldn't let us in her room because she feared our germs, and on and on. Suffice it to say, I have many memories of life at TPH; however, I will end with one short story.

Mr. A was an elderly gentleman mentally declining before the eyes of his heartbroken family in a private room at TPH. He had vivid hallucinations much of the time and was generally very depressed and not eating adequately. We students did everything we could to encourage his appetite and lift his spirits. One day I said, "Come on, Mr. A, let's go and visit the boys" (meaning the men in the open ward). I got him into his dressing gown and slippers, and he shuffled along beside me. When we turned the corner and entered the ward, about six of the men there were discussing the merits and shortcomings of their various doctors. "Hi, Joe," they called, for they liked this old man. "What's new Joe?" one asked. He looked at them for long minutes and then raised his hand and shook his finger in their general direction. "De ducturs," he paused before asking in accented English, "you know what de ducturs is?" He paused again and before giving his answer, "De ducturs is de squirrels, burying de nuts," and he turned on his heels and shuffled back to his room.

9

Nursing

Margaret L. Gorrie[*]

... The woman who is most successful in this work is the one who has complete possession of herself; one who understands and appreciates human nature; one who has a keen sense of her relationship to others, who has judgment, patience, observation and tact; who knows the great advantage of silence, but at the same time knows when to speak; the woman who has had the broadest culture acquired by reading or travel, who has added to her general education many accomplishments, thus making her interesting, versatile and resourceful—such a woman we crave for our mentally ill patients. When more of the type above described are in the mental hospitals...we may look for astounding results, even though the doctors are still debating over whether or not in dementia praecox there is a pathological change in the brain cell, or whether psychoanalysis is the proper method of treatment to employ in the functional neuroses. The nurse properly equipped herself, who cooperates with the physician and enters in to the life of her patients, can do more than anyone else to establish proper habits of thought.[1]

In 1915, Euphemia "Effie" Taylor thus described the characteristics of women who would be "successful" in psychiatric nursing. Her vision of the type of woman needed for care of the mentally ill was important to both the emerging occupational identity of nurses working in psychiatry and the education of the first two directors of nursing at TPH. Taylor,

---

[*]Margaret L. Gorrie, B.Sc., Nursing, University of Alberta, 1980; M.H.Sc., University of Toronto, 1984, is currently enrolled in the Ph.D. program in sociology at York University. She has worked in a variety of settings, including two Ontario provincial psychiatric hospitals. During her career, she has coordinated nursing education, researched in community health, and, most recently, assisted in teaching a course on the sociology of health and illness.

a Canadian-born woman, distinguished herself in nursing education in the United States. She was director of nursing services at the Henry Phipps Clinic at Johns Hopkins Hospital before and after World War I,[2] the first professor of psychiatric nursing at Yale University, and the dean of the School of Nursing at Yale.[3] The first director of nurses at TPH, Nettie Fidler, studied at the Phipps Clinic of Johns Hopkins and visited Yale University, and the second director of nurses, Eileen Ditchburn, was a graduate of Yale University's School of Nursing.[4]

In the opening decades of this century, women who were seen to excel in nursing were often described in terms of their character traits. They might be understanding, patient, tactful, versatile, and interesting, among other traits esteemed by Taylor. Personal traits, rather than a recognized body of knowledge as applied to care of the ill, were seen as key to the provision of quality nursing care. During the century, the emphasis on personal character traits as the foundation for good nursing care shifted as the work of nurses became based on specific types of knowledge and skills.

Nurses' work (quintessential women's work) requires skills which have been characterized as "general, complex, overlapping and invisible."[5] Many nursing skills may be learned and applied in a variety of settings, such as in the home as well as in the hospital, and are general rather than specialized in nature. Being "general" does not, however, connote simplicity; the skills required to communicate with a diversity of people are complex. Many different people (patients, staff, family members, and students) demand different qualities from nurses, who must set priorities and, often, cannot enjoy the luxury of doing one thing at a time. For example, as a patient in a hospital is being assisted to bathe, a nurse assesses his or her mood and other aspects of mental functioning. A large component of nurses' work is focused on achieving emotional and physical comfort for their patients. Much of this type of work is difficult to quantify.

Both nurses and their patients benefit if nurses have professional status. Nursing leaders worked to achieve this status by controlling the education and registration of nurses. Although some major changes in nursing education have occurred since the 1920s, nurses do not yet have a single vision of the preferred amount of educational preparation, nor is there a preferred educational setting between the university or technical college. Another option is unionization, but this began in a widespread manner in Ontario only during the 1960s, when TPH was closing. By this time, nursing educators viewed excellence in nursing as related to problem-solving skills (the "nursing process") and knowledge of patient care.

Historically, therefore, nurses have been the subject of some ambivalence: They often lacked extensive education, but nevertheless were known for their particularly good skills with patients. In psychiatric work, these might be the nurses who could defuse situations of incipient violence without denigrating patients' dignity. The profession continues to struggle to balance the value of formal education and knowledge gained from experience.

Psychiatric Nursing before the Opening of TPH

In the nineteenth century, nurses were brought into the asylums to care for patients and to lessen institutional brutality. Even before TPH in 1925, skilled nurses were sought out in psychiatric care.[6] This trend was not an outgrowth of Florence Nightingale's nursing reforms, but rather the result of physicians' work in asylums.[7] In Ontario, C.K. Clarke founded the first School of Nursing in an asylum in 1886 in Kingston.[8] In 1905, he played a role in opening the School of Nursing at the Toronto asylum, which prepared a number of nurses who went to work at TPH in its early years of operation, including one director of nurses, Myrtle Foley.[9]

In 1900, psychiatric nursing was a crazy-quilt of differing national traditions and provincial regulations and was not immediately accepted as a form of nursing. In England, a system of "State Mental Nurses," distinct from "Registered Nurses" developed, whereby graduates of psychiatric nursing programs were specifically prepared to work in psychiatry only.[10] In the United States, graduates of psychiatric nursing programs qualified to become "Registered Nurses" (like graduates of general hospital nursing programs), and became eligible to work in general as well as psychiatric settings. In Canada, individual provinces developed different approaches. In the western provinces, a register of psychiatric nurses, distinct from the register for general nurses, was created. In Ontario (the last province to pass legislation on registration of nurses), all graduate nurses from approved schools of nursing, whether located in psychiatric hospitals or general hospitals, were eligible to become registered and eligible to work in either kind of setting.[11]

These different approaches to the classification of psychiatric nurses reflect not only the degree to which mental problems were accepted as being within the jurisdiction of medicine, but also the degree of control exercised by physicians over nurses' education and organizations. While mental problems were considered illnesses, it was concern for treating the physical illnesses of people with mental problems that prompted the Graduate Nurses' Association of Ontario to include asylum care as appropriate work for its members.[12] Physicians actively worked to bring nurses to care for the mentally ill and thus aid in the medicalization of asylums. Nursing organizations, on the other hand, focused their energies on getting legislation passed to regulate the educational preparation of nurses and gain registration.

In the first half of this century, it was common for general hospitals to have training schools for nurses. These were virtually the only institutions through which one might become a nurse.[13] The passage of the *Ontario Nurses' Registration Act* in 1922 provided guidance for training schools for nurses and laid the groundwork for standardization of nurses' education. These schools existed to meet hospitals' needs for nursing services, as well as to educate student nurses. When conflict arose between students' learning and patients' need for nursing care, the latter took precedence. Thus, a nursing student could graduate from a hospital school of nursing after three years of working on the wards without having received much formal instruction. Graduates of these training schools might be knowledgeable, skilled nurses, or they might be little better than any untrained person.[14] Hospitals hired few graduate nurses. Graduate nurses would most likely seek employment from individual patients, do "private duty" in homes, or be employed by a hospital patient to provide one-on-one care (known as "specialling"). Hospitals employed graduate nurses to supervise ward work and oversee nurses in training. This method of occupational preparation meant pupil nurses were difficult to distinguish from graduates: Both were employees of the hospital (although only the latter received payment for their work), and there was great variance in the knowledge and skills of graduate nurses. Thus, long before TPH had opened its doors, the method by which women became nurses was firmly under the control of hospitals.

In 1910, 15 years before the opening of TPH, C.B. Farrar wrote that the advent of training schools for nurses in mental hospitals was "one of the most important steps in raising the mental hospital to a class equal to the general hospital."[15] Farrar viewed the work of psychiatric nurses as extending the work of physicians as well as complementing it. In describing the roles of physician and nurse, he believed it was, difficult to say which is more important... A capable physician with an inferior nurse, to carry out and supplement his work would surely be quite as much handicapped...as would a skilful nurse working with an incompetent doctor.[16]

Farrar fully supported the professional education of nurses, recognizing that improvements in patient care were dependent upon the knowledge and skills of those who provided continuous supervision and attendance upon the mentally ill.

In 1923, when Farrar asked his friend Sara May Parsons for her advice about nursing education, she wrote, "I think Miss Taylor's [of Johns Hopkins] way of preparing for psychiatric work was good."[17] Parsons was knowledgeable about the preparation of psychiatric nurses; she had been the superintendent of the Sheppard & Enoch Pratt Hospital Training School for Nurses, and advisor to the American Medico-Psychological Association on nursing education.[18] In suggesting that Farrar consider Taylor's work, Parsons was recommending a vision of nursing built upon Adolf Meyer's psychobiological approach to psychiatry.[19] Farrar took her advice, and arranged for the first director of nurses, Nettie Fidler, to attend programs developed by Taylor.

At the time TPH opened in 1925, the provision of nursing care for mentally ill patients was well accepted. The organizations that represented nurses viewed psychiatric work as separate from other types of nursing, such as infectious-disease nursing. At this time, however, learning the skills necessary for psychiatric nursing occurred, for the most part, through experience, although nurses-in-training in provincial mental hospital schools did receive instruction in psychiatry.

Nursing at TPH before World War II

Psychiatric nursing in the pre-World War II era relied heavily upon the ability of nurses to develop good rapport with patients, especially since there were so few therapies to assist the nurses in their day-to-day work. Nurses at TPH worked with a range of patients: Some had very limited intellectual abilities, some were highly intelligent, and others were intoxicated, psychotic, or may have been "of wholesome mind."[20] Patients of all ages, children, adults, and older people were mixed together on the wards. Sex was the basis for segregating patients, with one ward for females and one for males. Nurses were responsible for protecting vulnerable patients and containing the aggression of very disturbed patients. In addition to this work, nurses assisted physicians by noting information about patients which was relevant to their diagnosis and responsiveness to treatment. Nurses directed the work of attendants, particularly in the care of male patients.

The work of TPH nurses was not only invisible in character, but largely invisible to recorded history. There are few sources of information about nursing at TPH before World War II; the narrative nurses' notes from patients' charts were not kept, the personnel records were not retained, and because TPH did not have its own nursing school, there are no nursing alumnae. Fragments of descriptions of nurses' work at TPH do remain: some records of nursing education, some staff records from 1934, "flow" sheets in patients' charts, information on wages, and memories of some staff and students. Doris (Franks) Hueston was both a student at TPH and a staff member from 1932 to 1934. Her staff record from 1934 identifies her as the "Assistant Head Nurse, Male Ward."[21] In addition to this job, she recollects, "for a matter of a few days, it might even have been a week, I was superintendent" of nurses, as the director and assistant director of nurses were away.[22] On another occasion, she took over the operation of the switchboard: "It was an old-fashioned switchboard... Dr. McGhie was the Deputy Minister of Health and he was talking to Dr. Farrar and I unplugged him. I was better than nothing but that's about it."[23] Her work included "the outdoors" for a period of time, as well as time spent in what would now be described as a research assistant's role, searching patients' records for information for a study being conducted by Archibald Kilgour, a staff psychiatrist. An ability to learn quickly and work with very diverse people was necessary for nursing at TPH.

Psychiatric nursing throughout the 1920s and 1930s was dominated by considerations of patient safety and protection of patients from harm. On ward admission records nurses assessed the physical health of patients, noted their hygiene, nutritional status, the presence of vermin, and any bruising or scars. Flow sheets on patients' sleep patterns, temperature, weight, and menstruation were also maintained by nursing staff. The ward admission form had a section for describing patients' behaviour as "homicidal, violent, suicidal, depressed," but nursing staff did not use it.[24]

At TPH, Hueston recalls that occupational therapy was emphasized:

> Some people went for hours, some people spent a day and some people didn't go at all... That would be the depression ones...but

anybody who could went to occupational therapy and we tried to persuade them to do something.[25]

Nurses were involved in playing cards or other pastimes with patients, to develop rapport with them and to observe them. Hueston comments on this experience, "There was very little bedside nursing you see... You talked to them, you played checkers."[26]

The repertoire of treatments was limited. Nurses tried to calm agitated or violent patients by using packs and continuous water baths. "It was a sad business," says Hueston, "some of them were desperate... We used to give them those continuous hot baths and we wrapped them in sheets...and of course you didn't leave them."[27]

The care of patients who were in continuous water baths was intensive. In addition to monitoring the mental status of the patients, nurses tried to prevent the occurrence of any untoward effects which might result as a consequence of the enforced immobility and submersion in water. At the same time, nurses tried to calm the patients. Joan Karrick remembers attending patients in the baths,

> ... You would bring the patient in, and we had a special ointment that we put on their hands and a lotion that was put on the body. They were laid on the sling and there was another restraint over top of them—right over their body—and it was fastened around the neck, domed at the back. Their hands were free; there was a little place where their hands could splash...so they lay on the sling in the water, the water was kept at body temperature, and it was continually running in and out, so you got that soothing massage of water. You kept the lights low in there, so you decreased the stimulus, as you would for any patient who is upset. You checked the pulse, temporal pulse and you checked the temperature of the water and you offered the patient some fluids every fifteen minutes and you made a special effort to keep your voice low.[28]

Working with psychiatric patients was not without its risks for the nurses. Hueston recollects, "You were attacked frequently...we used to have trouble when they got violent and there were exciting times!"[29] Male staff, and occasionally the police, would be called to assist in subduing patients who became violent.

When TPH opened, Farrar believed the salaries for nurses offered by the province of Ontario (lower than those of other local hospitals, and lower than those in the United States) were too low to attract and retain suitably qualified nurses.[30] Qualified TPH nurses, one of whom had a postgraduate course from the Phipps' Psychiatric Clinic, were resigning to work for higher wages in the United States. This left TPH without qualified nurses to teach and supervise nursing students.[31] The deputy provincial secretary's response to Farrar's concerns paid no heed to pupils' needs for instruction and time to learn, nor to the fact that they did not come with the same skills as graduate nurses. Instead it was suggested to Farrar that he use student nurses.

> As a remedy for the situation do you not think it would be possible to make arrangements with some of the General Hospitals in this City to furnish you with pupil nurses to received [sic] a certain amount of training in Psychiatry... The general routine work on your wards would be taken care of by these young women...[32]

A further exchange of letters does not appear to have brought about the end desired by Farrar, as the deputy provincial secretary only offered sympathy for Farrar's difficulty, the cause of which he attributed to "the high scale of salaries paid in other hospitals."[33] Staffing problems related to low salaries remained a recurrent problem at TPH, although the shortage of nurses was never as severe as in the other provincial hospitals.[34]

Farrar believed qualified nurses were essential to improve care of mental patients. In later years, he supported the then somewhat unusual idea that hospitals ought to have a nurse heading up a single department, which would include all direct care staff (nurses, attendants, and ward aides) of both male and female patients.[35] In these aspects, his view of nursing was congruent with that of the contemporary nursing leaders. But Farrar was paternalistic toward the qualified nurses at TPH and had the authority not only to interfere in their personal lives, but to jeopardize their livelihood. For many years, staff of TPH resided on the upper floors of the hospital. Farrar complained to the deputy provincial secretary that nurses who lived at TPH were keeping irregular hours and suggested instituting a rule that nurses be expected back in their rooms no later than midnight. In this matter, unlike the matter of nurses' wages, the deputy provincial secretary concurred with Farrar:

> ...I think that this rule is entirely reasonable and that if a mistake is being made it is entirely on the side of leniency... You intimated that some of the Nurses were not willing to accept your judgment in this matter. If such is the case, I think it would be advisable for you to arrange to have such Nurses seek employment elsewhere, and if you find the slightest difficulty in making

replacements, I have no doubt that I shall be able to quite readily arrange for temporary replacements. These young women cannot expect to be allowed to wander into a public institution at all hours of the day and night.[36]

While Farrar wanted graduate nurses at TPH, he was not comfortable with permitting these women to behave as adults during their off work time.

The nurses employed at TPH in 1934 were a heterogeneous group, some of whom had only public school education. Of the 17 staff for whom there are records, 11 were assessed as not having the educational qualifications for the positions they held. This included the women in the positions of assistant director of nurses, head nurse of the male ward, head nurse of the female ward, as well as some staff nurse positions. Whether or not these staff members were graduate nurses from schools of nursing that waived minimal educational standards is not known. At this time, 12 years after the passage of nurses' registration legislation, it was not uncommon for hospitals to employ women who were regarded as full-fledged staff nurses and paid accordingly, but who did not meet a uniform standard of nursing knowledge and skill. The variability in the nurses' preparation may be a reflection of the difficulties psychiatric hospitals experienced in attracting staff who had the full qualifications when salaries were low and the work potentially dangerous. Alternatively, it may be that these staff, although lacking in formal qualifications, were skilled in managing patients' behaviour based on years of experience. TPH may have been reluctant to alter the mix of qualified and unqualified staff, as these nurses were essential to the safe operation of hospital wards.

The first director of nursing at TPH, Nettie Fidler, had many ideas about preparing women for nursing. Along with other nursing leaders, Fidler thought that high quality care depended upon reforms in nursing education. At TPH in 1931 Fidler organized the first course in psychiatric nursing for pupil nurses on "affiliation" from general hospitals[37] an arrangement that left TPH without the same type of organizational control over the pupil nurses that their home training schools possessed. Psychiatric nursing became a mandatory part of nursing education only in the 1950s, so the hospitals that sent their students to TPH for the three-month affiliation (the Toronto General Hospital, Toronto Western Hospital, Wellesley Hospital, Women's College Hospital, and Grace Hospital) were offering a more comprehensive program to their pupils than were most general hospitals. By way of comparison, at this time the "Minimum Curriculum for Approved Training Schools for Nurses" suggested four hours should be devoted to mental diseases.[38] (Fidler also started a course for graduate nurses from general hospitals who wanted to qualify for "public health work or other posts of responsibility requiring psychiatric knowledge and experience."[39])

Fidler spent only two years at TPH and was then asked "to reorganize the nursing service and take charge of the training courses" at the Whitby Ontario Hospital.[40] Whether this was Farrar's idea is not known. It is reasonable to believe, however, that he supported her leaving TPH, given the authority he had over the nurses.[41] Dorothy Riddell, former inspector of nurses' training schools, emphasized how much Fidler's work did to improve patient care in many Ontario provincial psychiatric hospitals. She commented, "There was a whole nucleus of people that she trained who became directors of nursing in the Ontario Hospitals and they stood out for years and years—the mainstay of the hospitals."[42] Fidler's contribution to nursing education did not stop there. In 1936 she resigned from the services of the provincial government and joined the University of Toronto School of Nursing. In 1952 she succeeded Kathleen Russell, its founder and dean, in directing the School of Nursing. She remained in this position until her retirement in 1962.

One of the most important contributions Fidler made to nursing education was demonstrating that it could be completed in two years, if the pupils were recognized as students, and the time was used to meet their learning needs. This contrasted with the apprenticeship system in which pupil nurses served three years under the control of hospitals. In Fidler's words,

> Hospital nursing schools have been created not as educational institutions but as money-saving devices. There is no attempt to distinguish between the differing purposes of a hospital and a school; the two institutions are entangled in a most confused and confusing manner. It is taken for granted, and admitted, that the object in conducting the school is to obtain cheap and relatively stable nursing service from the 'students.'[43]

Her work in this area prompted the move in Ontario away from hospital-based schools of nursing into schools under the control of educators. Whether her views on the organizational aspects of nursing education were established at TPH is not clear. Certainly the nursing education programs she developed at TPH did not assert TPH's control over student labour to the same degree as did other hospitals. Affiliate students remained under the control of their home hospitals, and TPH never opted to develop its own nursing school as a means of enlarging its control over student labour. It is clear, however, that when Fidler assumed the leadership of the University of Toronto's School of Nursing, her education in psychiatry influenced her vision of nursing education. She was described as,

> aware of the new approach to sickness that must be grasped, put into practice, and passed on to incoming students—the recognition of emotional stress and mental upsets as factors in dealing with so-called physical medicine.[44]

She worked actively with professional associations as well as the University of Toronto to promote the integration of psychiatric concepts into general nursing education.[45]

After Fidler, Eileen Ditchburn was head of nursing at TPH for two years. Then came Edith Dick, in 1935, followed by Myrtle Foley, who remained in the position until 1943 or 1944.[46] These women were responsible for both the supervision of the nursing staff and the teaching of nursing students. While this dual role linked nursing education and practice, care for patients preceded (and could detract from) care for students' learning needs. From the outset, the case study method was used to teach students, complemented by lectures and seminars from nurses, physicians, occupational therapists, and psychologists. Rather than learning by concept or method, students learned as apprentices on the job.[47] We don't know what TPH nurses taught their students, but in a different psychiatric hospital (Ponoka Hospital for the Insane in Alberta) in the early 1930s, Hilda Bennett taught nurses, and her recollections may represent the emphasis of nursing instructors in this era:

> It was most important that the students understood the difference in the conditions of the patients. We were most particular about the young students getting into the admitting ward and knowing how to receive a patient and how to treat and understand the new patient. We got a great many patients, as you can understand, from the north. Those women had gone north with their husbands, they were lonely, lost souls. They would be brought in, really breaking down because they were so lonely. And the students had to understand that. It was one of our greatest emphases, was to try to understand the conditions from which that person arrived.[48]

The nursing instructors often reminded students of the importance of their patients' social circumstances. Student nurses were expected to learn all they could about their patients. Hueston recalls the challenge of preparing case histories.

We did do these case studies. I had a patient, you had them from the beginning and you sort of wrote a case history. It was old-fashioned foolscap and it was several pages and we were marked on it...we interviewed the relatives and their friends and we did the whole business... It was hard to do. It took us a long time to know the difference between bedside nursing and psychiatric nursing.[49]

Margaret Allemang points out,

What was emphasized very much was protection of the patient and safety and recording our observations. I remember being specifically assigned to the baths for a certain period of time and I know we had to keep very detailed observations about the temperature of the water, the temperature of the patient, the pulse and everything that was said. We took general care of the patients...we sat with the patient.[50]

Students took away from their experience at TPH a fuller understanding of people. Doris Hueston remarked, "It certainly broadened me. I got as much out of it as I put in."[51] "When I was there, I thought more deeply about emotions than I had previously. It made you think more deeply about patients and yourself,"[52] mentioned Margaret Allemang in retrospect. In subsequent decades, an explicit objective of nursing school curricula became the development of self-awareness among students as a means of improving the interpersonal skills of nurses. The emphasis on the interpersonal skills among nurses would, however, be overshadowed by the therapeutic developments during and after World War II.

Nursing at TPH during and after World War II

By the end of the 1930s, two changes occurred that affected nursing at TPH; one was the beginning of World War II and the other was a dramatic change in psychiatric treatments.

In the provincial psychiatric hospitals, the years leading up to World War II were marked by nursing shortages; wartime conditions greatly exacerbated these shortages. Male nursing students, for example, were encouraged to sign up for war service.[53] To attract more women, hospital nursing schools deferred a planned increase in their entrance requirements. Married graduate nurses were actively recruited back into the work force, and advertising presented nursing as a patriotic duty. Work conditions and wages improved somewhat during the war years to attract more women.

During the war large numbers of married women streamed into the workforce, making a more mature nursing work force. Until this time, nurses who married were "retired" from nursing.

The Civil Service Commission, responsible for staffing TPH and the other provincial psychiatric hospitals, moved cautiously in this new inclusion of married women. In a memorandum addressed to Ontario Hospital superintendents, C.H. Lewis, acting director of the Hospitals Division, wrote:

> The Civil Service Commissioner has advised that, due to the shortage of nurses at the present time, it will be quite in order to accept applications from married nurses on the understanding that they are to be appointed to the temporary staff only.[54]

It was decided that graduate nurses might be employed on a part-time, rather than full-time basis only, to further relieve the shortages.[55] The implementation of this policy, however, ran into obstacles, and D.J. Foster, Civil Service Commissioner, limited its application only to previously hired nurses. In 1942, Foster wrote B.T. McGhie:

> I have discussed with the Prime Minister the numerous applications being made by married nurses in the service to work half-time. The purpose apparently is to avoid income tax, and the Government does not wish to lend itself to any such policy. These requests, therefore, will not be granted, and if such nurses resign it should be indicated to them that they cannot expect re-employment on a half-time basis later on.[56]

For these married nurses already employed in the civil service there were considerations other than tax evasion. For example, they had families and household work. Though attempting to attract nurses back into hospital nursing, the government was unable to provide the kind of flexibility in work arrangements that many women required. Nursing shortages in the psychiatric hospitals continued.

Throughout these years, psychiatric nurses in Ontario were leaving for nursing positions in the United States, as well as for more remunerative general hospital positions in the province.[57] There was also war service. It is known that at least two TPH nurses left nursing to work in war plants.[58] The impact of wartime on the TPH nursing department was severe, although it was the other Ontario Hospitals that were most harshly affected. Beginning in 1939, when TPH opened the research department,

... There was a staff of 50 nurses, including both students and graduates. By December, 1942, this number had dropped to 33 and at this time [1943] the staff consists of 19 Registered Nurses, including the Superintendent of Nurses.[59]

Such staff shortages could do nothing but compromise both the care patients received and the educational experience nurses obtained at this time.

The wartime shortage of nurses alarmed government officials, necessitating an increase in wages in 1941.[60] B.T. McGhie supported a wage increase, noting, "The unrest in our female nursing staff, which now exists, can, I think, only be evaded by the action I propose." It was during the war years that the eight-hour day for graduate nurses was begun[61] (although a six-day work week continued).

In these years, the department of nursing at TPH was headed by Myrtle Foley. She had been a nurse at TPH from as early as 1926 and had worked as a staff nurse and assistant director of nursing before becoming director.[62] She was a graduate of the Ontario Hospital in Toronto and had taken one year of further postgraduate education from the School of Nursing at the University of Toronto.[63] She had one of the longest tenures of the nursing directors at TPH. A nursing consultant from the American Psychiatric Association reviewed the nursing services in April 1943 and described the educational program as "one of the best seen anywhere" for both "the formal instruction and clinical assignment."[64] She noted,

... This hospital represents the highest in teaching and research and is, therefore, the life line for the promotion of the welfare of mental patients in Ontario, with influence extending even beyond these borders.[65]

The shortage of nurses meant the TPH nursing instructor had to work directly with patients rather than students. Foley had assumed some student teaching, as well as retaining the administrative aspects of her role. In the face of severe nursing shortages, Foley managed to maintain standards of psychiatric nursing education that were regarded as superior to any other.

Just before the Second World War, psychiatric nursing at TPH was altered by the introduction of a series of physical therapies. Until this time, physical therapies (such as continuous water baths [CWBs] or packs) were used not with the expectation of effecting a cure, but to calm and contain agitated and aggressive patients while permitting the illness to abate. While CWBs and packs continued to be used, late in the 1930s physical therapies began to be introduced that offered the possibility of actually altering the illness trajectory, potentially effecting a cure. These therapies created a need for more skilled physical care of mental patients by nurses, thereby increasing the overall need for nursing care. Coma therapy (induced by insulin injections), convulsive therapy (induced by Metrazol or electricity), and the surgical excision of brain tissue (known as psychosurgery, leucotomy, or lobotomy) all necessitated the close monitoring of patients' physical and mental status.[66] During the 1940s and 1950s, these forms of treatment altered the work of TPH nurses, making it more similar to general hospital nursing.

The nursing staff tried to minimize treatment risks by carefully monitoring patients. Doris Gibney recollected working with patients who received electroconvulsive and insulin coma treatments.

> I know that some people were frightened. There's no doubt about that, there's no question. I used to be the nurse who was involved in the giving of ECT. Patients were in the treatment room, on a stretcher. We used to put a firm pillow under their neck and the small of the back. There were two other attendants, one to support the shoulders and one at the hips. My job was to put a padded tongue depressor between the teeth and kind of talk to them. They were never left alone. We always tried to bring them back to a single room. They could be a little confused, almost like a patient coming out of anaesthetic.[67]

> Insulin therapy was another treatment that we were involved in. You developed a good relationship with the patient because you spent a lot of time with them and supported them and tried to encourage them. They would receive large doses of insulin and then they would start to perspire and sometimes go into shock and convulsions. You would have to watch them. You would leave them in that for a certain period of time and then start giving them glucose. The coma was terminated by intravenous glucose usually. We would give them lemonade and gradually they would come out of it. This would go on most of the morning and then by noon the treatment would be terminated. They would be watched very carefully. Their pulse rate would be checked every fifteen to twenty minutes and if there were any undue signs it would be terminated. And then they would get up, dress and have their noon meal. They would be watched that evening too because they could have a delayed [hypoglycaemic] reaction.[68]

These forms of treatment relied upon nurses monitoring patients closely, for the treatments themselves could cause physical harm, such as bone fractures from ECT, or insulin shock as an aftereffect of coma treatment. Such vigilance was more labour intensive and increased nurses' work pressures from previous years, when only general information about patients' physical status would be monitored.

TPH was the provincial centre for lobotomy surgery. Doris Gibney recalls:

> They brought them in from all around the province. I remember going with them to the Toronto General Hospital and then they were brought back when they were stable and 'specialed.' Some of them made what seemed to be a very good recovery. They were not as aggressive. They were more aware of their surroundings. Their behaviour was more appropriate.[69]

Joan Karrick was a TPH nurse who also worked with the patients admitted for lobotomy, and recollects,

> They were long-term patients, usually ones that had histories of violence. [Lobotomy] helped to make them an easier nursing management, not to turn them out to the community. Although there was one did go back to the community...[70]

While lobotomy and insulin-coma therapy have since become the focus of controversy, if not outright dismissal as ineffective measures, it is significant that the nurses of the 1940s and 1950s emphasized positive rather than negative results. Patients who were transferred to TPH for lobotomy assessment impressed the nurses with their responsiveness to the environment of TPH and to the nurses themselves. Gibney remembers: "People from the back wards were usually able to adjust. If you expect a certain level of behaviour, they would usually live up to that."[71] Eileen Mitchell reflects that "often the severely psychotic person has some control, if you can just reach them."[72] The nurses saw patients, even those who had been very institutionalized, as capable of learning and benefiting from appropriate kinds of stimulation and nursing care.

Somewhat paradoxically, the intensive nursing that was integral to the performance of ECT, insulin coma, and lobotomy therapies encouraged a new closeness in dealing with patients. This was accelerated by the introduction of psychotropic medications in the 1950s. The new drugs lessened the psychotic symptoms of patients and broadened the range of patients for whom interpersonal therapy became possible. At TPH, it was Elizabeth ("Betty") Bregg who first introduced the newly articulated emphasis in nursing on interpersonal relationships.

Bregg became director of nursing at TPH at some point in the mid-1940s.[73] She had originally graduated from the Ontario Hospital at New Toronto in 1940.[74] After assuming the position of director of nursing at TPH, Bregg took educational leave in the early 1950s, and completed a B.Sc. in nursing at Columbia University in New York. While there, her thinking about psychiatric nursing was influenced by Hildegarde Pepleau, whose work with Harry Stack Sullivan was the foundation for her vision of nursing, now recognized as the first theory of nursing.[75] When Bregg returned to TPH, she began to articulate this embryonic theoretical basis of a distinct nursing role among health care providers. As Gibney recollects, "It was in the 1950s that we started trying to look at behaviour rather than at disease and tried to deal with it from a behavioral point of view and deal with it therapeutically."[76]

While working therapeutically with patients was not entirely new to nurses in the 1950s, the conception and description of nursing was shifting. As one of many disciplines involved in patient care, nurses were becoming more self-conscious and articulate about the independent aspects of their role in patient care.

Others did not always agree with this new view of nursing. For example, in one patient's chart the following entry by William Mitchell conveys a different understanding of the nurse's role. "A program of total push and active socialization has been asked of the ward personnel for this patient, and it is hoped that she will be assigned a single nurse who will pester her back into reality."[77]

Bregg was seen as being ahead of her time. She was important for nursing at TPH as she initiated a different vision of nursing. She was admired for her teaching abilities and compassion for patients. As one handwritten note to Jean [Wilson] at the University of Toronto School of Nursing relates, "The great thing that you give them is their awareness and appreciation of the individual. We think that nothing else is as important as that."[78] The rather conservative environment of TPH was not receptive to the new ideas she articulated and after having been back a few years she moved on to a teaching position at an American university.

Assistant director of nursing and longstanding TPH staff member, Grace Sagert, became director of nursing and remained in this position until her retirement in 1962. She was succeeded by Marion Clarke, who was the director of nursing until TPH closed. While capable directors of nursing, neither Sagert nor Clarke seemed to combine their leadership skills and knowledge of psychiatric nursing into a highly visible profile of nursing at TPH.

From the earliest years at TPH until its closure, the hospital was a centre for psychiatric nursing education. Student nurses on affiliation from nearby hospitals spent three months at TPH. Students from the University of Toronto School of Nursing also had their psychiatric nursing experience during the summer months. For the young women attending nursing schools, contact with psychotic individuals and persons sent from the courts was new and a bit frightening. A graduate of the early 1950s from Women's College Hospital recollected feeling anxious about being a student at TPH.

> The keys to locked doors and the anxiety of being sure the door was carefully locked behind me, lest a patient "escape" was a major concern. I recall the odour of paraldehyde that permeated the air. The atmosphere of the wards was often times electric— never being able to anticipate just what might take place next.[79]

Being at TPH was not, however, solely a fearful experience, as the same Women's College Hospital graduate recollected. "The meals were really great, particularly breakfast!" Affiliate nursing students were taught by TPH nursing staff, while the University of Toronto students were taught by their own teacher.

The wave of specialization following World War II gave rise to a number of new health care occupations. For some nurses, this meant opportunities for further learning and a move into occupational areas that were opening up, such as laboratory work. The predominant effect on nursing as an occupation, however, was limiting. In the pre-World War II era in which generalists dominated health care, nurses worked in diverse settings and did diverse tasks with patients. For example, at TPH the social service work and work in the outdoors was done by nurses. However, as disciplines such as social work and psychology gained increased recognition, nursing found itself vulnerable to encroachment.

It is hard to say who was right in these turf struggles. While nursing educators believed it was essential for student nurses to work with outpatients, social workers did not necessarily share this view. From a nursing perspective, the outpatient setting helped nursing students learn about people with mental illnesses as they coped with their day-to-day lives. As Eileen Mitchell describes, "They saw people as very disturbed but still very much a person and making their own decisions about treatment. There was a kind of awareness that this might be themselves or might be a relative."[80] Nursing educators believed student nurses could not work well with patients unless they saw them within the fuller context of their lives, beyond being inpatients, but without impinging upon the territory of social workers.

During the 1950s, nurses were not, however, simply passive heirs to the residue of other occupations. They maintained control over some of the conditions of their work, resisting changes that they thought might endanger patient care. Mitchell remembers these differing views:

> I know that it was a bit of a jolt to some of the young psychiatric interns when certain things would be insisted on from the standpoint of nursing and they didn't think it was necessary. There was a little bit of professional friction at times. But safety was always paramount in the nursing division. It had to be. We weren't experimenting to see what would happen.[81]

Friction between disciplines, and within nursing, arose over the issue of nurses wearing uniforms. This issue symbolized differences of opinion about the place of nursing in the hospital hierarchy. In the 1950s, nurses resisted working in civilian clothes. As Mitchell recollects,

> One of the medical people thought that it would be more homey if the nurses didn't wear uniforms. And trying to defend our position when we'd always been in uniform was a bit difficult. We felt that there was a certain respect for nursing and we felt that was important to the person who was frightened and shaky and perhaps approaching panic. That they knew that this person was this professional person. We continued to wear uniforms at that time.[82]

A reluctance to embrace changes may have been related, in part, to the fact that many nurses believed they had "learned the hard way" about work with psychiatric patients, and they saw experimentation in nursing approaches as not in the best interests of the patients. Nurses were not hasty to implement suggestions made by medical staff when they saw any possibility of adverse consequences for vulnerable patients.

In the 1960s, the nurses working on the female ward stopped wearing uniforms and dressed in civilian clothing. This symbolized a new treatment philosophy, a new therapeutic milieu. There was less rigidity in the divisions of labour between the varied health care providers. Phillip Melville, the psychiatrist on the female ward, is credited as "the one who had all of these ideas, introducing these new approaches to treatment."[83] Many TPH nurses were proud of the new approaches being used on the female ward, and noted that not even the Allan Institute in Montreal, a benchmark for TPH staff during the early 1960s, had completely abolished some form of nurses' uniform.[84] This move to discontinue the wearing of uniforms was not supported by all of the nurses, including Marion Clarke, the director of nursing.

The head nurse who introduced the change, Joy Rogers, remembers it as a very difficult time. "We were instituting a lot of the Maxwell Jones and other milieu approaches to treatments. It was very much a multi-disciplinary model that we were initiating."[85] This approach to patient care turned traditional assumptions of care around 180 degrees. Some relaxation of hospital security had occurred before the therapeutic milieu began, with doors being unlocked and visitors permitted more ready access to patients. Therapeutic milieu, however, moved the philosophy of care on the female ward from a hierarchial system based on medical and professional authority toward a more equal sharing of power in the relationships between disciplines, as well as between patients and caregivers. Taking the nurses out of uniform on this ward at TPH resulted in the loss of half of the nurses, who found they could not work within the ambiguity of the milieu approach.

In the early 1960s psychiatric nursing came to encompass a broader range of skills. Moving away from the earlier focus of care to individuals, nurses became involved in learning about group processes. Nurses led patient groups and worked almost interchangeably with colleagues from other disciplines. Nurses went, said Rogers, "from the lowest on the totem pole to being a colleague and being invited to participate in presentations. Our whole awareness was being raised about what we could possibly be."[86] Milieu therapy was a well-entrenched component of TPH nursing at the time the hospital closed. For nurses, the 1960s witnessed great optimism about psychiatric and mental health care, as the traditional boundaries governing occupational jurisdictions came under question and began to loosen.

In 1966, TPH closed and the nursing staff moved on: some to the Clarke Institute of Psychiatry, some to Queen Street Mental Health Centre. Some staff remained at the same site to work with the mentally handicapped at Surrey Place.

Conclusion

Between 1925 and 1966, the work of psychiatric nurses changed as circumstances changed. Yet it remained much the same in terms of the day-to-day interactions between nurses and patients. There is a continuous thread in the description of psychiatric nursing at TPH: the emphasis on the nurse/patient relationship. In the 1920s and 1930s, nurses attempted to develop rapport with patients through recreational and occupational diversions. In the 1940s and 1950s, nurses provided reassurance and support to patients undergoing treatment, and tried to diminish patients' anxiety through the development of a supportive relationship. In the 1960s, nurses became more expert in creating an interactional environment. Whether the terminology is that of rapport, interpersonal relations, or empathy, there is similarity in the focus of nurses' work throughout the years.

When TPH opened, excelling in nursing meant possessing certain character traits. At the time of TPH's closure, it meant the ability both to relate to patients in an empathic manner and apply a body of knowledge based on the interpersonalist tradition in psychiatry. Yet throughout there was continuity too: nurses always saw their mission as fostering communication and providing emotional support. This work has always been women's work, and as such is characterized by the need to meet the emotional needs of others.

The contributions of TPH nurses were twofold: to the well-being of patients and to the education of nurses about psychiatric nursing. Whether in the early years, when very limited therapeutic options existed, or in the postwar era of intensive physical therapies, or during the rise of interactive therapies such as milieu therapy, nurses with clinical acumen were the mainstay of hospital care. They were relied upon to maintain patient safety and to help psychotic patients find some control. Nurses who were able to work well with very disturbed, aggressive patients, were recognized, although not always well appreciated or rewarded. TPH staff nurses have contributed to patients' ability to gain control over their lives and look with hope to the future. Upon recovering from a lengthy, psychotic episode, one patient wrote to TPH staff that she felt like shouting, "Stop the world. I want to get ON!" Nurses were an important part of a patient's recovery.

In addition to the role played by nurses in patient care, TPH nurses helped demystify mental illness and promote knowledge about psychiatry throughout Ontario. TPH nurses taught a large number of affiliate nursing students from a variety of general hospitals in Toronto. The work of Fidler, while she was at Whitby Ontario Hospital from 1932 to 1936, preparing nurses for leadership positions in the other provincial psychiatric hospitals, was an important contribution to the increasing knowledge about psychiatric nursing and the care of the mentally ill. Fidler led the way, but a whole generation followed close behind.

Endnotes

[1] Euphemia "Effie" J. Taylor, "Nursing in the Henry Phipps Psychiatric Clinic," *Johns Hopkins Hospital Bulletin*, 26: 9 (1915); quoted in Olga Church, "That Noble Reform: The Emergence of Psychiatric Nursing in the United States, 1881-1963" (Unpublished Ph.D. dissertation: University of Illinois, 1982), p. 75.

[2] Kathleen C. Buckwalter & Olga Church, "Euphemia Jane Taylor: An Uncommon Psychiatric Nurse," *Perspectives in Psychiatric Care*, 17 (3): 125-31 (May-June 1979).

[3] Olga Church: "Emergence of Training Programs for Asylum Nursing at the Turn of the Century," *ANS Advances in Nursing Science* 7 (2): 35-46 (January 1985).

[4] Province of Ontario, Hospitals Division, Department of Health, *Toronto Psychiatric Hospital: Report covering period 1926-1932* (Toronto: Queens Printer, 1932), pp. 8-9. Hereafter *TPH Report 1926-32*.

[5] Ontario Pay Equity Commission *Pay Equity in Predominantly Female Establishments: Health Care Sector,* Report to the Minister of Labour, prepared by Pat Armstrong (1988), p. 8.

[6] C.K. Clarke worked to combine some of the content and form of general hospital and asylum nurses' training. The journal of organized nursing, *The Canadian Nurse*, published information on the progress of this project. See C.K. Clarke, "Some Remarks Upon the Nursing of Cases of Mental Disease," *The Canadian Nurse* 2 (3): 11-14 (1906) n.a.; "Post-Graduate Work," *The Canadian Nurse* 2 (3):27-28 (1906), noting the "new course in mental diseases" added to the Toronto General Hospital Training School; R.W. Bruce-Smith, "Training Schools for Asylum Nurses in Ontario," *The Canadian Nurse* 2 (4): 23 (1906); Edward Ryan, "The Relation of the Work of Hospitals for the Insane to that of General Hospitals," *The Canadian Nurse* 3 (5): 251-53; 319-20 (1907).

[7] Mich Carpenter, "Asylum Nursing Before 1914: A Chapter in the History of Labour," In Celia Davis, ed., *Rewriting Nursing History* (London: Croom Helm, 1980), pp. 123-46.

[8] Dorothy Jean Sillars, "The Development of Community Mental Health Nursing In Toronto From 1917 To 1947" (Unpublished M.Sc.N. thesis, University of Toronto, 1983), p. 15.

[9] Archives of Ontario RG 10 107-0-423 container #65, "Laura Fitzsimmons Survey 1943-44."

[10] Robert Dingwall, Anne Marie Rafferty, Charles Webster, *An Introduction to the Social History of Nursing* (London: Routledge, 1988), pp. 123-44.

[11] Helen Mussallem, "The Changing Roles of Professional Nurses' Associations," in Alice Baumgart and Jenniece Larsen (eds.), *Canadian Nursing Faces the Future* (Toronto: C.V. Mosby, 1988), pp. 399-419.

[12] Report of meeting held in Toronto on December 28, 1905 "to discuss a draft of the proposed bill for Registration." "The Graduate Nurses Association of Ontario," *The Canadian Nurse* 2 (1): 64 (1906).

[13] Following World War I, seven universities offered nursing education; the impetus for creating these programs was the public health movement and interest in scientific management of hospitals. These programs cannot be seen as offering a real alternative to the hospital-based programs, as their admission requirements and costs created insurmountable barriers for the majority of women who sought nursing preparation. See Alice Baumgart and Rondalyn Kirkwood, "Social Reform Versus Education Reform: University Nursing Education in Canada, 1919-1960," *Journal of Advanced Nursing* 15 (5): 510-16 (1990).

[14] Problems in the educational preparation of nurses related to their employee status within the hospital were noted early in the century by nursing leaders. See M.A. Nutting, "Some Problems of the Training School," *The Canadian Nurse* 4 (12): 582-96 (1908). The Weir Report, released in 1932, recommended nursing education occur in educational institutions rather than hospitals; however, it was not until after World War II that these changes took place.

[15] Farrar to Geo. A. Pope (president of the trustees of the Sheppard and Enoch Pratt Hospital), dated March 16, 1910. All correspondence with Farrar, unless otherwise noted, is in the Farrar private archive.

[16] Ibid.

[17] S.M. Parsons to C.B. Farrar, October 4, 1923.

[18] Olga Church, "That Noble Reform: The Emergence of Psychiatric Nursing In The United States, 1882-1963" (Unpublished Ph.D. dissertation: University of Illinois, 1982), p. 67.

[19] Olga Church, "From Custody to Community In Psychiatric Nursing," *Nursing Research* 36 (1): 48-55 (1987).

[20] A sample of TPH patients' case books was taken. One carton of case books for each decade was sampled; a total of ten case books were reviewed for 1926, 1936, 1946, 1956, and 1966. One patient was admitted in 1926 for assessment following a four-year hospitalization at the Ontario Hospital, Hamilton, for "alcoholic dementia." This patient had brought legal action against the superintendent of the hospital and was transferred to TPH for an independent assessment of his mental status. C.B. Farrar found him to be "of wholesome mind" and he was released. (Case Book #497.) TPH Case Books are the property of the Clarke Institute of Psychiatry.

[21] Staff record, March 1934. Farrar private archive.

[22] Interview with Doris (Franks) Hueston, August 27, 1992.

[23] Ibid.

[24] In the sample of charts reviewed from 1926 and 1936, none of the ward admission forms had this section completed.

[25] Interview with Doris (Franks) Hueston, August 27, 1992.

[26] Ibid.

[27] Ibid.

[28] Interview with Joan Karrick, August 19, 1992.

[29] Interview with Doris (Franks) Hueston, August 27, 1992.

[30] Farrar to H.M. Robbins (deputy provincial secretary), February 26, 1926.

[31] Farrar to H.M. Robbins, February 26, 1926, and March 25, 1926.

[32] H.M. Robbins to C.B. Farrar, March 30, 1926.

[33] H.M. Robbins to C.B. Farrar, April 9, 1926.

[34] During the 1930s, the ratio of nurses to patients decreased. In 1935, thirty-seven nurses and attendants cared for fifty-five patients. In 1936, thirty-three nurses and attendants cared for fifty-eight patients. In 1937, twenty nurses and twenty-two maids and attendants cared for sixty-one patients. Archives of Ontario RG 10 107-0-188, container #26, "Establishment Staff & Patient Ratios 1935-36." This situation was

accompanied by recognition of low remuneration as causing nurses to emigrate to the United States. "Dr. McGhie insisted that the nurses here have no grievance other than the wages and hours." As in the 1920s, the provincial government initially refused to adjust wages; furthermore, a policy was formed which prohibited the rehiring of nurses who resigned to accept positions in the United States. Conditions were such that wages for nurses employed in Ontario Hospitals were increased in 1937. Archives of Ontario RG 10 107-0-164, container #22 "Nurses (Training Schools) 1936–1937."

[35] Farrar to Dr. R.C. Montgomery (director, Hospitals Division), August 24, 1944.

[36] H.M. Robbins (deputy provincial secretary) to C.B. Farrar, March 8, 1929.

[37] TPH Report 1926–32.

[38] Archives of Ontario RG 10 107-0-179 "Male Nurses 1932-38."

[39] TPH Report 1926–32.

[40] Ibid.

[41] Interview with Dorothy Riddell, August 19, 1992.

[42] Ibid.

[43] Nettie D. Fidler, "Demonstration School of Nursing in Ontario, Canada," *Nursing Mirror* 49: Supplement between 444–445: (February 17, 1950).

[44] *University of Toronto Alumni Bulletin*, 52: 18-19 (1952). University of Toronto Archives Accession #P78-0334, file 1.

[45] Fidler chaired a committee of the Canadian Nurses Association looking into nurses' education. The committee looked at the need "to lay more emphasis on the integration of psychiatric concepts with general training" and the Association passed a resolution that "every effort be made to establish practice fields and to encourage the inclusion of psychiatric experience in the basic professional course." Archives of Ontario RG 10 107-0-178 "Nurses 1952."

[46] TPH Report 1926–32.

[47] Ontario Department of Health, Toronto Psychiatric Hospital, *Post-Graduate Course in Psychiatric Nursing*, January 1935.

[48] Interview with Hilda Bennett, August 28, 1992.

[49] Interview with Doris (Franks) Hueston, August 27, 1992.

[50] Interview with Margaret Allemang, October 9, 1992.

[51] Interview with Doris (Franks) Hueston, August 27, 1992.

[52] Interview with Margaret Allemang, October 9, 1992.

[53] Archives of Ontario RG 10 107-0-181 "Male Nurses 1939-41."

[54] C.H. Lewis (acting director, Hospitals Division) to Ontario Hospital Superintendents, July 11, 1941. Archives of Ontario RG 10 107-0-167, container #23, "Nurses (salaries) etc. 1941."

[55] Ibid.

[56] D.J. Foster (civil service commissioner) to B.T. McGhie, September 3, 1942. Archives of Ontario RG 10 107-0-168, container #23, "Nurses (salaries) etc. 1942."

[57] H.J. Kirby to the civil service commissioner, July 31, 1941. Archives of Ontario RG 10 107-0-167, container #23, "Nurses (salaries) etc. 1941;" Memorandum from C.B. Farrar, April 13, 1942.

[58] Memorandum from C.B. Farrar, July 13, 1944. Archives of Ontario RG 10 107-0-171, container #23, "Nurses (salaries) etc. 1944."

[59] Archives of Ontario RG 10 107-0-423, container #65, "Laura Fitzsimmons Survey 1943-44."

[60] H.J. Kirby to the civil service commissioner, July 31, 1941. Archives of Ontario RG 10 107-0-167, container #23, "Nurses (salaries) etc. 1941."

61 Archives of Ontario RG 10 107-0-423, container #65, "Laura Fitzsimmons Survey 1943-44." In her recommendations to the American Psychiatric Association, Fitzsimmons suggested an eight-hour day. In a review of her report, C.B. Farrar commented "the eight-hour plan for graduate nursing staff was first inaugurated at the Psychiatric Hospital."

62 The actual dates upon which Myrtle Foley began her varied positions are not known. Foley signed one of the ward admission records sampled from 1926, and the department had another identified director and assistant until 1934. The Ontario Department of Health, Toronto Psychiatric Hospital "Post Graduate Course in Psychiatric Nursing," January 1935, cites Myrtle Foley as the assistant director of Nursing. She was responsible for demonstrating hydrotherapy. In 1939, she was the director of the department, as recollected by Margaret Allemang, a nursing student at TPH on affiliation (interviewed September 1992). See also Baskett chapter, Chapter 4.

63 Laura Fitzsimmons Survey of the Toronto Psychiatric Hospital, done April 19, 1943. Archives of Ontario RG 10 107-0-423, container 65, "Laura Fitzsimmons Survey 1943-44."

64 Ibid.

65 Ibid.

66 See also Baskett chapter, Chapter 4.

67 Interview with Doris Gibney, September 10, 1992.

68 Ibid.

69 Ibid.

70 Interview with Joan Karrick, August 19, 1992.

71 Interview with Doris Gibney, September 10, 1992.

72 Interview with Eileen Mitchell, September 11, 1992.

73 When Doris Gibney began work at TPH in 1949, Betty Bregg was the director of nursing. Interview with Doris Gibney, September 10, 1992.

74 Elizabeth Bregg is included in the graduation photo of the 1940 class of the Ontario Hospital, Toronto. QSMHC Archives (Greenland-Griffin Collection.)

75 Afaf Ibrahim Meleis, *Theoretical Nursing, Development and Progress* (New York: J.B. Lippincott, 1985), pp. 7-34. Meleis states Pepleau "developed the first articulated concept of nursing as an interpersonal relationship."

76 Interview with Doris Gibney, September 10, 1992.

77 Case Book #21,020.

78 E. B[regg] to M. Jean Wilson, School of Nursing [May 1956]. University of Toronto Archives A73-0053, box 007, Faculty of Nursing correspondence with TPH.

79 Letter to author from Bev Andrews, September 19, 1992.

80 Interview with Eileen Mitchell, September 11, 1992.

81 Ibid.

82 Ibid.

83 Interview with Joy Rogers, August 24, 1992.

84 Ibid.

85 Ibid.

86 Ibid. Rogers recollects presenting a paper she wrote about the nursing transition to a milieu approach to the TPH Journal Club. This was the first time a nurse had presented in this academic forum at TPH.

10

Psychology

Hugh McLeod and Andrew Boyd[*]

The beginning of clinical psychology[1] at TPH in 1930 coincided with its establishment in Ontario Hospitals.[2] In order to improve diagnosis and assist such non-governmental organizations as the Children's Aid Society and the Christian Brothers, psychologists joined the staffs of Brockville, Whitby, London, and Orillia psychiatric hospitals.[3] Each hospital received one psychologist, drawn mostly from recent graduates of the University of Toronto masters program in psychology.[4] At TPH, the psychologist was supposed to be stationary, linked to the receiving function of TPH, while psychologists at the other four hospitals would be mobile, performing psychometric testing in regions surrounding their hospitals.[5] Yet for Jean Brown, TPH's first psychologist, that definition would prove to be more of an ideal than a reality.

It was an ideal job for Brown. During its candidate search, Ontario's Department of Health consulted Earle MacPhee, an educator in applied psychology who was one of five members of the graduate faculty in psychology at the University of Toronto. MacPhee recommended Brown, who had been a stellar student, for a position.[6] With her M.A. thesis[7] and courses in applied psychology, three years of practical experience, and expertise in psychometric testing of hearing-impaired clients, Brown was an ideal candidate for the position. Initially scheduled to go to the London Ontario Hospital,[8] Brown joined the staff at TPH in 1930.[9]

---

[*]Hugh N. McLeod, Ph.D., University of London, Professor Emeritus, Lakehead University, Thunder Bay, Ontario. Born in Wolseley, Saskatchewan, Dr. McLeod was employed for many years as a clinical psychologist in various hospitals in Canada and the UK, and was Professor of Psychology at the University of Saskatchewan and Lakehead University. Now retired, Hugh McLeod lives in Scarborough, Ontario.
Andrew Boyd, M.A., History, University of Toronto, 1992, is currently enrolled in the Ph.D. program at the University of Toronto, specializing in aviation history.

Brown was already familiar with the range of tasks she would undertake at TPH. Having worked in the Toronto area testing children and educating parents, she became an expert in clinical psychology (referred to simply as "applied psychology" by the medical profession in 1930). To the general public, however, the mechanical tests and cardboard squares that were Brown's tools of trade were curious and arcane instruments. Between 1927 and 1930 she was one of the few psychologists employed through the Mental Hygiene Division of the Department of Public Health, directed by Edmund Lewis (who later became director of outpatients at TPH). Although she was part of the division, she essentially worked alone, testing at Toronto's public schools.[10] Brown recalled,

> I drove my father's car to the tests. The test equipment was in a small suitcase that was broken into by some young boys. I had to go to court to get it back, and as the judge went through my suitcase he kept asking, "What is this penny for?" and "What is this shoelace for?"...[11]

Unveiling the mysteries of "modern" applied psychology would unfortunately prove problematic. She encountered resistance on all fronts; physicians, academics, and institutional administrators would seek to limit her work, acting upon the traditional prejudices of professional chauvinism, elitism, or misunderstanding and distrust of her occupation. Fortunately, however, Jean Brown possessed the resiliency to outmanoeuvre her detractors and do pioneering work during her first lonely 16 years as the sole psychologist at TPH.

TESTING

Brown performed diagnostic procedures inside and outside the hospital. She viewed her job as:

> three-fold. It sounds a bit grandiose, but—service, research and teaching... I had to teach the post-grads and tell them about mental tests, their application and limitations. And then the government got word of this, and they asked me to give lectures to Department of Public Health doctors, and then they asked me to publish it...[12]

Her inpatient duties centred upon diagnostic psychometrics, assisting the psychiatrist's diagnosis of a patient. Although a complete test regime could comprise six performance and three aptitude tests, time allotted for testing each patient limited her primarily to the Stanford-Binet Intelligence Test (also known as an IQ test). A host of developmental, memory, and performance tests could have rounded out her evaluations. Annual reports indicate IQ tests comprised 78 percent of the inpatient tests and 84 percent of the outpatient tests administered between November 1, 1931, and October 31, 1932.[13] Yet these numbers do not necessarily reflect the true nature of Brown's job. For example, although an interview accompanied each battery of tests, interviews were reported as just over one percent of administered tests.[14] This figure only represents subjects who could not respond to the conventional test situation. During this period, Brown performed a total of 836 tests (an average of 3.2 per day) and was paid an annual salary of $1,300.[15] It seems clear that the department was getting its money's worth!

The preponderance of aptitude testing within Brown's total work provides an interesting insight into the position of applied psychology in the early 1930s. It was held in low esteem. A significant example of this appears in the 1932 departmental report for TPH, where Brown's name is listed fourteenth out of nineteen officers of the hospital, ranking below all the physicians and most of the nurses.[16] When questioned about this Brown said, "It was a medical setting and I was a psychologist... The inner group of nursing staff were conscious of their authority."[17]

Applied psychology's first major step forward occurred during World War I when aptitude testing was used to stream inductees into appropriate positions within the American armed forces.[18] Thanks to applied psychology, administrators suddenly had what appeared to be a rapid and accurate method of quantifying the skills of large groups of people. Psychometrics could be used to establish the mental capacity of individuals and ensure their appropriate placement within the educational system and work force.

In diagnosis, however, the utility of psychometric numbers was limited. While aptitude testing may measure a subject's ability to perform on a specific test, it remains a matter of debate within the profession as to whether it measures a subject's actual intelligence. Additionally, in a medical environment the establishment of an IQ level was and still is meaningless unless combined with the subject's specific age, background, and ailment. Developmental scoring was still new in psychometrics at the time of Brown's arrival at TPH, and the establishment of guidelines for relative scores at given age levels placed further qualifications on test data.[19] Yet those raw data had to be interpreted. Who would do it and who would follow up with treatment became fundamental issues of disagreement between the psychological and psychiatric communities.

Which members of the medical team at TPH contributed to a diagnosis depended largely upon the judgment of the attending physician. While many approached Brown as a partner in the treatment process, others discounted her input and viewed applied psychology as a technical trade rather than as a profession.[20] With regard to Edmund Lewis, her superior at TPH, Brown stated:

> He gloried in raising my blood pressure. In 1930 I wrote an honest report on a child and he said I might as well write "damn" on the sheet (the child got a lower IQ score than Lewis wanted). So, I put on my hat and went home for three months... Dr. Lewis wouldn't have psychology rise above what he wanted it for.[21]

While each psychologist who served at TPH has a collection of similar stories, it is important to consider these difficulties as prejudices of individual physicians, rather than a monolithic professional bias. Similar affronts were mitigated somewhat by the cooperation Brown received from many inpatient psychiatrists.[22] Most inpatient doctors would provide her with a detailed briefing on the patient's history and current status before she gave her tests, and allowed her to interpret the test results.[23] This input improved the overall diagnosis of a patient, and TPH's role as a receiving hospital placed a premium on the accuracy of a rapid diagnosis. The sooner the nature of a patient's problem could be determined, the sooner the patient could be placed in an appropriate stream of treatment.

Psychometrics was not, however, any more of an exact science than psychiatry. While Brown had a number of tests at her disposal in her first years at TPH, there was still no systematic scoring methodology. In a paper written shortly before she joined TPH, Brown discussed the scoring of the Kohs' Block Test, a performance test based on spatial arrangement: "There is an urgent need for single performance tests or sets of tests for clinical use. A careful study of available performance tests had indicated that few show consistent age or grade increments over any period of years."[24]

She concluded that, while it generally correlated with the Stanford-Binet intelligence test, the wide range of arithmetic deviations within specific age groups precluded establishing a developmental scoring system for the Kohs' Block Test.[25] Solipsism, and its insistence that reality is subjective, was the bugbear of psychology. It both frustrated psychologists and justified their existence. Some differences between individuals could not be quantified, making sensitive interpretation the more necessary.

Jean Brown's first 16 years at TPH saw the recognition of applied psychology's value as a profession. Yet she had constantly to test the limits, adjusting her level of interpretation to the willingness of the attending physician to receive it. She commented, "At the beginning we [psychologists] were just trying to establish ourselves in the hospitals, and I think that the psychiatrists were also attempting to establish themselves in the medical profession."[26]

The growing pains of both professions created a fair amount of territorial conflict as they each sought to define their roles in the delivery of health care. In a medical setting, however, psychology was fated to lose the battle for credibility. The structure and hierarchy of the hospital is determined by the relative level of an employee's medical qualifications and not by one's academic knowledge or unofficial practical experience. Until well into the 1960s, psychologists were non-medical professionals attempting to operate within an area the physicians had reserved for themselves. Predictably, they suffered the torments any profession endures when it attempts to occupy what another profession views as its own turf. In 1930, however, this conflict was yet to come; Jean Brown understood her role, and attempted to do as much as she could within the narrow boundaries allowed her.[27]

When asked if her gender played any role in her treatment at TPH, Brown stated: "We found in psychology that differences were due more to our degrees than our gender. I never felt like a second class citizen because of that; other girls who got their Ph.D. like Mary Wright in London were fine."[28]

One instance of professional chauvinism arose when both Brown and a psychiatrist were called to testify as witnesses in the early 1940s. When she was placed on the stand, her quantitative data and straightforward delivery gave the reporters something concrete to print in the next day's newspaper. When her testimony was reported in *The Globe and Mail* and the psychiatrist's was not, a stir was created that reached up into the Department of Health and it was firmly indicated to Brown that such an incident should never occur again.[29]

Other instances arose when Earle MacPhee of the psychology department sent students to Brown for practical experience. Lewis, director of the outpatient service, found out that MacPhee had been hanging his hat and coat in the director's office at the hospital and one day had a lackey come over and remove them. The implication was, of course, that MacPhee was not of sufficient medical stature to allow such behavior.[30] Perhaps unaware of his "lowly professional status," MacPhee later became vice-president of finance at the University of British Columbia. In a similar vein, Toby Levinson stated,

> I can remember when Bunnie Wilshire, who was the executive director of the outpatient department, would bring in these young girls from Cobourg training school, and put them in the office, and you were supposed to do revised [Stanford-Binet Tests] but if you weren't finished when Lewis wanted the results, she'd put her head in the door and say "Have you got a number yet?"[31]

On the outpatient side, Jean Brown's duties revolved around psychometric testing for a wide range of governmental and non-governmental social welfare organizations.[32] TPH served as a psychometric resource center for institutions within the Toronto area and, in 1932, over 80 percent of her tests were performed on outpatients.[33] Her clients ranged from unwed mothers to the occasional arraigned murder suspect and covered most social welfare institutions in between.[34] Her weekly schedule during these years indicates the nature of her outpatient work:

> Monday was called "Unmarried Mother's Day" and I tested women from the Infant's Home and the Victor Home. Thursdays and Fridays Brother Cyril and Brother John [Christian Brothers] would bring the boys down for testing, and whenever I went to the Good Shepherd, a nun would sit behind a screen while I did my tests, listening to every word.[35]

The rest of Brown's week was filled with testing wards of the Children's Aid Society and an occasional trip to the Don Jail to test its inmates. Although Lewis eventually managed to have this practice discontinued, she tested a number of violent offenders in the 1930s and described it as one of the most distasteful parts of her job.[36]

In another outpatient service, Brown also cooperated with a number of institutions in a study of illegitimate mothers. Unfortunately, the results were inconclusive, and it was becoming apparent that straight psychometrics might not hold the answers for modern society's ills. Brown said, "The conclusions were disappointing to a novice like me. I tried social class, intelligence, patterns of repetition, but there was no common factor contributing to illegitimate motherhood."[37]

In a way, this study reconfirmed the bankruptcy of the euphoria about applied psychology in the interwar years. Failures of this type would have a dual effect upon the profession. The stature of the psychologist would be gradually enhanced in a clinical setting, as it became clear to all concerned that test results were not definitive. Yet academic psychologists would increasingly denigrate applied psychologists, believing them to be essentially street vendors practising a lowly craft. This division would not become apparent until after World War II, however. As applied psychology gradually evolved into clinical psychology during the 1930s and 1940s, Brown tested away on her weekly cycles, occasionally being called out of Toronto to perform tests on hearing-impaired clients (a specialty she developed early in her career and refined through regular correspondence with James Drever and Mary Collins at the Department of Psychology in Edinburgh, leaders in this field).[38]

Brown's "department of one" finally doubled in 1946 when Toby Levinson joined TPH as an intern "straight out of [the psychology program at] the University of Toronto."[39] Levinson's arrival afforded Brown an opportunity to spend a summer at the New York Psychiatric Institute, acquiring new techniques and having a closer look at the new process of projective testing. When Zygmunt Piotrowski, department head at New York Psychiatric, left for holidays that summer, Brown remained in charge of their department which, she says, "...showed what a high opinion they had of Canadian clinicians."[40] Levinson spent four years at TPH while she completed her M.A. at the University of Toronto and then later returned on a part-time basis in 1952 for another four years. The growth that started with Levinson in 1946 turned into a mini-explosion by the end of the decade as both the numbers of practitioners within the profession and their role within TPH blossomed.

In 1947, the structure of clinical psychology at TPH slowly began to alter as Brown's many roles were compartmentalized and separate areas of activity set up for different types of psychology. With the departure of Farrar and the arrival of Stokes as director, a reorganization at TPH occurred. Brown remembers Farrar with fondness, for it was he who arranged for Brown to go to New York that summer. While she was working there, he wrote her an encouraging letter. She related: "He was behind me. He sent me a couple of books to review, and he brought in people from different disciplines to speak to us during our Saturday morning full-dress conferences in the lecture hall."[41]

The arrival of Stokes coincided with a fundamental change in the culture of the psychology group at TPH. In 1947, an outpatient department was established off the TPH premises at the northeast corner of College Street and University Avenue (where the Best Institute now stands), and a separate child and adolescent outpatient unit was added in 1948.[42] The establishment of a forensic unit completed the reorganization of TPH's services and new arrivals came to staff these divisions. Harley Wideman arrived in fall 1949 with a recent M.A. in psychology from the University of Toronto and remained until early 1954, when he went to Wellesley Hospital as staff psychologist. During this time he completed his Ph.D. at the University of Toronto.[43] Stokes was interested in acquiring an experienced "community oriented" psychologist, and Bruce Quarrington followed Wideman in 1950, assuming the position of chief psychologist as an appointee of the University of Toronto.[44] At this point, distinctions began to emerge among the different types of psychology at TPH. In Quarrington's words:

> In inpatients, the psychologist's role was still narrowly circumscribed to assessment. In outpatients, assessments were also done, but the emphasis was on behavioral therapy—particularly in the children's unit and the outpatient clinic.[45]

Toby Levinson said: "At that time, I think that to be a psychologist meant that you would grind out psychological tests, more specifically, you would come up with an IQ."[46] Stokes and Quarrington brought a different style to psychiatry and psychology at TPH. Levinson continued,

> I think ultimately it was Bruce's influence that made psychiatrists realize that psychologists had some special functions with regard to research. I think that was the beginning of some serious considerations of psychologists as research scientists.[47]

The psychology group liked Stokes. When interviewed in 1992, its members were unanimous that his clinical skills were unsurpassed.[48] Stokes' changes were not, however, limited solely to the outpatient department. While psychology's role in inpatients did remain limited, new additions to other groups influenced the culture of some of the wards. Frank Rubinstein, a social worker with a recent Ph.D. from the University of Pittsburgh, had a significant impact on the women's ward of the inpatient department. Rubinstein was very interested in the idea of a social community; he and psychiatrist Phillip Melville proceeded to organize the ward along those lines. Rubinstein suggested that the staff dress casually, that perhaps they should live in the hospital full-time and that they meet more or less continuously with the patients. Groups were set up and the patients were persuaded that they, together with staff who were members of the groups, would determine whether such and such patient should have medication, what kind of medication and how much they would have. These innovations on the women's ward lasted well into the 1960s, but the men's ward, under Alec Bonkalo's direction, continued along more traditional lines.[49] Modifications similar to those implemented by Rubinstein and Melville could not have occurred without the support Stokes brought to experimentation with alternative forms of treatment.

Bruce Quarrington described Stokes' attitudes towards patient evaluation:

> His attempt to express his very profound commitment to what psychiatry should be employed the analogy of a bull's-eye. The inner core represented the genetic foundation of the patient, the next ring was the physiological elements of the patient's condition, and the next ring was the psychological condition of the patient and the outer ring was the social forces affecting the individual.[50]

From the psychology group's point of view, Stokes' multi-factorial approach to treatment engendered an eclectic and "laissez faire" research culture. Harley Wideman compared it to contemporary institutions in the United States: "The discussions among residents at Boston State and residents in TPH were miles apart."[51] Describing the hospital atmosphere, Wideman commented, "Stokes was very non-directive himself, and Bruce had never really wanted to take direction from anybody, and he didn't want to give anybody direction himself."[52] Elaborating on this theme Quarrington stated, "At lunch time at TPH, the talk would go in all different directions and rarely touch upon work, whereas lunches at Wayne State and other institutions I visited were informal research reviews and discussions."[53]

The geographical location of the outpatient units may have contributed to a sense of alienation. TPH annexed a church at the corner of Elizabeth and College Streets, in which Quarrington established an office for a while. Hugh McLeod recalled,

> We were setting up machinery for the testing of patients there, and I had some machinery which had been suggested to me by Professor Raymond Catell of Illinois. Late one night Owen White was setting up some machinery and at eleven-thirty there was a knock on the College Street door of the church. Owen thought he'd ignore it but the rapping continued and finally he

opened the door. There was an inebriated man at the door who said, "This is a church, and I need help," and Owen said, "No, this is a psychological laboratory and we don't help anybody."[54]

There were also vagaries of treatment. When psychologist Hugh McLeod first arrived at TPH in 1955, he was assigned to research being conducted by Daniel Cappon, a psychiatrist attempting to correlate patients' dreams immediately prior to surgery with their rates of recovery. This research eventually made it to publication, but, in the words of McLeod,

> Dr. Cappon came to my desk when I first came to the hospital and he threw all kinds of papers on the desk, tissues, old envelopes, toilet paper with dreams written down on them, just a complete maelstrom of cacophony, and he said "figure this out." ... One of the disconcerting things was that we would set up a procedure to see the patients at the Toronto General Hospital pre-op, and we had a format to follow, but Dr. Cappon, after a few weeks, decided that he would change it and there would be a constant change of formats.[55]

McLeod also remembered a treatment initiated by Rolv Gjessing from Norway that harkened back to Farrar's early adaptations of Silas Weir Mitchell's rest cure: "I remember Mr. L. was an archetypal catatonic and therefore he was treated via Stokes via Gjessing on this porridge diet...for months at a time he had nothing but porridge."[56]

Quarrington and Wideman believed that part of the problem at TPH was a lack of a concerted research focus, unlike Wayne State where, for a time, most resources were dedicated to studying schizophrenia.[57] This was simply one of the inevitable costs of pushing knowledge forward in as many directions as possible within the confines of one institution.

The psychology group continued to grow in the late 1940s, providing a stable place of employment for some psychologists and a whistle stop for others moving onto doctoral work or into different areas of the profession. A constant flow of newcomers characterized the group throughout the late 1940s and the 1950s.[58] Quarrington explained this phenomenon: "Turnover was slightly higher because TPH looked more appealing as a training ground than as a place to work. Those who left were looking for a more coherent set of responsibilities and a more ordered life."[59]

Barbro Biringer came in 1952 with an M.A. from Stockholm and some studies in Chicago. She worked in outpatients from 1952 to 1954, left for two years to have a child, returned to the inpatients from 1954 to 1956, and then went to the psychology department at St. Michael's Hospital. She later worked at the Addiction Research Foundation.[60]

Hugh McLeod came in 1955 as senior inpatient psychologist and stayed until 1964, when he went to the University of Saskatchewan and later to Lakehead University in Thunder Bay, Ontario. For his first two years at TPH he worked with Daniel Cappon on a dream research project; for the remainder, he was on the inpatient service. Harry Silverman came to the adolescent outpatient unit in 1958 and stayed until 1960, when he went to the University of London to do Ph.D. work. When he returned he went to the Etobicoke school board as chief psychologist (where he remained for five years) and, after that, joined the faculty at the Ontario Institute for Studies in Education, where he continued teaching.[61] This was just the beginning.[62]

The arrival of a number of new psychologists coincided with a major change in psychological tests, especially projective testing.[63] Projective techniques such as Thematic Apperception Test (TAT) allowed psychologists to examine qualitative aspects of their clients' personalities, in addition to traditional quantitative measurements. This increased the level of interpretation required of psychologists during testing and subsequently enhanced their credibility within the medical environment. The studies of the reliability of the Rorschach and the validity of other clinical instruments occupied the majority of the psychology group's research time at TPH in the 1950s. Its members published over 15 papers during this period, either jointly, singly, or in collaboration with members of the psychiatry, speech pathology, or social work groups.[64]

Psychology's process of professionalization was accelerating. The first meetings of the Ontario Psychological Association were held at the Big Brother offices on Jarvis Street in 1947.[65] As its membership grew, the OPA engendered a new concept of psychology. Another important way station was the establishment of the Ontario Board of Examiners in Psychology in 1960, which would register psychologists in Ontario. In several ways, therefore, psychology would advance rapidly at TPH.

In addition to offering graduate training in psychology, in the early 1960s the psychology group was involved in the formal teaching of psychiatric residents, nurses, and undergraduate medical students. As applied psychology evolved into what William Line later termed "community psychology,"[66] and into "clinical psychology" in the early 1960s, it remained narrowly circumscribed within the graduate department. In the 1930s and early 1940s, there was no clinical training of psychologists at the University of Toronto. The only instruction particularly relevant to future clinical work was a course in psychological testing given by Mary Louise Northway and Reva Appleby Gerstein of the psychology department.

The establishment of an M.A. specialty in clinical psychology had its roots in the appointment of Bruce Quarrington in 1953 as assistant professor of psychology. Yet, in the 1950s, others in the department plumped for an academic program.[67] Clinical psychology was also a fairly expensive specialty to teach.[68] Yet to the chagrin of the Department of Psychology, clinical work was becoming increasingly attractive to graduate students. Many of them found it more relevant than laboratory work and that, on the whole, it paid more than academic psychology.[69] Pressures to establish a specialization in clinical psychology mounted in the late fifties and culminated in a four-person teaching and supervisory group consisting of Bruce Quarrington, Mary Hackney, Harley Wideman, and one other instructor.[70] Yet the venture failed. In the words of Bruce Quarrington,

> The clinical option attracted people with academic promise, and by doing so diverted them from the academic program... Roger Myers' [the head of the psychology department] clinical interests were weaker than his sense of the achievable.[71]

Myers believed mainstream academic experimental psychology was the route to developing a large, prestigious university department. Although successful in his efforts, the cost was felt by the applied psychology department at the Ontario Institute for Studies in Education (OISE).

The University of Toronto never actually offered a clinical M.A. in psychology, but simply allowed students to specialize in clinical studies in addition to their core M.A. courses.[72] Funding was gradually cut for the clinical field of the program and it shrank from its initial base of four instructors, losing roughly one per year until it was fully terminated in three years after its foundation.[73] Toronto ran against the academic trend set by other Canadian and American universities by failing to develop a formal clinical doctoral program. McGill and the University of Montreal both established clinical programs at the masters level after the Second World War.[74] McGill also offered a Doctor of Applied Science (D.Ap.Sc.), but never graduated anyone in that program.[75] Ironically, the levels of enrollment for the University of Toronto's clinical specialty were exceptionally high. Harley Wideman explained, "At one point twenty-one out of twenty-five graduate students were taking the clinical options."[76]

The brief life of the clinical specialty underscores some of the barriers clinical psychology encountered well into the 1960s. Despite its broadening role, clinical psychology was still sandwiched between a fairly well circumscribed mandate within TPH and a lack of credibility with its academic associates. This is rather puzzling in the context of the contribution University of Toronto psychology professors made to the war effort and to initial conceptualizations of community psychology.

The Second World War produced a significant, if somewhat brief, change in the focus of academic psychology at the University of Toronto. A burst of interest in psychological testing arose from the need to stream and train armed services inductees for specific duties. Several University of Toronto professors were seconded by the services: William Line became chief of personnel services for the Canadian army; Edward Bott and Roger Myers were also in England associated with the war effort; Sperrin Chant became head of personnel services for the air force; and Ed Belyea, a graduate of the Toronto program and future professor at the University of British Columbia, headed up personnel services for the Canadian navy.[77]

With the end of hostilities, there was a keen interest in establishing psychology training facilities in Canadian universities for practical work, particularly in the health field. The Department of Veteran's Affairs (D.V.A.) of the federal government was eager to have people work with returnees who were in the various D.V.A. hospitals across the country. Line received overall responsibility to establish psychological services in D.V.A. hospitals,[78] and a number of clinically oriented courses were introduced postwar at Toronto and other Canadian graduate schools. At Toronto, Mary (Salter) Ainsworth taught a course in projective techniques and went on to become a world renowned developmental psychologist at Johns Hopkins University in Baltimore. Magda Arnold taught a graduate course in personality theory. She achieved international recognition while a professor at Chicago's Loyola University and published widely in the area of emotion and motivation. The departure of these two women from the faculty was a great loss for the University of Toronto, but was viewed as a predictable outgrowth of chauvinism and conservatism at the Department of Psychology.[79] Robert Jackson taught a course in statistics. He later became the first principal of the Ontario Institute for Studies in Education in Toronto. Roger Myers taught a graduate course in psychotherapeutic methods, and William Blatz, director of the Institute of Child Study associated with the University of Toronto, taught a course in abnormal psychology. These offerings were echoed at other Canadian and American universities, but Toronto failed to maintain its lead in the teaching of clinical psychology.

The demise of the masters program in clinical psychology is symbolic of the relationship between TPH and the psychology department at the University of Toronto. Unlike medicine, whose mandate was to graduate both practitioners and researchers, psychology centred on research, and despite all of William Line's rhetoric about community psychology, the department was simply not dedicated to strong cooperation with clinical units. When viewed in the context of Line's career, this paradox deepens. From the psychology group's point of view, Line's much vaunted commitment to applied psychology evaporated after the war. Displaying little interest in his graduate students' doctoral research, he withdrew from active clinical involvement, published and spoke frequently, but demonstrated little concrete commitment to the ideals he was espousing.[80] For the psychology group at TPH, Line became the fisher king of community psychology; he was willing to discuss its great promise, but, for reasons best known to himself, he was unwilling or unable to help it grow.

Despite its short life, the masters program was a success from its graduates' point of view, and served to erode further the boundaries between psychology and psychiatry. Practical training for the program occurred in the outpatient clinic and a night clinic staffed exclusively by graduate students in psychology and teaching members of the psychology group. Bruce Quarrington recalled:

> We at the psychology [group] operated an evening clinic in the outpatient just to teach students, M.A. students, from the university, and we staffed the whole thing, I mean there were no psychiatrists...and it was fine, as a matter of fact I still run into students who think of that as the golden time, and there they were, psychologists, diagnosing and treating and doing it all on their own with not a physician in sight.[81]

In the postwar era the profession was thus moving from tight constraint within a psychometric role, to a somewhat more loosely defined role, where therapy often occurred as a collaborative process between physician and psychologist or was performed exclusively by the psychologist.[82]

The range of this latitude, however, continued to be determined by the psychiatrist, and many physicians still viewed psychologists as technicians. Hugh McLeod recalled a set of instructions given to him by a psychiatrist at Sunnybrook Hospital prior to his arrival at TPH:

> If a psychologist sees a patient, he says good morning, and then you give them a test, and you say good-bye, and if I hear that you have said anything more than good morning and good-bye you are fired, because anything more than good morning and goodbye is therapy and you are not allowed to do it.[83]

Harley Wideman overstepped the prescribed boundaries in his early years at TPH. He noted, "I...wasn't interested in simply an IQ score, I wanted to know something about the personality of the people, and I also wanted to start treating them."[84] Wideman got into trouble in the early 1950s for administering psychotherapy when one of TPH's nursing trainees encountered some emotional difficulties. By the end of the decade, however, psychotherapy by psychologists was common in units outside the hospital proper and was generally accepted. With a series of collaborative papers initiated by Quarrington and a steadily increasing level of professional credibility, TPH had become a more friendly place for the psychology group.

As the psychology group moved into the 1960s and plans for the Clarke Institute began to emerge in 1965, a new psychiatric director took over from Stokes: Charles Roberts. Roberts behaved very much like a new broom, putting each employee through a highly confrontational interview upon his arrival. Bruce Quarrington stated,

> In many cases people decided their future on the basis of that single interview. It was a change in administrative climate that no one could miss and many people feared the imposition of a bureaucracy that Stokes had managed to obviate.[85]

This perception of Roberts' attitude, combined with the severe financial loss that many employees in the psychology group would have suffered if they had transferred their careers and pension plans to the Clarke Institute,[86] produced an exodus from the psychology group in 1965 and 1966.

In the early 1960s, approximately ten full-time psychologists were employed at TPH, four in the adult outpatient unit, three in the child and adolescent outpatient unit, and three in the forensic unit.[87] Bruce Quarrington's transfer to the Clarke marked the exception, rather than the rule, for the psychology group. Some of the other departees left for academia or joined full-service hospitals as staff psychologists. For example, Stephen Neiger went to Lakeshore Hospital in Mimico, Jean Brown left earlier for Women's College Hospital, and Alan Hutchison went to the provincial forensic services. Quarrington, after initially transferring to the Clarke, soon left for a professorship at York University. McLeod went to the University of Saskatchewan, and Al Slemon went to the University of Western Ontario in London.

Each path leading away from TPH's clinical environment entailed an increase in professional status for members of the psychology group. Jean Brown made a telling comment: "When I went to Women's College [Hospital], I was treated like an equal."[88] For the departees from TPH, prestige lay in academics, private practice, or in medical situations where they would be the most highly ranked professionals in their field.[89] TPH provided a liberal research haven for a core group of inquisitive and motivated psychologists, and the hospital's postwar culture allowed them to pursue their own research agenda in relative peace. The spatial separation among the various outpatient units and the hospital helped foster a spirit of eclecticism established by the hospital's director. Psychologists who stayed at TPH thrived in this environment; the ones who left, or simply passed through, sought a different climate from that provided by Stokes, McLeod, and Quarrington. For the majority of the psychology group, TPH's closure marked the end of that peculiar brand of freedom. The clinical setting at TPH was unique; in an age of increasing accountability in both research and administration, the psychology group knew their culture could not be duplicated.

Appendix: A who's who of TPH psychologists

Bill Currie was a psychologist at the inpatients for a number of years before he transferred to Lancaster Hospital in Saint John, New Brunswick and later to Dartmouth, Nova Scotia. *Joseph Rubin* was with the inpatients for a period before going to the University of Maine for Ph.D. work. He later transferred to the Hawthorne Children's Center in Detroit, Michigan. *Harry Hutchison* was with the inpatients and later became chief psychologist of forensic services. These latter three were all Ph.D. students at the University of Toronto at the time of their appointments.[90]

Lydia (Senyshyn) York was with the inpatients for a period before transferring to the day care unit under Arthur Jones and, later, to Mt. Sinai

Hospital. *Bill Otto* came from Leyden, Holland, with a doctoral degree and was with the inpatients for a number of years before transferring in 1962 or 1963 to Mt. Sinai Hospital. *Evangeline (Scraba) Munns* took Brown's office upon her departure for Women's College in 1962, and was there for a number of years before going to York University for Ph.D. work. *Birute (Petrulis) Jonys* took over from Hugh McLeod in 1964 after obtaining a Ph.D. from the University of Chicago. She stayed at TPH briefly before transferring to the North York school board. *Stephen Neiger* came from Innsbruck, Austria, with M.D. and Ph.D. degrees to head up the outpatient unit in the early 1950s where he remained until 1966, transferring to the Lakeshore Psychiatric Hospital. *Bill Lawrence* was with the inpatients in the early 1960s on his way from the Hamilton Ontario Hospital to further studies.

Tom Mallinson, with a new Ph.D. from Columbia University, was at the outpatients unit in the late 1950s and acted as chief psychologist for one year while Bruce Quarrington was away at the Institute for Advanced Studies at Berkeley, California. Mallinson left for Simon Fraser University in the early 1960s. *Al Slemon* headed up the children's unit on Grosvenor Street in the late 1950s, before going to the Faculty of Education at the University of Western Ontario. *Douglas Quirk* worked briefly at the outpatients before transferring to the Queen Street Mental Health Centre. *Daniel Paitich* was with the forensic services for many years before transferring to the Clarke Institute. These latter three were all Ph.D. students at the University of Toronto during their tenure at TPH.

Owen White, statistical genius, was also at TPH during the late 1950s and early 1960s. He later transferred to the University of London (England) to work with Professor H.J. Eysenck.

Interviews and Transcripts
TPH Hospital Psychology Group Focus Group: February 7, 1992.
Interview with Harley Wideman: September 23, 1992.
Interview with Bruce Quarrington: September 29, 1992.
Interview with Jean Brown-Fuller: October 2, 1992.

Government Publications
Province of Ontario, Department of Health, Hospitals Division, *Toronto Psychiatric Hospital: Report Covering Period 1926-1932* (Toronto: Queens Printer, 1932).

JOURNAL PUBLICATIONS

Paul Barbarik, "Psychologists in Profile: William Line (1897-1964)," *Ontario Psychologist* 8 (5): 57-62 (December 1976).

Ernest Douglass and Bruce Quarrington, "Differentiation of Interiorized and Exteriorized Secondary Stuttering," *Journal of Speech and Hearing Disorders* 17 (4): 377-85 (December 1952).

Leonard Gelfund, Bruce Quarrington, Harley Wideman, and Jean Brown, "Inter-Judge Agreement on Traits Rated from the Rorschach," *Journal of Consulting Psychology* 18 (6): 471 (December 1954).

BOOKS

Mitchell G. Ash, and William R. Woodward, eds., *Psychology in Twentieth Century Thought and Society* (Cambridge: Cambridge University Press, 1987).

Joseph Brozek, ed., *Explorations in the History of Psychology in the United States* (Lewisburg: Bucknell University Press, 1984).

Claude E. Buxton, ed., *Points of View in the Modern History of Psychology* (Orlando: Academic Press, 1985).

Wayne Dennis, ed., *Readings in the History of Psychology* (New York: Appleton-Century Crofts, 1948).

W.M. O'Neill, *Beginnings of Modern Psychology* (New Jersey: Harvester Press, 1968).

Robert D. Romanyshyn. *Psychological Life: From Science to Metaphor* (Austin: University of Texas Press, 1982).

Duane P. Schultz, *History of Modern Psychology* (New York: Academic Press, 1969).

ENDNOTES

[1] Clinical psychology was known as applied psychology until well into the 1940s. These terms are used interchangeably within the context of psychology at TPH.

[2] Interview with Jean Brown-Fuller, October 2, 1992.

[3] Ibid.

[4] Ibid.

[5] Ibid.

[6] Ibid.

[7] Jean Brown. *Standardization of the Fergusson Form Board Series* (Toronto: University of Toronto M.A. thesis, 1926).

[8] Ibid.

[9] Ibid.

[10] Ibid.

[11] Ibid.

[12] Ibid.

[13] Province of Ontario, Hospitals Division, Department of Health, *Toronto Psychiatric Hospital: Report Covering Period 1926-1932* (Toronto: Queens Printer, 1932), p. 19.

[14] Ibid.

[15] Staff record of Jean Brown in TPH Archival Papers. QSMHC Archives.

[16] Ibid.

[17] Interview with Jean Brown-Fuller, October 2, 1992.
[18] Michael M. Sokal, "James McKeen Cattell and American Psychology in the 1920s," in Joseph Brozek, ed., *Explorations in the History of Psychology* (Lewisburg: Bucknell University Press, 1984), pp. 273-323.
[19] Interview with Jean Brown-Fuller, October 2, 1992.
[20] Ibid.
[21] Ibid.
[22] Ibid.
[23] Ibid.
[24] Jean Brown, "An Inquiry Into the Standardization of the Kohs' Block-Design Test," *Journal of Applied Psychology* 14 (2): 178-81 (April 1930).
[25] Ibid.
[26] Ibid.
[27] Ibid.
[28] Ibid.
[29] Ibid.
[30] Ibid.
[31] TPH Psychology Focus Group, p. 4.
[32] Interview with Jean Brown-Fuller, October 2, 1992.
[33] TPH Report 1926-32.
[34] Interview with Jean Brown-Fuller, October 2, 1992.
[35] Ibid.
[36] Ibid.
[37] Ibid.
[38] Ibid.
[39] TPH Psychology Focus Group, p. 2.
[40] Ibid.
[41] Ibid.
[42] Interview with Bruce Quarrington, September 29, 1992.
[43] TPH Psychology Focus Group, p. 1.
[44] Interview with Bruce Quarrington, September 29, 1992.
[45] Ibid.
[46] TPH Psychology Focus Group, p. 4.
[47] Ibid., p. 30.
[48] Ibid., p. 13.
[49] TPH Psychology Focus Group, p.17 for entire Rubinstein-Melville anecdote.
[50] Interview with Bruce Quarrington, September 29, 1992.
[51] Interview with Harley Wideman, September 23, 1992.
[52] TPH Psychology Focus Group, p. 14.
[53] Interview with Bruce Quarrington, September 29, 1992.
[54] TPH Psychology Focus Group, p. 26.
[55] Ibid., p. 21.
[56] Ibid., p. 21.
[57] Interview with Bruce Quarrington, September 29, 1992, and interview with Harley Wideman, September 23, 1992.

[58] Interview with Bruce Quarrington, September 29, 1992.
[59] Ibid.
[60] TPH Psychology Focus Group, p. 4.
[61] TPH Psychology Focus Group, pp. 1-3 for all dates in this paragraph.
[62] For a list of psychologists involved with TPH see appendix.
[63] Projective testing required the client to read into generic images their personal interpretation of the images' meaning or a story behind them. Ideally, the answers and arrangement of elements would provide insights into a client's psychopathology. To coax projective responses from clients, psychologists entered the realm of therapy.
[64] Hugh McLeod published eleven papers; Bruce Quarrington published approximately six papers in collaboration with other members of Toronto Psychiatric; and Jean Brown published two papers and a number of book reviews during her period at TPH. The psychology group was also involved in a number of off-site studies, the most notable being the Forest Hill Project. In addition to this, a number of masters theses and doctoral dissertations were constructed around new tests being experimented with at TPH, including those of Toby Levinson, Donald Hawser and Harley Wideman. Despite its difficulties with academicians, the psychology group was quite prolific in its publications.
[65] Ibid.
[66] Paul Barbarik, "The Buried Canadian Roots of Community Psychology," *Journal of Community Psychology* 7 (4): 362-67 (1979).
[67] Interview with Bruce Quarrington, September 29, 1992.
[68] Ibid.
[69] Ibid.
[70] Ibid.
[71] Ibid.
[72] Ibid.
[73] Ibid.
[74] George A. Ferguson, "Psychology at McGill," and Luc Granger, "Psychology at Montreal," in Mary J. Wright and Roger C. Myers, eds., *History of Academic Psychology in Canada* (Toronto: C.S. Hogrefe, 1982).
[75] To the best of Hugh McLeod's knowledge.
[76] Interview with Harley Wideman, September 23, 1992.
[77] C. Roger Myers, "Psychology at Toronto," in *History of Academic Psychology in Canada*.
[78] Bruce Quarrington also came from this venue. In his September 29, 1992, interview, he said of his experience in the D.V.A. hospital for tuberculosis victims: "it was largely the psychologist's terrain by default; the psychiatrists tended to avoid the wards because they were scared of catching tuberculosis."
[79] Interview with Bruce Quarrington, September 29, 1992.
[80] Interviews with Drs. Wideman and Quarrington contradict the portrayal of Line presented by Professor Babarik in his previously cited article. Wideman characterized Line as a performer-dreamer, who did not like to organize or implement his ideas. Roger Myers' portrayal of Line in his previously cited work also supports this interpretation, describing lecture notes scribbled on the back of cigarette cases and how Line did not live up to "his early scientific promise." Thus, William Line, whose career spanned both scientific and applied psychology, does not seem to have pleased either of the communities. When viewed in the context of the TPH Psychology Group interviews, his failure appears to be due not to a lack of support from his peers, but rather from a lack of organization and persistence on his part. A more detailed study of his career would shed light on the complex relationships among

governmental, clinical, community, and academic psychology during the formative years of the profession.

[81] TPH Psychology Focus Group, p. 13.

[82] Interview with Bruce Quarrington, September 29, 1992.

[83] TPH Psychology Focus Group, p. 13.

[84] Interview with Harley Wideman, September 23, 1992.

[85] Interview with Bruce Quarrington, September 29, 1992.

[86] Ibid.

[87] Ibid.

[88] Interview with Jean Brown-Fuller, October 2, 1992.

[89] For example, where they either headed psychology teams, or worked without the supervision of a psychiatrists.

[90] All dates in this paragraph collated by Hugh McLeod.

11

Social Work

Mora Skelton[*]

with sections by Jane Smith and Lorraine Williams
and special assistance from Barry Katz, Janet Churnin
and Cyril Greenland[1]

When I first climbed the wooden front steps of the house on College Street to report for work in the Spring of 1947, there was nothing to show that it was not someone's fairly grungy three-storey red brick home. Actually, it was the outpatient clinic of TPH. Inside were John Dewan, the clinic director, Edward Rosen, who was interested in children's psychiatric problems, a few postgraduate medical students studying psychiatry (known to all as PGs), psychologists, and one social service nurse (whose function is discussed in the chapter on nursing). There were *no* social workers as we know them today at TPH at that time or any of the Ontario hospitals treating mental illness.

---

[*]Mora Skelton, M.S.W., University of Toronto, was chief social worker at the TPH mental retardation clinic and at Surrey Place Centre. She became assistant executive director of the Ontario Association for the Mentally Retarded from 1970-1983 (now the Ontario Association for Community Living). Currently retired, she has written a number of articles on mental retardation. Jane Smith, M.S.W., University of Toronto, 1959, worked at the Clarke Institute of Psychiatry from 1966 until her retirement in 1991. A long-time field instructor for the University of Toronto School of Social Work, she has authored a number of articles related to psychiatric social work. She is currently working on housing for persons with psychiatric problems. Lorraine O'Connell Williams, M.S.W., University of Ottawa, established social work at the TPH Forensic Clinic in 1956. She has worked in the psychiatric, correctional, and family casework fields during her career. Author of three books, several articles and pamphlets, she has taught and consulted in Toronto and now has a private practice in marital and individual counselling and runs sessions for marriage preparation courses.

When I returned to work at TPH a second time, in 1962, there were five thriving outpatient clinics connected with the hospital. Hospital and clinic staffs had been increased and there were 24 social workers.

In this chapter, we will try to show you how some of these changes came about. But first, an answer to a frequent question: "What do psychiatric social workers DO?"

Mort Teicher, TPH's first chief social worker, wrote the "Role of a Psychiatric Social Worker"[2] in 1952, but his words are still relevant:

The job of the social worker falls into two broad categories:

1. Intake: The social worker helps the patient and his relatives express feelings about the hospital and clinic services (they may have to work through feelings of anger, shame, panic, before they can really use treatment) and assesses the family's attitude toward the patient as well as the extent to which they and the patient are able and willing to participate in treatment.

2. Continued Service: The social worker helps the patient move into and use the psychiatric hospital or clinic and helps him find his way in the community after discharge.

Social workers were hired in Teicher's time to work on discharge planning and rehabilitation, and thus (hopefully) cut back on recidivism into hospital. The social worker was the member of the treatment team who focused on the world in which patients lived—the world in which they had become mentally ill and to which they would return on discharge. This world might include relatives' attitudes, job pressures (or the pressure of no job), finances, a place to live. With the patient's permission, the social worker would start early in the period of hospitalization to plan with the patient for discharge. Relevant community resources would be used, help sought from relatives or other important persons, and a supportive, continuing follow-up by the social worker planned, so that the patient need not face the stress of return to the community alone.

Later, extensions of this basic service appeared. We worked with groups of various kinds: patients, relatives, or a patient and family together in an effort to harness group strengths. In some settings, there was even an assumption of a primary treatment role.

The Teicher years: 1948–1956

In 1947, the Canadian government established a grant-in-aid program to help universities in Canada expand their education programs for people in mental health disciplines. One reason for this move was concern about the fact that psychiatric patients tended to improve after going to a hospital or clinic, then relapse after returning to an unfavorable environment and be admitted to hospital again. This indicated the need for more attention to rehabilitation, discharge planning, and follow-up.

As part of this program, the University of Toronto obtained a grant to be used jointly by the Department of Psychiatry and the School of Social Work to train postgraduate medical students and social workers—a most forward-looking and unusual pairing of disciplines at a time when no psychiatric or mental health facility in Ontario employed social workers.

In 1947, I was the first social worker to be hired by TPH, and Helen Levine was hired soon afterwards. Modest forerunners of the new look in psychiatric treatment in Ontario, we were relegated to two tiny cubbyholes on the third floor, reached by a winding wooden stair. The fire department decreed that "there must be a fire escape from the third floor," but there was no way of adding one, it seemed.

A strong young man arrived with a rope, knotted at intervals, to be dangled out of our third floor window in case of fire. However, while demonstrating how easy it would be for us and our clients to climb down to the ground outside, the strong young man fell and broke his arm. Helen and I coiled the rope in a corner and prayed for rain.

Things started to roll in 1948 when Aldwyn Stokes, director of TPH, and Harry Cassidy, director of the School of Social Work at the University of Toronto, recruited Morton I. Teicher, a social worker, to help expand the training in mental health disciplines. Teicher set up shop in a large ground-floor room at the outpatient clinic. He was to be our boss, chief social worker for the in- and outpatient departments at TPH. He was young; he was outspoken; he was American, and was soon known to one and all as Mort.

Harry Cassidy had arranged for Teicher's appointment as an assistant professor at the School of Social Work. On the medical side, Aldwyn Stokes obtained an appointment for him in the Faculty of Medicine (unusual at that time for a non-medical person), where Teicher taught in the Department of Psychiatry.

With a foot both in social work and medical camps, and with the continued backing of Stokes (who, according to Teicher, was always open to new ideas), the new man was in a position to expand the social work department in the hospital and clinic and to establish it on a new basis. More than that, he had the funds to do it.

Teicher quotes Stokes as saying: "If you are going to have a good education program, you must have an 'exemplary service' program on which to base it. You must demonstrate high quality patient care and treatment in order to teach it."

Teicher started with the outpatient clinic. He hired Caye Campbell as supervisor of the social work staff. She was an excellent person, loved and respected by her colleagues and students. Together with Ted Rosen and Caye, Teicher developed a child guidance approach. This approach featured a therapist (psychiatrist or psychologist) who saw the child for a series of interviews or play therapy sessions while the social worker saw the family. Using this approach, the clinic grew and prospered.

The Inpatient Social Work Department: 1950–1956

In 1950, Margaret Burns took up her position as supervisor of inpatient social service. Teicher said recently that one of his greatest contributions in those early days was bringing Caye Campbell and Marg Burns to TPH to head up the two departments. Elizabeth (Locke) Morin was imported from Ottawa to serve on one of the two inpatient wards, and I was seconded from outpatients to work on the other. Marg, Elizabeth, and I focused on rehabilitation, discharge planning, and follow-up (the areas of greatest need), and we tried to see all relatives at the time of the patient's admission.

Those were the days before tranquillizing drugs. Patients were given paraldehyde "cocktails," wet packs, or hydrotherapy (continuous running water baths) to control outbursts. Lobotomy was a treatment of last resort, but was still used. Even in a well-run hospital, there was much to disturb a newcomer.

Meanwhile, at the outpatient clinic, Teicher was busy formulating his thoughts and putting them down on paper. One of his most effective articles was "Let's Abolish the Social Service Exchange,"[3] which appeared in 1952 and brought recognition to the TPH social service department. Concerning this article, Teicher says:

> There used to be an institution called the social service exchange. If a social agency or hospital sent in the name of a client, they would get back the names of other agencies to whom the client was known, and they could ask for information about the client... We did it routinely (without the client's consent) at TPH, and, therefore, TPH was listed on the patient's record. In those days— even today—the stigma of the mental hospital was significant.
>
> The more I thought about this, the more upset I became about it. I sat down and wrote an article and I had a hell of a time getting it published. Finally, a very brave editor named David French published this article in the *Social Work Journal*. It was as if the sky had descended upon him. Protest letters poured in to the editor and the board wanted to fire him...
>
> Well, one of the great achievements of my eight years at TPH was that there is no longer a social service exchange in North America. It was really abolished on the basis of that article. That was a great contribution of TPH. The atmosphere that surrounded us at TPH was such that you could do this sort of thing and get support for it. It was a really marvellous atmosphere.

In his spare time, Mort wrestled with the American Association of Psychiatric Social Workers to get them to recognize the University of Toronto School of Social Work program in psychiatric social work. He won.

THE PERRETZ YEARS

by Jane Smith

Edgar Perretz was director of social work at TPH from 1956 to 1960. In addition, he was a professor at the School of Social Work at the University of Toronto and social work advisor to the mental health branch of the Ontario Department of Health. During his time as director, he concentrated on building up the Department of Social Work at TPH by ensuring that each section had an adequate number of trained social workers. The department expanded greatly during his years to approximately 20 (the largest number of social workers employed by a hospital in Toronto at that time).

He also accomplished a great deal by promoting mental health field placements for social work students, as well as helping students obtain mental health grants to pay for their training. Only students in their final (second) year of postgraduate study who were placed for supervised field training in a mental health setting could apply for these grants, which came from the provincial government as part of the Canadian grants-in-aid program. It was understood that the students, in return for a grant, would work in a mental health setting for two years. This was an excellent way to make sure that there were always new, adequately trained graduates available for employment in psychiatric and mental health facilities. As a director, Perretz was well respected by both students and staff for his knowledge, dedication, and warmth.

The Greenland years

by Mora Skelton

From 1960 to 1966, TPH secured the services of a quite unusual man as director of social work.[4] Cyril Greenland was born in Wales, and obtained training and social work experience in England and Scotland. He emigrated to Canada at Edgar Perretz's invitation and worked for two years as chief social worker at the Ontario Hospital at Whitby. In 1960, he was appointed social work advisor to the mental health branch of the Ontario Department of Health and part-time director of social work at TPH. There is some reason to think that this was an unfortunate combination of jobs.

For over 20 years Greenland's "true love of his life" has been studying the phenomenon of violence—perhaps the fatal flaw in our species. He has worked in this field and written extensively about it, giving particular attention to child abuse and neglect, criminal violence, dangerous sexual offenders, family violence, and history of psychiatry.

In his own words, Greenland describes the rewards and difficulties involved in his work at TPH:

> Although I was not appointed social work advisor (at the mental health branch of the Ministry of Health of Ontario) and director of social work at TPH until 1960, my contact with TPH preceded that by about two years. At that time I was the director of social work at the Ontario Hospital at Whitby—since 1958. Since my mandate included research relating to social psychiatry and social work, I lost no time in contacting TPH in search of advice

and contacts. I was, for example, very fortunate in securing the interest and support of Tom Mallinson and Bruce Quarrington, psychologists at TPH.

Tom Mallinson became a partner in my Total Push project which involved the remotivation and rehabilitation of a chronic ward known as Pavilion 2B at Whitby. He helped construct the research and measurement aspects of the study and he also obtained the services of psychology intern Ann Adams (now Alvirez) to work on the project. Pavilion 2B at the Ontario Hospital, Whitby, was an incredibly bleak place. The patients who were not permanently in bed paced up and down pissing in the corners and often naked. Many were emaciated and looked like concentration camp victims. Some were starving because stronger patients were eating their food...

Total Push was carried out over a period of three months. In that time, we did everything in our power to upgrade the ward: physical environment, staffing, cleaning, etc. We approached relatives and relevant community agencies seeking their help. The task was basically concerned with trying to reorient chronic patients to the real world.

This was one of several projects started at that time. Another, concerned with the history of Canadian psychiatry, was a study of Ernest Jones (Freud's disciple and biographer), who lived in Toronto from 1908-1913. The project brought me into touch with Aldwyn Stokes, a fellow Welshman. His interest and support opened many otherwise closed doors. With his encouragement, I presented a paper, titled "Social Class and Schizophrenia"[5] to the TPH Journal Club. This paper was eventually published as a supplement to *Canada's Mental Health*, February 1961.

Since I worked full-time as social work advisor and half-time director of social work at TPH, my contact with the TPH social workers was mostly limited to administrative matters. Also, since my provincial mandate was to recruit social workers for the Ontario Hospitals and to establish social work departments there, the social work supervisors at TPH saw me as a threat to their flock of workers who enjoyed the "hot-house" atmosphere of TPH. Very few of them were interested in roughing it in the bush. The exception was Vincent Castellano, who was courageous enough to go to the Ontario Hospital at Goderich, where he became director of social work.

One anecdote worth recording is the time I organized a chess tournament at TPH. With the support of Professor Stokes, about 20 players, staff and patients, played simultaneous chess against a grand master, whose name I have forgotten. One game was won by TPH, one drawn, and the rest lost. The winner and the drawer were both patients. All the staff, including myself, were quickly defeated.

In summary, my position as part-time director of social work at TPH, was that of a temporary caretaker. When Rita Lindenfield returned from getting her Ph.D. and was nominated as director of social work (after the move to) the Clarke, I resigned as social work advisor to become a research scientist at the Clarke Institute in the social pathology section with Hans Mohr. So ended my brief career at TPH.[6]

Social services 1958–1966

by Mora Skelton and Jane Smith

The inpatient department

Several themes emerge as highlights of this department during the final decade leading up to the move to the Clarke Institute in 1966. By 1966, when the transfer to the Clarke came about, TPH might be said to have come within sight of Stokes' goal: offering exemplary service to patients on the one hand and becoming an outstanding teaching hospital on the other. The social work department was part of it all.

Louise (McDonald) Ellis worked on the women's ward from 1964 to 1966. She remembers "patients were admitted on a day when the social worker was free to see the relatives." Ellis also notes that,

> The social workers were an enthusiastic group and we worked hard. We interviewed patients and relatives routinely and we saw them all. We worked Tuesday and Thursday evenings and one Saturday a month... TPH holds many fond memories for me.

Doreen Cullan, who worked on the women's ward from 1961 to 1964, remembers the prime importance of the interprofessional team at TPH. In her work, she felt responsible to the team first of all and recalls relatively few professional meetings of social workers. Her memory is full of the names of occupational therapists, nurses, and physicians with whom she worked closely. Often they met in the coffee shop in informal case conferences where real decisions were made.

Fairs with picnics and outdoor games were held on the hospital lawn in the summer, when patients and staff mixed together. TPH was small enough for staff to get to know all the patients on the ward. Even people from the business office and the cheery little elevator man greeted patients when they met in the halls.

Both Ellis and Cullan were responsible to Frank Rubinstein, who was in charge of the service side of social work at that time. He was an American, and Cullan remembers that on the day President Kennedy was killed, Frank spoke for his fellow citizens when he said: "This is a personal tragedy for us all."

Aideen Nicholson tells a story about the very first conference she attended after joining the staff at TPH in 1957. She was a social worker, straight from England. At the TPH case conference, with the patient sitting up front and all the staff in attendance, she heard a senior psychiatrist say to the patient: "If you were my son, I would want such and such done." "So, I sat up very straight," says Aideen, "because I wasn't accustomed to clinical discussions getting so personal and my first thought was: 'Look, he has a father who was there... What he wants from a professional is something different.'" In England, the hospital staff had prided themselves on keeping a professional distance, but, after some thought, Aideen decided that she liked the difference at TPH.

Physical expansion of TPH was limited by the size of the hospital building (70 beds) and staff had felt the pinch long before the move to larger quarters in 1966. Yola Kossak, a social work student at TPH from September 1959 to May 1960, recalls that she and another student shared a desk with two part-time staff. A hasty retreat was required of the other three if anyone was to have an interview in privacy.

Everyone interviewed remembered Stokes fondly and spoke of his gentleness and scholarly approach. He seemed to know all the staff by name, and had an intimate knowledge of the programs being carried out, both inside the hospital and in the various clinics attached to it. "He was the Great White Father," says Doreen.

RITA LINDENFIELD 1956–66

An outstanding figure at inpatients during those ten final years was Rita Lindenfield. From 1956–59 she had been supervisor of inpatient social service. She left to obtain her Ph.D. at the University of Chicago and returned to TPH from 1961–66 as consultant on social work education and research. She was also a clinical teacher at the Department of Psychiatry and assistant professor at the University of Toronto. After the move to the Clarke, she became social worker-in-chief there.

At TPH in those final years, Rita was head of the teaching side of social work. Almost everyone was either teaching or being taught, often both at once. Rita, with senior psychiatrist Mary Jackson, was engaged in teaching the residents (PGs) as well as nurses and social work students, and supervising the teaching of social work staff. Airi (Leppanen) Giffen, a social work student at TPH at that time, says Rita was patient and generous in her help to students. Lindenfield was also a writer and her articles, which have stood up well for more than 20 years, speak clearly for her.

One of the best is "The Teaching Program in a Psychiatric Hospital: Implications for Patients, Trainees and Staff."[7] In it, she takes time to consider what it must mean to a patient to be interviewed before a group of students. She states that patients should be *asked* to take part, not merely *told* that such a session will take place, and asks what effect the frequent turnover of trainees has on a patient who may have painfully learned to trust one person now removed. (All this was written in 1965, before the day of patients' rights, patient advocacy, and the threat of litigation.) Similarly, she considers the problem of trainees (for TPH taught postgraduate doctors, nurses, social work students) who have a desire to succeed and help, but are handicapped by their lack of knowledge.

Stokes recruited the White Cross Guild, a volunteer group, around 1959. In an article titled "Our Volunteers—Dilemma or Delight,"[8] Lindenfield suggests that if an organization plans to use volunteers at all, it should be frank with them and include them in planning. She writes, "Let us, staff and volunteers alike, credit each other with as much good will, as much common sense and high motives as we claim for ourselves."

Fay Aldridge, a group worker, joined the TPH social work staff from 1957–1959. She established a group program where she put Lindenfield's theory into practice by including volunteers in psychodrama, art therapy, and recreation groups.

In "Working with Other Professions"[9] Lindenfield says: "Some social workers seem eager to break with their past and take on a range of tasks and responsibilities normally seen as the province of other [helping] professions." (This was a trend I well remember.) Lindenfield felt any crossover of skills and responsibilities without the support of appropriate training was an error. "The helping professions (teachers, social workers, clergymen, Public Health nurses, psychiatrists) do overlap," continues Lindenfield. She adds,

> Our skills tend to become a blend...the danger is that knowledge may be annexed rather than integrated and as a result, our skills may resemble a synthetic (product), rather than a synthesis. Basically what is needed is an honest exploration and clarification of the concerns, knowledge and responsibilities of all the helping professions...then, and only then, can we work with those professional people whose contribution is different—but no less worthwhile—than ours.[10]

It must have taken Lindenfield real courage to express an opinion so unpopular among some of her colleagues.

THE CHILDREN'S OUTPATIENT CLINIC

by Jane Smith

Thirty-four Grosvenor Street was the location of the children's unit of TPH, which opened as a separate clinic in 1958. It was an old, three-storey red brick building not far from the firehall, which kids coming to the clinic loved to pass and see the fire engines inside.

I arrived at the children's unit in October, 1959, at which time Edward Rosen was the director and Catherine ("Caye") Campbell was the social work supervisor. In addition to Campbell, there were four social workers when I arrived (three caseworkers and one group worker—Charles ["Chuck"] Fine, a classmate of mine). Little did I know that I would soon get involved in doing group work myself, as group work was just starting at the clinic.

Customarily, a psychiatrist would see the child, and the social worker would see the parents. A condition of treatment was that the family got involved. This model made the roles very clear and the roles were seen as equally important, which nicely took care of interprofessional rivalries. We also saw a number of children from the Children's Aid Society, both for assessment and treatment. At one point, a group was set up for Children's Aid kids, with a worker from the Children's Aid and the clinic group worker, Chuck.

Many things stand out in my mind about my six years at the children's clinic, including the respect and dignity with which everyone was treated and the exciting and innovative new approaches which were tried. There was a psychodrama group for kids, several children's activity groups, and a mothers' and fathers' group, although these were not all run at the same time. As well, two of the social workers were involved with Rosen in running a group for parents of children with learning disabilities. He worked with the kids and the social workers with the parents. The emphasis was on assessing and diagnosing learning disabilities and recognizing this group as a distinct clinical entity. This was probably the first group treatment of its kind in Toronto.

When Paul Steinhauer, a psychiatrist, joined the staff, he instituted family therapy. He had received extensive training in the United States in this type of treatment, which was new in Toronto at that time. Two residents and two social workers were involved initially, though the number was expanded later. Nora Wilson (who worked at the clinic from 1963 to 1966) and I were the first two social workers to get involved.

This program consisted of three hours per week for one year. One resident and one social worker would interview the family, while the other resident and social worker were behind a one-way mirror, with Steinhauer. Then we would switch for the second hour, and in the final hour we would all meet and discuss what had happened, with Steinhauer as supervisor. Sometimes Steinhauer would come into the room in the middle of an interview to tell us what we were doing wrong. All of us found this quite traumatic, and so it was stopped. All the same, I will always be grateful to Steinhauer for his excellent teaching, which helped me immensely in my career at the Clarke Institute later on.

Most of us had the opportunity, after three years' experience, to become field instructors for the School of Social Work, which was another giving and getting experience. Teaching by Caye Campbell, the social work supervisor, was outstanding. Not only was she a brilliant clinician, but she had a great capacity for challenging and supporting staff at the same time. In fact, it was because of her reputation that I applied for the job.

Several anecdotes stand out in my mind. One concerns a patient of child psychiatrist Edward Rosen. The child had left his pet fish in the doctor's office on a Friday afternoon, so Rosen took the fish home to look after until the child returned for his appointment the next week. Someone found this a bit odd, but when asked about it Rosen said, "What kind of a doctor would I be if I couldn't even keep a fish alive?" Rosen also helped generate thought and conversation at our educational seminars by reading *I and Thou* by Martin Buber,[11] after which we would sit around and discuss it.

Then there was our little orchestra with banjos, guitars, bongo drums, etc., for lunchtime recreation either in the basement or, in the summer, in the park. Most of us have happy memories of the basement where we went for coffee breaks or lunch time if desired. We all took turns being responsible for supplying the coffee and cookies.

The six years were indeed pleasant ones, with the high staff morale which allows one to be free and creative in one's job because one's energies are focused on the work at hand. It was an exciting time to be in social work, with lots of innovative and new treatments being tried, in an atmosphere of respect and encouragement.

Adult outpatients' clinic

Barry Katz was supervisor of social work at the adult outpatient clinic from 1958 (when the adult and children's clinic separated) to 1966 (when TPH and its clinics moved to the Clarke). Don Coates was in charge, and referrals were accepted from physicians, family and child care agencies, and nursing services. The clinic was located at the corner of College and Elizabeth Streets, near to TPH.

Said Nora Wilson:
> I had my second-year student placement at the old outpatient department at TPH. At the end of my first year, my one request was that I not go into a psychiatric placement for my second year...because I was scared out of my wits. But that is where I ended up, with Barry Katz as my supervisor and was just absolutely enthralled... I lost my fear of the mentally ill somewhere during the year and ended up working in that field for the next 20 years...

Barry said: "I think that I'm being honest when I say that I consider this one of the highlights in my social work career. It was a time of great learning for me." He added,
> ...what impressed me most was the relatively classless nature of the place. There was a real sense of equality among the various professions as they worked together in the OPD clinic. Social workers ran group therapy sessions, saw patients on an individual basis, and saw families. Social workers were part of the

training process, not only of social work students, but of postgraduate doctors and others.

The other thing that impressed me about the place was the erudition and intelligence of the staff. I don't think that I ever worked with so many bright people anywhere, before or since. I am thinking, for example, of Stephen Neiger, a psychologist with a medical degree. When he was a psychologist on our staff, one of his major interests was the study of sexuality. I still remember that because he was coming out with stuff which is common knowledge now, but this was back in the 1960s. We were not so liberated about these things then.

One of the most interesting cases I can remember was that of a young man with Gilles de la Tourette's Syndrome. We always knew when this young man walked into the clinic because the air would turn blue with his swearing—a symptom of his condition. One day his mother came to see me. She said that her son had been hired as a disc jockey at a radio station. She was scared stiff because if he was presenting a program of music...all of a sudden his condition might take over and he'd be in trouble with the Radio Commission. I don't remember what I did (about the job), but eventually he was not hired.

Don Coates had a great interest in the social part of psychiatry. He was very much involved in what was going on in the community, and we had weekly seminars where we actually brought in (speakers) from the community.

Barry expressed an opinion about the move to the Clarke in 1966 which was echoed again and again by people we interviewed—particularly by staff who had been working in the small, semi-isolated clinics of TPH:

We lost a great deal when we moved over to a much larger site at the Clarke Institute, because [the clinic] had been like an extended family... Once [your workplace] reaches a certain size you lose the informality, the ease of communication, that we used to have at TPH.

I was so upset [that last day] at the clinic that when I got up to leave I ripped my pants—a great big rip. The only way I could leave the place was by borrowing a raincoat from one of my students.

Otherwise, Barry would still be there, in the building at the corner of College and Elizabeth streets.

Daycare

The TPH daycare clinic opened in 1958 in an old church building on College Street, just a few steps from TPH itself.

Janet Churnin, a young social worker from England, joined the staff later that year and stayed till 1962. Janet says that she started work "in a daze" because she was new to Canada and new to the field of psychiatry, though she had had experience in a hospital setting. She learned on the job.

The clinic was a small operation, headed by Arthur L. Jones, and assisted by one other psychiatrist, Marvin Miller. There were two nurses, plus occupational therapists. Jones saw patients and families at intake then called in other staff members as seemed appropriate. As Janet recalls it, the atmosphere was friendly and informal, with staff members working well together. No one wore a uniform.

The clinic served approximately 20 patients at any one time. Patients were referred by TPH or one of its clinics, or a variety of outside agencies. Most patients attended five days a week from 9 to 4, although a few came less often. Luncheon was served and sometimes staff and patients ate together. Insulin therapy (thought at the time to be helpful) and ECT were used, as well as psychotherapy. Janet remembers that, due to shortage of staff, she was often required to restrain patients during ECT.

The day program was planned by occupational therapists, but once a week Janet would take a group of patients to the art gallery or to the museum, or she would hold a discussion group on books. Her chief job was counselling patients and families, or assisting patients to find work or recreation.

Once a week, all staff met together for case discussion, and all staff attended rounds at the hospital at twelve o'clock. When indicated, daycare staff attended other case conferences and both in- and outpatients.

Setting up social work at the forensic clinic

by Lorraine M. Williams

It was 1956 and I was deeply satisfied with my revolutionary position as the only full-time member of a treatment team for the rehabilitation of women offenders. I worked out of a converted gardener's residence on the grounds of Toronto's sombre Mercer Reformatory for Women.

However, I knew that marriage and the ofttimes 24-hour-a-day work with female inmates would not be compatible. With a September 1956 wedding date getting close, I began searching around for a more nine-to-five position. By sheer luck, as I was doing some research at the University of Toronto School of Social Work Library, an ad on its bulletin board seemed to offer everything I was looking for:

> Wanted—Social Worker with Master's Degree...

That was me, an energetic 1955 grad of the University of Ottawa's (St. Pat's College) widely respected School of Social Welfare.

> ...to set up Social Work Department in new outpatient clinic of Toronto Psychiatric Hospital...

My social work career up to then had been exactly that—setting up new services that didn't exist before.

> ...to work with patients who have been in conflict with the law and/or have problems in the sexual area...

My two previous positions had been working with delinquent young boys and then women serving sentences under two years. With both sets of clients, problems in sexuality cropped up.

> a knowledge of psychiatric theory...

My theoretical classroom instruction plus fieldwork in Brooklyn, New York, and Toronto had included heavy indoctrination in Freudian psychoanalytic theory—with Adler and Jung thrown in.

> Male applicant.

The one qualification I didn't have, but that wasn't going to stop me.

I sent a letter to a Mr. Peter Thomson (I didn't realize he was a doctor at that time) in August 1956 outlining my qualifications. After a relaxed interview, in which I was impressed by his total unpretentiousness, he admitted he'd specified a man because (to paraphrase) he was concerned that the symptomology of some of the cases referred to us could be too indelicate for a woman to hear. Since most of my clients were in prison for prostitution, there wasn't much I hadn't heard at that stage. However, Peter Thomson's gentleness, thoughtfulness, and sensitivity, as revealed in that concern—plus my sense that it reflected more his British experience than any knowledge of 1950s North American womanhood—convinced me that the forensic clinic was the next setting for me.

And it all turned out the way I anticipated! Peter Thomson, the first director, was open to listening to and learning from staff members who were definitely wet behind the ears, but were also articulate, intelligent, and compassionate. Every six months we got a new crop of PGs who, by being immersed in the treatment of patients with sexual disorders, had to encounter their personal understanding of human sexuality. In their eagerness to learn, they refreshed and renewed those of us on the core staff. This new creation, the forensic clinic, was making history. Scores of nursing ("second-year students only," their protective instructors mandated) and medical students, social agencies, and other "community resources" (as social work parlance had it) visited and sat wide-eyed in our conference room as we described our polymorphously perverse patients in cool clinical terms—many of which were utterly foreign to these products of the conservative 1950s.

The outpatient forensic clinic was a rarity in its day: a multi-disciplined therapeutic setting where the traditional hierarchical structure of psychiatrist, psychologist, and social worker held little sway. Our research director, Gordon Watson, held a postgraduate degree in divinity (not your normal appointee in any setting heavily oriented to Freudian interpretation of reality). Peter Thomson consulted with all of us, both when the clinic first opened and later on when new approaches were introduced.

This openness to all our ideas and faith in us tapped our productivity and imaginations. For me it was a revelation, having come from an authoritarian institution where change was seen as undermining the establishment. Thomson left to me, his 23-year-old chief social worker, such foundational tasks as devising an intake system, developing a questionnaire which the research director would later use to obtain a profile of our patient population, and initiating some experiments in group therapy for different patient populations such as adolescents (he was aware that I was probably the only staffer at that time who had experience in conducting therapeutic groups).

He endorsed the practice of weekly team conferences after initial assessments, where every team member shared findings and made specific treatment recommendations. Assignment of patients to particular staff members was based on the patient's needs, not on any closed concept of "The Doctor treats the patient, the Psychologist does the testing, and the Social Worker arranges for financial assistance or other environmental resources." That's not to say that those traditional assignments didn't occur. They often did, but nobody was stuck in some stereotypical role. Often the social worker or psychologist was selected as the prime therapist.

One of my most colourful patients was a female impersonator-transvestite (an activity forbidden by the criminal code at the time). Married to a committed lesbian, he seemed to have a perfect equation to an unusual life style. Treatment with this client consisted mainly in listening to very unusual stories about his unusual clientele, trying to teach him some discretion about where and when he made his sorties in drag, and listening to all the pain underneath. More often, I worked with spouses, children, or relatives of patients. Often, I'd go to court to give testimony (something I was used to from my Mercer Reformatory days) or would collaborate in pre-sentence reports.

After our first year, Thomson obtained funding to hire another part-time social worker (Airi Giffen) and then another full-time one (Val Hartmann). Airi joined the staff early in 1957 and worked with us for approximately one year. Val came at the beginning of 1958, took over as supervisor of social work when I left the clinic at the end of that year, and continued in this post until his untimely death in the early 1980s.

As my staff grew, so did other departments. Ed Turner, who had been one of our postgraduate medical students, came on staff full-time, and was eventually to succeed Peter Thomson as director. Harry Hutchison bolstered psychologist Daniel Paitich, who initially had been holding the fort alone. Harry introduced us to the intricacies of the polygraph machine, of which most of us were highly sceptical (and may be to this day). Many of the new staff had backgrounds in criminology and other areas, so our pool of knowledge deepened.

We tapped that pool quite often. Thomson instituted our own Study Club. I think it met once every two weeks. We each took turns preparing a particular topic of our choice, and could invite guest specialists if we wished. Thus, our "in-service training" was rich and personal. Thomson himself was involved in his training analysis at the time, as he neared the completion of his psychoanalytic training, and gave many enlightening presentations on Freud's selected papers and case studies.

For a clinic working with both sexual and forensic issues, Freudian theory gave us a conceptual framework. One part-time psychiatrist relished presenting patient histories with the most bizarre symptoms imaginable. Psychologist Dan Paitich digested research papers, presenting findings of projects we would normally never have known about. Coming from an undergraduate background in philosophy, I had a particular interest in the ethical implication of our patients' behaviour, so I often used my turn to bring in experts with humanistic backgrounds.

Finally, I recall the patients. They were mainly men. Some were in trouble with the law, some privately sought help. Some, for whom outpatient treatment was part of their court sentence, were initially resentful. Outside colleagues warned us: "Compulsory treatment never works." We learned that wasn't true. Patients learned to trust us, to know we cared, that we weren't voyeurs of their symptoms, but often as puzzled as they were, that we were determined to help them if that's what they really wanted. And help them we did, from young men with homosexual panic desiring to be heterosexual, to men seemingly unable to break the hold of exhibitionistic urges, to badly shaken parents (mostly mothers) of adolescents convicted of making obscene phone calls. These people persevered through long and painful therapeutic processes to attain some degree of "normality." It was their perseverance that gave staff the conviction that the forensic clinic was a service not only needed for the good of society, but more importantly for the restoration of those patients who, until the founding of the clinic, had no place else to go for help.

CONCLUSION

That was TPH as we remember it. Everyone was learning and teaching and trying to solve problems: staff and patients alike. The hospital with its clinics resembled a strong tree with sturdy branches, each at a comfortable distance one from the other, balancing the others. I do not know how much was gained by pulling everyone together under one roof at the Clarke Institute, but I do know that something seems to have been lost.

ENDNOTES

[1] Unless otherwise indicated, all quotes from former TPH staff are taken from personal communication with Mora Skelton during summer 1992 and a transcript of a Social Workers Focus Group convened May 1992. Those present were Fay Aldridge, Jane (Jackson) Bright, Louise (MacDonald) Ellis, Cyril Greenland, Barry Katz, Aideen Nicholson, Mora Skelton, Jane Smith, Morton I. Teicher, Nora Wilson. Other former TPH students and staff who contributed their time to producing this chapter are Vincent Castellano, Janet Churnin, Doreen Cullan, Airi (Leppanen) Giffen, Yola Kossak, Rita Lindenfield, Elizabeth (Locke) Morin and Lorraine M. Williams. The work

of Catherine Campbell, Chuck Fine, Val Hartmann, Helen Levin and Frank Rubinstein was remembered by their colleagues. All assistance has been greatly appreciated.

[2] Morton I. Teicher, "The Role of the Psychiatric Social Worker," *Canadian Welfare* 27 (8): 14-20 (March 1952).

[3] Morton I. Teicher, "Let's Abolish the Social Service Exchange," *Social Work Journal* 33 (1): 28-31 (January 1952).

[4] Some idea of his important and varied career can be gained from an interview reported in *Pioneers of Mental Health and Social Change, 1930-1989*, by Djuwe Joe Blom and Sam Sussman (London, ON: Third Eye, 1989). This book features a series of interviews with four persons of importance in the field of mental health and social change in Canada. Greenland's subject was "Strategies of Social Change."

[5] Cyril Greenland, "Social Class and Schizophrenia," *Canada's Mental Health* 9 (6): supp. 1-12 (June 1961).

[6] Letter from Cyril Greenland, August 28, 1992. Greenland's literary output has been considerable. In his book, Sam Sussman mentions thirty-five articles and reports written by Greenland. I have come upon a listing of one hundred and fifty reports, book reviews, articles, books written by him between 1945 and 1985. Of those, thirty-nine were written during his tenure at TPH.

[7] Rita Lindenfield, "The Teaching Program in a Psychiatric Hospital: Implications for Patients, Trainees and Staff," *Canadian Medical Association Journal* 92 (14): 752-55 (April 1965).

[8] Rita Lindenfield, "Our Volunteers — Dilemma or Delight?" *Ontario Mental Health Services* n.v.: 21-22 (November-December 1964).

[9] Rita Lindenfield, "Working with Other Professions," *The Social Worker* Centennial Issue: 175-81 (September 1967).

[10] Ibid.

[11] Martin Buber, *I and Thou*, 2d ed. (Edinburgh: T. and T. Clark, 1937).

12

Occupational Therapy

Judith Friedland[*]

There was certainly something extraordinary about occupational therapy at TPH. When asked what made it so unique, people have been hard pressed to respond; a look of puzzlement comes over their faces. However, the look is soon replaced with a knowing smile and eventually the words come out. "It was just a very special place to be in. You knew you were in the best place for psychiatry, and in the best place for psych OT."

When asked to elaborate on what made TPH "the best," many common themes emerged. For one thing, it was a small teaching hospital, adjacent to other important teaching hospitals and to the University of Toronto itself. In addition, the patients were generally at an early stage in their illness and so there was great hope that a difference could be made. There was a chance to help them get well before they became chronically ill and had to be sent elsewhere. As a teaching institute, the environment provided a great learning experience for all its staff. Throughout most— but not all—of TPH's history, psychiatry was itself a much revered specialty area and the staff that had been hired to work at the hospital (including the occupational therapists) were considered to be among the brightest in their fields. So it was likely this mix of geography, of people, and of status that was responsible for the special ambience that was TPH.

"Psych OT" (as it continues to be called) was a very prestigious field to be in at that time (in contrast to the situation today, when more people choose to work in the area of physical medicine). There was a tolerance and respect for the ambiguity and the lack of concrete principles in

---

[*]Judith Friedland, Ph.D., O.T. (C) is an Associate Professor in the Faculty of Medicine, University of Toronto and is Chair of the Department of Occupational Therapy. She was an occupational therapist in the day hospital at TPH from 1961 to 1963.

psychiatry, or as Farrar put it: "...that there are no absolute standards in psychiatry."[1] There was an implicit challenge in the need to think each case through. There was also a definite pride in the contribution made by OT to the care and treatment of people with psychiatric disorders. One reason for the preferential position of psych OT lay in the endorsement and promotion of the profession by influential psychiatrists, particularly Adolf Meyer in the United States and C.K. Clarke in Canada.

Meyer, who was professor of psychiatry at Johns Hopkins University, was responsible for disseminating the practice of occupational therapy in the United States. In 1922, he told the Fifth Annual Meeting of the National Society for the Promotion of Occupational Therapy: "The proper use of time in some helpful and gratifying activity appeared to me a fundamental issue in the treatment of any neuropsychiatric patient".[2] He was a great proponent of "occupation" therapy (as he termed it) and saw it as a means of promoting the patient's adjustment through modifying unhealthy adaptations and developing healthy habits. He also saw that one of the by-products of occupation was that it decreased the need for physical restraint.

Closer to home and in the same year, C.K. Clarke was advocating occupational therapy in the Ontario Hospitals for the Insane. Clarke was much influenced by Richard M. Bucke, superintendent of the asylum in London, Ontario, who had very strong views on the value of occupation, and by Joseph Workman, the earlier superintendent of the Toronto Asylum, also a forceful advocate of occupation.[3] Writing of his experiences at the Rockwood Asylum in Kingston, Clarke noted that non-restraint had become an established practice and credited this fact to the use of occupation. Clarke was careful to state that:

> No one comforted himself with the belief that occupation was a panacea for all the ills that the mind is heir to, but we did realize that intelligently supervised occupation was a tremendous factor not only in aiding cure in recent cases, but in making happy and improving the most unfortunate class in our community.[4]

Indeed, early records of occupational therapy attendance at TPH suggest that it was considered a panacea for almost all of the patients. A 1934[5] report noted that 85 percent of all patients admitted to the hospital received occupational therapy.

When Farrar became the first superintendent of the Toronto Psychiatric Hospital in 1925, he likely brought with him a conviction of the importance of occupation. Indeed, when Farrar wrote about treatment for war neuroses and psychoses, he had stated that "Congenial and systematic occupation should be given foremost place in any scheme of treatment. Idleness...should be reduced to the uttermost minimum."[6] And in his paper on *Rehabilitation in Nervous and Mental Cases Among Ex-Soldiers*, he noted that

> There is the benefit of occupation as such, common to practically all cases; and there is the possible benefit of an awakened and sustained interest in an employment which is new, and which affords a pleasing relief from a former distasteful or humdrum occupation. Here we have occupation-therapy passing over into vocational re-training, with the latter perhaps completing the cure begun by the former.[7]

Psychiatrists and neurologists helped to establish the profession of occupational therapy. The first course to train war aides in occupational therapy was set up in Toronto at the behest of Herbert Haultain in 1918.[8] The first president of the Canadian Association of Occupational Therapists was Goldwin Howland, a prominent neurologist.[9] Howland, together with the then dean of the Faculty of Medicine, Alexander Primrose, helped set up the first two-year course at the University of Toronto. For many years, the Honourary Advisory Council of the Canadian Association of Occupational Therapists had on its roster such illustrious names as Clarence Hincks, C.B. Farrar, and Wilder Penfield.[10]

At an open meeting of the Occupational Therapy Society at Government House in 1925, Farrar was among those who spoke and *The Evening Telegram* reported his comments the following day:

> Next to proper housing and proper feeding, occupational therapy is the most important factor in the cure of nervous patients. The rest cure, so long ordered for these patients, has been supplanted by work, and occupational therapy provides this most necessary employment and effects the cure.[11]

In 1933, Herbert A. Bruce, lieutenant governor of Ontario, in his address to the third annual convention of the Canadian and Ontario Occupational Therapy Associations[12] cited Plato's view that in every man and woman is born the instinct to make and to do. Veterans of two world wars had shown that, though maimed and suffering, men still aspired to make and to do. Waxing still more eloquent, Bruce went on to quote Voltaire who said that "Not to be occupied and not to exist amount to the same thing. One must give oneself all the occupation one can to make life supportable in this world."[13]

Thus it was no surprise to find that when TPH was established, OT was among the first of the departments to be created.[14] The purpose of OT was to provide a living laboratory where behavioral observations could be made, occupations engaged in, and new skills taught. The observations would be used to contribute to diagnosis, to complement other assessments (e.g., in psychology), to monitor progress, and to influence discharge plans.

The OT department at TPH was apparently established on March 1, 1927, but it is unclear who the first "occupationalist" was. It may have been a Marjorie Hoch, a woman who would likely have trained in the war aides program provided by the University of Toronto in 1918 to treat returning war veterans.[15] When the need for services to veterans diminished, the aides were dispersed to various mental hospitals in the province (including TPH). Kathleen Robb (Reed) was appointed in 1929 and Gwynneth Schofield (Thompson) in 1930.[16] Both had been graduates of the two-year course in occupational therapy which had been newly established at the University of Toronto in 1926 in the Department of University Extension. Kay Robb remembers interning at TPH while Hoch was in charge. At the end of the internship, Farrar, who took a great interest in all of his staff, called her in and asked if she would like to come back after she graduated.

There was a quick turnover in staff during the Depression years as most women did not continue to work after they married; for some, this was by choice, for others it was because they were not allowed to work in a government job if their spouses had work.[17] As employees of the Ontario Department of Health, these women could be transferred to any Ontario Hospital as needed, for example, to Brockville, to London or to Kingston, etc. In many cases, they stayed only a year in any one place before being sent on or leaving of their own accord. However, in 1933, Helen Primrose LeVesconte was appointed director of the department of occupational therapy at TPH and she remained for 12 years. The staff record for 1934[18] indicates that her duties included: "direction of the occupational therapy department, provision of instruction in OT to postgraduate affiliate nurses, and assisting in the supervision of Occupational Therapy in the Ontario Hospitals"—all for the sum of $1300 per annum! (It is nice to know that in the same report she was recommended for an increase in pay.) Peg Langley (Lewis) joined Helen in 1935 and remained with her until she entered the army and went overseas in 1941.[19] It was during this extended period of leadership by Helen LeVesconte that the standards and tone of the department at TPH (and indeed, most would say, of the whole profession) were set.

A certain dignity and sense of purpose seemed to permeate all that Helen LeVesconte did. Perhaps it had something to do with the privilege of her class which had encouraged her to think broadly, to be creative, and to engage those who could be helpful to the cause. Her ancestors were among the Huguenots who fled to the Channel Islands in the 17th century. Her great-great-grandfather had been an officer in the Royal Navy and fought in the Battle of Trafalgar. When her great grandfather emigrated to Canada, he was given 500 acres of crown land on the Trent River. Her grandfather served as a justice of the peace, and her father was a graduate of the University of Toronto and Osgoode Hall.[20] (The social origin of LeVesconte's mother is unknown.)

LeVesconte was educated in Toronto at Havergal College and the Margaret Eaton School (for domestic science) and upon graduation she taught physical education. Always something of an activist, she realized the dearth of athletic opportunities available to girls at that time and soon organized girls' championship intercollegiate basketball.[21] During this period she was also working in the Voluntary Aide Dispatch (VAD) at the Spadina Military Hospital. Here, she struck up a friendship with Amelia Earhart who had come to Toronto during World War I in order to engage in work for the war effort.[22] It was through her work at the Spadina Military Hospital that LeVesconte became interested in the value of occupation as therapy. Thus she was more than ready to enroll when the first program in occupational therapy at the University of Toronto opened its doors in 1926.

Within months of graduating, LeVesconte assumed the position of director of occupational therapy at the Ontario Hospital, Kingston. Here, she would have enjoyed something of the legacy of C.K. Clarke's days at Rockwood (which by then had changed its name to Kingston Hospital). Clarke had remarked upon the nature of the therapists who carried out this work, that the best "possessed intelligence, education and enthusiasm..."[23] Each of these qualities could be applied to Helen LeVesconte, who even then served as a strong and dedicated leader of her profession.

As director of OT at TPH, LeVesconte had an office on the fourth floor. The office evidently had only one chair; apparently when you came into LeVesconte's office—you stood! One former student reported that "When you worked under Helen you never sat down, so she didn't need any more than one seat. If you came in with creases in the back of your skirt [it meant] you'd been sitting down, so we quick fast pressed our skirts if we could before she saw us."[24] Coming from a military family, Helen LeVesconte had a strong sense of order, discipline, and thoroughness, but at the same time she was warm and compassionate and had a fine sense of humour. When she left TPH in 1945, LeVesconte had developed a strong and loyal following, particularly among the many students who had attended lectures and fulfilled their internship requirements at TPH. She left the hospital to become the full-time supervisor of the course in occupational therapy at the University of Toronto—a position she had already held part-time since 1934. In her letter of resignation[25] she acknowledged Farrar's support and stated that: "The encouragement and cooperation which is given here is a constant inspiration."

Peg Langley (Lewis) joined LeVesconte in 1935. She remembers being thrilled to be at TPH and finding the work very interesting,[26] leaving in 1941 for a posting overseas. Mary (Clark) Ray, who had served overseas during the war, took over from LeVesconte in 1945 and was in charge for a short time until she left to join her husband in Peace River.[27] Myrtle Mackey (MacArthur) was then asked to be director and she remembers calling LeVesconte to ask for reassurance that she could do the job, since in her eyes it was *the* job to have.[28] Her respect for the position was due primarily to her respect for LeVesconte; she simply could not imagine herself sitting in LeVesconte's chair. Sheila (Dunn) Irvine took over as director in 1946. Sheila had interned at TPH and knew that was where she wanted to work. She remained as director for 20 years, moving the department from the fourth floor to the ground floor, then to the "old church," and finally to the Clarke. Looking back she says, "I adored the work. I just loved it... It was *the* place to be."[29] Soon after Irvine took over, Aldwyn B. Stokes was appointed professor of psychiatry and director of TPH. His experience in England, and in particular his work at Mill Hill during World War II, had made him another strong supporter of occupational therapy. When he addressed the 19th annual convention of the Canadian Association of Occupational Therapists in 1949, he spoke of the prisoners of war from Dunkirk and pointed out that "it was for the occupational therapists to return them to useful places in society."[30] Mary Jackson also joined TPH during this period. She had a profound respect for OT and supported the department when she had management responsibilities.

In LeVesconte's day, OT was carried out at the bedside and in the two sunrooms on the fourth floor. Throughout the 1930s and most of the

1940s, male and female patients were treated separately in their respective sunrooms, the men having access to a carpentry workshop in the north sunroom. There was some mixing of the two groups for certain activities until eventually the OT department, which had begun to take over the hallway between the two sunrooms, was no longer segregated on the basis of gender. In her efforts to occupy patients as fully as possible and to simulate real life, LeVesconte insisted that therapists plan programs for evenings and weekends, take turns running dances, keep the department open on Saturday mornings, and help to serve Christmas dinner. This extensive programming continued throughout the years at TPH.

Toward the end of the 1950s, the OT department moved to the "old church" and, along with the new day hospital, the building took on a lively and welcoming presence. Although OT was still offered on the wards and in the sunrooms, patients were now eager to "get their clothes and be able to go over to OT"—if not for the sake of OT then at least just to get off the ward! Most patients seemed to enjoy their daily outings to the department and the opportunity it afforded them to engage in a more normal day.

Over the years a great variety of activities were carried out in OT. Although all therapists regarded the use of purposeful activity as essential, in much the way that Clarke and Meyer did, they were often not very skilled in crafts. Some therapists used this deficiency to advantage in working with clients who were themselves skilled craftworkers; those patients showed the therapists what to do. Other therapists developed new programs: they organized sports, set up pre-vocational tasks, or ran socializing programs. Some of TPH's best therapists were actually urged *not* to attempt certain crafts (e.g., weaving) with their patients as it only led to more work for others when they had to undo the mess that was created![31]

In the early days, crafts were often used in very specific ways. For example, repetition of the same action in weaving was thought to be calming, working with clay was (and still is) a good medium for projection; good concentration was needed to do leatherwork or carpentry. Although therapists never felt particularly threatened and none were ever harmed, everyone remembers being very careful with the tools they used, always taking a "count" before patients left to go back to the ward, and being sure that no potentially dangerous tools were missing.

The quality of what the patients produced was not of great importance. Good work, of course, boosted a patient's self-esteem, but developing a therapeutic relationship and motivating the patient to become engaged in activity generally took priority. Crafts were used precisely because they were different—that is, they were *not* something that the patient had done before. In this way, the therapist and patient worked together in a somewhat conflict-free arena (without carrying any baggage from the past) to form their relationship for the future. Once the relationship was formed and the patient's interest had been sparked, the work in OT could move on to developing skills.

Skills in the activities of daily living (ADL) were often a focus of treatment for the women, as most of them would be going home again to care for themselves, their homes, and their families. Men, by contrast, often did not need these skills, as most would be going home to be looked after by someone (e.g., a wife, mother, or daughter). As for work skills, some activities did provide a form of pre-vocational testing, but there was no vocational rehabilitation at TPH. The relatively short length of stay made such a program neither feasible nor, in many cases, necessary.[32] Almost all patients were deficient in social interaction skills. No matter how successful the "medical" treatments were, most patients still needed to regain the social skills lost during their illness, and many patients needed to learn skills the illness had prevented them from developing in the first place.

Outings into the community were a good way for therapists to help patients to work on social skills. For the patients, it was almost always something to look forward to, a chance to take on all the trappings of normalcy, if only for a brief period of time, and to test themselves in the world to which they would soon return. Blocks of tickets to Famous Players Theatres were easy to come by; there was always window shopping at Eaton's College Street store, swimming at the YMCA, walks through Queen's Park, bowling, visits to the Royal Ontario Museum and the Art Gallery of Ontario, and outings to the Orange Parade or Santa Claus Parade. Kathleen Reed remembers taking a group through Eaton's College Street and having to cancel an order placed by one of her patients for a 96-piece set of dinner dishes.[33] Therapists always worried about "losing" patients on outings. Myrtle Mackey (MacArthur) remembers losing a patient one very hot summer day. Worrying that she shouldn't waste a minute in looking for him, she grabbed a heavy coat to cover her uniform, and then ran off to search the automobile stores that lined Bay Street near Grenville.[34] There was also the story about a young boy with schizophrenia who seemed to blend in, wax-like, with the figures in the Royal Ontario Museum and was, therefore, difficult to find.[35]

With the advent of antipsychotic medications, the atmosphere in occupational therapy changed somewhat. Therapists were somewhat less directive and did not need to structure activities to the same degree. They could be a bit more relaxed because patients were less impulsive, could be reasoned with, were not as likely to "take off," and could look after each other. But overmedication decreased patients' ability to apply themselves to a task, and in some ways they were not able to work as well. While the medication certainly helped to control symptoms, it also seemed to take away some measure of the patients' spontaneity and sense of personal involvement.

There was always interesting research going on at TPH, and some projects (e.g., insulin coma therapy) counted on the involvement of the occupational therapists. Patients received their insulin in the morning. The OTs were asked to keep them active in the afternoon, but to keep a close watch that they didn't go back into shock. If these patients were taken on outings, therapists always carried glucose in some form. The vigilance and the responsibility were considerable. When lobotomies were carried out, the OTs were asked to help reactivate the patients, to push them since ambition and drive were now reduced. As soon as patients had recovered from their surgery they were expected to be dressed and active. Sheila Irvine remembers helping to draw up the chart which was to be used for assessing patients' behavior before and after their surgery so that this information could be used in making discharge plans.[36]

The day hospital opened in 1961 in an effort to provide care for patients not ill enough to be admitted and not well enough to be totally discharged. These patients received their medications, saw a psychiatrist (and often the social worker or psychologist), but the major part of each day was spent engaged in the occupational therapy program. By this time, the "therapeutic community" was very much the vogue and all of the patients' interactions were considered opportunities for learning.[37] Community meetings were held on a regular basis and patients planned their own activities together with the staff. Boundaries between hospital and community were diminished. For a period of time, local artist Jack Pollock came in to provide art lessons to one of the patient groups in OT. His "students," who had often visited his gallery on outings, built him a flower box in return.[38] In an effort to flatten the hierarchy within the setting, and to simulate a more natural environment, occupational therapists in the day hospital were the first to come "out of uniform."

A story could be told about TPH through the uniforms worn (and not worn) by the occupational therapists. In the 1920s, they wore white uniforms with a red crest that said "Occupational Therapy" and they had long flowing veils; sometime in the 1930s they began to wear the trademark green uniform, brown oxfords, and brown leather belt, with a white nurse's cap trimmed in green velvet; and in the early 1960s they stopped wearing uniforms altogether. Nancy (Cornish) Sidle remembers that the desire of inpatient therapists to come out of uniform was hastened along when she left a ballpoint pen in her uniform pocket and then sent it off with the other uniforms to the laundry—and the laundry did the rest![39]

Under Sheila Irvine's leadership, the occupational therapy department at TPH continued to be a much sought after place of employment for occupational therapists. What attracted them into psych OT (and what kept them there) was their fascination with psychiatry, their interest in people, and their belief in the value of occupation. The OT department was so good, in part, because of the *esprit de corps* of the people in it. It was a family, albeit a somewhat elitist family, a group that everyone wanted to be a part of. The OTs were by and large a fine lot: many had come from "good" families; they were very bright, and always won the prizes at school. On one occasion, there were four OTs working at TPH, all of whom had graduated from the combined program in physical and occupational therapy, and each one of them had won the prize for leadership in *physical therapy*![40]

The OTs got along well with the rest of the staff at the hospital and were part of its larger family. From the kitchen staff to the psychologists, social workers, nurses, and psychiatrists, the OTs had good relationships with almost everyone. Their opinions were sought and their voices were heard. Case conferences provided a forum for all those involved with a patient to present their observations for consideration and discussion. In many instances, it was the OT who had seen the most of the patient, in the most natural environment available, and had worked with the patient beyond the point of assessing. As a result, the OT had important information to share.

Case conferences at TPH always provided an excellent learning experience, and, in a way, are perhaps the single best example of what was so extraordinary about being at TPH. For that hour or so at midday, a case was presented, information was shared, the patient was interviewed, and discussion ensued. For everyone present, there was a sense of being on an intellectual odyssey, and at the same time, those same people were anchored in the reality of trying to do their utmost to help their patients to get better. At that time, as now, a health professional could not ask for a better environment in which to work.

Acknowledgements

Many people gave generously of their time and their memories to help me reconstruct this picture of TPH and put it into the context of the times. I would like to thank: Nancy Cornish Sidle, Sheila Dunn Irvine, Thelma Cardwell, Isobel Robinson, Mary Clark Ray, Marge Luckett Murphy, Peg Langley Lewis, Edith Clavir Kaplan, Jenny Lewis Goodman, Gwynneth Schofield Thompson, Myrtle Mackey MacArthur, Kathleen Robb Reed, Marion Sanderson, and Freda Dancey Finley.

Endnotes

[1] See Farrar, in the *Physician's Handbook*, as cited in Edward Shorter's chapter on Farrar (Chapter 3).

[2] Adolf Meyer, "The Philosophy of Occupation Therapy," *American Journal of Occupational Therapy* 31 (10): 639-42 (November/December 1977). [Reprinted from the *Archives of Occupational Therapy*, 1: 1-10 (1922).]

[3] C.K. Clarke, "Statement re Occupational Therapy in Ontario Hospitals for the Insane," January 13, 1922, p. 13. Farrar private archive.

[4] Ibid.

[5] Province of Ontario, Hospitals Division, Department of Health, *Toronto Psychiatric Hospital Report covering Year which ended 31st October 1934* (Toronto: Queens Printer, 1934).

[6] C.B. Farrar, "War Neuroses and Psychoses," *Canadian Journal of Occupational Therapy* 7 (1): 5-16 (1940).

[7] C.B. Farrar, "Rehabilitation in Nervous and Mental Cases Among Ex-Soldiers," *Canadian Journal of Occupational Therapy*, 7 (1): 23 (1940).

[8] Isobel Robinson, "The Mists of Time," *Canadian Journal of Occupational Therapy* 48 (4): 145-52 (October 1981).

[9] Ibid., p. 147. Dr. Goldwin Howland, father of the former Chief Justice of Ontario, William Howland, was a staunch supporter of, and active contributor to, the profession.

[10] See members of the honourary advisory council listed in early volumes of the *Canadian Journal of Occupational Therapy*, for example, 1933 and 1934. Prominent men and women from across Canada, the United States and Europe served in this capacity.

[11] *The Evening Telegram* (Toronto), May 1, 1925.

[12] Herbert A. Bruce, "An Address," reprinted in the *Canadian Journal of Occupational Therapy* 1: 6-9 (1933).
[13] Ibid. Voltaire as quoted by Bruce, p. 7.
[14] Province of Ontario, Hospitals Division, Department of Health, *Toronto Psychiatric Hospital Report Covering Period 1926-1932* (Toronto: Queens Printer, 1932).
[15] Personal communication with Margaret ("Peg") Langley (Lewis) and Kathleen Robb (Reed).
[16] TPH Report 1926-32.
[17] Personal communication with Kathleen Robb (Reed).
[18] Department of Health, Hospitals Division, Staff Record, February 5, 1934.
[19] Personal communication with Margaret ("Peg") Langley (Lewis).
[20] Many honours were bestowed upon Helen P. LeVesconte during her career and upon her retirement. She was made a life member of the Canadian Association of Occupational Therapists in 1965 and received honourary doctorates from the University of Western Ontario and the University of Alberta following her retirement.
[21] Ibid.
[22] Personal communication with Margaret ("Peg") Langley (Lewis).
[23] C.K. Clarke, "Statement re Occupational Therapy in Ontario Hospitals for the Insane," January 13 (1922), p. 12. Farrar private archive.
[24] Personal communication with Mary (Clark) Ray.
[25] H.P. LeVesconte to C.B. Farrar, 1945.
[26] Personal communication with Margaret ("Peg") Langley (Lewis).
[27] Personal communication with Mary (Clark) Ray.
[28] Personal communication with Myrtle (Mackey) MacArthur.
[29] Personal communication with Sheila (Dunn) Irvine.
[30] *The Ottawa Journal*, November 7, 1949.
[31] Nancy (Cornish) Sidle claims that she was so bad at crafts that Sheila Irvine asked her not to use them because of the problems that resulted.
[32] Personal communication with Marjorie (Luckett) Murphy.
[33] Personal communication with Kathleen (Robb) Reed.
[34] Personal communication with Myrtle (Mackey) MacArthur.
[35] Personal communication with Kathleen (Robb) Reed.
[36] Sheila (Dunn) Irvine, personal communication. The chart appears in Abe Miller's book *Lobotomy* [Toronto: Ontario Department of Health, 1954].
[37] J. Stuart Whiteley and John Gordon, *Group Approaches in Psychiatry* (London: Routledge & Kegan Paul, 1979).
[38] Artist Jack Pollock had his gallery nearby on Elizabeth Street and was a marvellous teacher.
[39] Personal communication with Nancy (Cornish) Sidle.
[40] Ibid.

13

The Outpatient Department

Donald Coates[*]

This account of the Toronto Psychiatric Hospital outpatient department (OPD) follows three stories: first, the historical development of the OPD taken largely from records; second, what happened in the teaching program during my residency in 1957; and third, a fuller account of some of the OPD in the 1960s from my viewpoint as director. The outpatient department was established just after the hospital was founded and played a significant role in the growth and development of specialized clinics. My personal contact was restricted to two brief periods, the second of which was dominated by plans for the Clarke. Yet these recollections may shed light on the development of psychiatry in Toronto and in Canada.

Outpatient department history

From the beginning, TPH was to have an outpatient department accessible to all. The 1932 hospital report[1] (first to describe the work of individual departments) suggests that the demand was large from the opening and that it continued to grow, so that, in only four years, the department required a full-time staff. In contrast to the 1960s, during those initial years over half the cases were under 20 years of age. While a large majority were retarded and referred to care-providing agencies for behavior problems requiring advice, the majority of adults were psychotic. Like the TPH inpatient service, only a small proportion of those

---

[*]Donald B. Coates was a resident at TPH in 1957 and directed its adult outpatient department from 1963-65. From 1966-70, he directed the Community Studies Section of the Clarke Institute. In his career he has served as director, consultant, and staff psychiatrist in Vancouver hospitals and clinics and as associate professor of psychiatry at the University of British Columbia.

seen required continuing treatment or transfer to Ontario Hospitals for a longer stay. Most were followed up in the community. From this modest beginning the OPD grew, not only in size, but in specialization, and over the succeeding 40 years was superseded by many specialized services. At TPH, these included a children's service, forensic services, and a daycare program. Elsewhere, alternate services sprang up to provide care for retardation, alcoholism, and addictions.

Outpatient services began in March 1926 with a Wednesday afternoon clinic for schoolchildren, conducted by Edmund P. Lewis of the mental hygiene service, Toronto public health. He was soon joined by a visiting psychiatrist from family court.[2] Over the next few years, sessions were developed by both inpatient staff and visitors from Ontario Hospitals. The emphasis remained predominantly on children, with special attention given to assessing their intelligence. In late 1927, a full-time stenographer was engaged, followed in 1930 by full-time psychologist Jean Brown. In 1931, Lewis became the first full-time medical director. Bernice Wilshire, RN, was appointed full-time clinic director, a position she would occupy for 30 years until she retired, when John Dewan left to become TPH director in 1960.

"Speech training" was the only specialized treatment program continuous throughout the department's history. Starting in 1931, a volunteer therapist intermittently gave a program of "speech training" to children, adolescents, and adults, many of whom were stutterers. Treatment consisted of

> mental hygiene, relaxation and speech therapy. Social activities were also arranged, and vocational placements for adults. Very often it was found best to help the parents to understand that their child was stuttering because of emotional maladjustment.[3]

This describes an eclectic approach to treatment; unfortunately, we have not been provided with a similar account of the treatment given to the remaining cases. The 1932 report does tell us that the social service department: "functioned very effectively in facilitating the disposal of cases [and] included placement, improvement in living conditions, assisting in recreational, relief and educational programs." Despite the satisfaction expressed in the 1932 report that so many cases were discharged to the community, of the 775 new cases seen in the clinic in 1932, 31 percent went on to other institutions (half were transferred to the Ontario Hospital Orillia and the remainder to training schools or other Ontario Hospitals).[4]

Who then were the patients in 1931? In contrast to the voluntary patients seeking help or treatment in the 1960s, 67 percent of patients in 1931 were referred by welfare agencies (principally child care agencies), with a further 20 percent sent by family agencies and industrial schools. Hospitals, clinics, and doctors referred most other cases, and, indeed, many children showed poor health (as evidenced by bad teeth, undernourishment, and chronic infections). But the overall reasons for referral were behavioral difficulties or social problems, as follows: stealing (116), illegitimacy (112), advice regarding placement (112), suspected mental defect (86), sex (52), inability to hold a job, inadequate home supervision, vagrancy, and backwardness at school. Six people were assessed for Canadian Immigration as a basis for being deported from Canada, reflecting an era which practiced both sterilization and deportation of people with mental retardation and the mentally ill for eugenic purposes.

THE DEPRESSION AND WAR YEARS

After the 1932 report, little is available on the development of the OPD until the next internal landmark, the move to a renovated house at 112 College Street in November 1946. Adult psychiatric services had been greatly curtailed during the war (for example, Queen Street Hospital, despite its size and importance, functioned with only two doctors). Yet the child guidance movement gained acceptance during these years.

The years following World War II commenced a period of growth. The Canadian Mental Health Association (formerly the CNCMH), encouraged by psychiatrists who had wartime experience in personnel selection and early treatment of traumatic disorders,[5] started to train mental health consultants to go into schools and industry and apply some of these lessons to civilian problems. In Forest Hill, a Toronto suburb, this took the form of a large scale study focussed on mental health, the Crestwood Heights Project.[6] Many general hospitals opened psychiatric inpatient and outpatient services during this era.

THE ADULT OUTPATIENT DEPARTMENT IN 1952

By 1952, when the OPD moved to its third and final location at 241 Elizabeth Street, major changes had occurred both in the clinic and in the available services, particularly children's services, in Toronto. The development of child guidance centres had continued. The mental health association helped set up a consultation service in 1952, which became the Toronto Mental Health Clinic in 1953. This clinic, along with the TPH consultation service to Children's Aid (starting circa 1950) and the Toronto Board of Education Child Adjustment Service (from 1951 onward), provided rich new community resources. Children's services were further decentralized by setting up local child guidance clinics under the auspices of public health departments in Toronto, York Township, and East York-Leaside. As well, adult psychiatry in general hospitals was beginning to be a force, with in- and outpatient units in several general hospitals.

All these additions were reflected in the OPD, which continued to grow and to tax severely the available facility at 112 College Street. By 1948, the caseload had risen to 4,257 patients, with a corresponding growth in staff. In contrast to the 1932 pattern, in 1948 only 16 percent of referrals were aged 14 or under, and the rest were widely distributed in age. Although cases were referred by community agencies (35 percent), hospitals and private physicians (30 percent), a full 30 percent were either self- or family-referred. This dramatic shift in patients reflects the change from a child-oriented to an adult-oriented service, and the even greater shift from a consultation service to a primary treatment service. Many patients were carried in treatment over longer periods. Although some attended for medication review, the majority were being treated with a new therapeutic modality: psychotherapy. To meet this extraordinary demand, the staff had grown by 1948 to include four full-time psychiatrists, six part-time residents-in-training, two psychologists, five social workers, and a nurse teacher-supervisor; all these were in addition to a full-time medical director, a clinic organizer, and four secretarial staff. Moreover, the program was now focused on training a wide variety of mental health professionals to meet the demand for therapists in a rapidly expanding network of mental health centres throughout Ontario. In particular, the OPD responded to an incentive program for the training of physicians as psychiatrists; at first a one-year program, later it expanded to two. Not only did the majority of Ontario psychiatrists train at TPH OPD, but residents also came from Saskatchewan, Alberta, and British Columbia. This shift in emphasis necessitated not only a major increase in teaching staff, but also affected the type of cases selected for treatment and caused waiting lists to grow.

Personal recollections as a resident

My own formal training in psychiatry began in July, 1956 at Queen Street Hospital, a historic moment. Around this time a formal University of Toronto resident program was started up, directed by Abe Miller and situated in the newly-built admitting wing (the first renovation of the old building). I was one of five residents at Queen Street who, along with another ten residents in other hospitals, commenced the two-year diploma in psychiatry and four-year program in the specialty. At that time, all training began in inpatient settings, with a considerable emphasis on history-taking. Queen Street offered rich investigative resources, both physical and psychological. The teaching tended toward diagnostics, but included a weekly case seminar with Martin Fisher, an analyst who whetted the appetite for a dynamic approach (and later founded a school of art therapy). Though insulin coma and ECT were mainstays, there was an air of therapeutic optimism and much interest in the still undefined role for neuroleptics. There was little organized follow-up for discharged patients. Frequent readmissions occurred.

I next spent six months at the Wellesley Hospital unit, staffed largely by neuropsychiatrists (distinguished neurologists Herbert Hyland and J. Clifford Richardson, neuropsychiatrist Allan Walters, and psychiatrist James Grant). It dramatizes the changes that have occurred since 1957 to note that Hyland and Richardson were world authorities (on the basis of their series of 22 cases) on the then strange and exceedingly rare phenomenon of anorexia nervosa. At the Wellesley the patients were for the most part neurotic and depressed, "breakdowns in living" (as Professor Stokes would have characterized them), rather than psychotic as at Queen Street. A lot of minor tranquilizers and ECT's were ordered in that very busy unit and patients were discharged after relatively short stays. The orientation was primarily neurological, and I recall the great interest shown in the early neurochemistry of depressions and in Wilder Penfield's direct stimulation of the cerebral cortex as a model for obsessive-compulsive behavior.

My days as a medical student yield little recall of TPH. The medical school calendar states that 100 hours of instruction in psychiatry were given in the final year, but this must have been entirely lecture demonstrations held in the TPH conference room, which did not accommodate a class of 150 students. Many of these I skipped under the pressure of concerns. I do recall one early morning case conference at which two patients were assessed for lobotomy as part of a major research study,[7] but only later did I understand this.

Because I was an indifferent medical student and also very anxious, particularly in my final year, I went seeking help (or, at least, reassurance) from the University of Toronto health service. This led to my being assessed by John Dewan and assigned to Bob Arthurs for psychotherapy, never dreaming they would later become my teachers and still later my associates. Another and more significant encounter with John Dewan occurred when I was a resident for three months on the psychiatry service at Sunnybrook Veterans Hospital. I had great respect for his subtle interviewing skills, particularly in gaining the trust of very suspicious, paranoid, or schizophrenic young men. Later I came to respect him for his administrative skill, but I never watched him interview patients again. At TPH, staff meetings could involve considerable wrangling, but when Dewan (as chair) summarized with a simple comment, there was often a surprising consensus reached.

OPD MEMORIES AS A RESIDENT: 1957

The OPD of 1957, with a staff of 30, was very large as outpatient departments go, so that even absorbing 6 new residents at a time did not upset its rhythms. As far back as 1952 there were 33 well-utilized interviewing rooms.[8] When the clinic moved around the corner to occupy the building abandoned by the Hospital for Sick Children at 241 Elizabeth Street, the offices were strung out in a long line off a dark hallway leading from the single street entrance, past the reception and records desk. First, came areas of speech therapy and the social work department, followed by a central area composed of group therapy rooms, and a medical examining room opposite a large conference room, where most teaching sessions took place. Beyond the offices of the director and clinic manager was a large waiting room with institutional (i.e., Ontario Hospital) furniture, which also served as the site of the weekly psychosomatic conference. Off this were 10 or 12 tiny cells, 2 larger offices for psychologists, and the OPD's own telephone switchboard and operator.

The atmosphere was dingy and undecorated except for large, faded prints of the Group of Seven (*de rigueur* in banks and government offices). All the offices were claustrophobic, and staff welcomed conferences as a chance to gather in a larger space. Everyone took their lunch hour or any other chance to leave the building, though coffee breaks morning and afternoon were used to catch up on shared cases with other staff. The offices were each so small that there was room for only two chairs, a tiny desk, a single patient, and one resident therapist. Any outer clothing or galoshes had to be left outside. Almost all the staff smoked, as did most of the patients, either in self-defense or as an expression of their tension, and it remains a wonder there were no suffocations. In any case, it made for psychotherapy of a physically intimate, if not always totally empathic, kind. After they entered the clinic and signed in with a receptionist, most patients had to navigate the long hall and then wait in the large and exposed common area. This made for congestion and noise on the hour as we all tried to start our appointments promptly, the 50-minute hour being one aspect of therapy we novices had confidence we could fulfill.

Since the partitions between cubicles were only ten feet tall and open above, as many as ten therapeutic conversations occurred simultaneously and could readily be overheard from the next cubicle. This, at times, was a source of great concern to novice therapists who felt responsible for the therapeutic atmosphere. More remarkable was that the patients, particularly when practically sitting in their therapists' laps, were so absorbed with their own preoccupations that they were unaware of their neighbours' cries.

The teaching program was rich and highly organized. Daniel Cappon would preselect three illustrative cases and prepare extensive case notes on each. These three patients were assigned to three of the eight residents for six months of ongoing weekly therapy. I felt lucky to be assigned a 30-year-old, single librarian with obsessive and depressive symptoms, who was both articulate and a "good reporter." Each week at a conference attended by the entire clinic, one and only one phase of personality development would be reviewed, the data coming from the three study cases as seen in the residents' interviews, from psychologists' testing and social workers' meetings with relatives, plus a literature review of the topic by yet another resident. In the course of six months, this process provided a rich clinical picture without resorting to analytic dogma. In addition, I had weekly supervision by Dan Cappon, with content ranging from detailed review of my treatment of cases to broad theoretical interests. Cappon at that time was one of two Jungian therapists in Toronto and eager to spread the Jungian view. He impressed me by his scholarship, in particular a series of three articles describing mental mechanisms and psychophysical parallels, and his series of public lectures given in the late fifties on the family of gods and the family of man, which reflected both his empiricism and a grander view of psychiatry.

Patients with physical disorders were presented at a weekly psychosomatic conference conducted by John Lovett-Doust. After discussion the patients were interviewed by him in front of a large audience.[9] I recall these as lively meetings, frequently attended by staff from other TPH units. The discussion reflected the astonishing gulf between two competing schools of theory. On the one hand, there was organic psychiatry (neuropsychiatry), an example being the classic *Clinical Psychiatry* by three British authors, which guided my way through first year.[10] Their viewpoint was so neurophysiological, ignoring any social or psychological interpretations, that even in their discussion of school delinquency and school phobia they expressed concern that epilepsy, tumour, or other lesion might be the cause. In sharp contrast, during my 1957 training in TPH outpatients, the landmark publication of the three-volume *American Handbook of Psychiatry*[11] represented a completely new perspective. It was so psychoanalytically oriented that all disorders, whether manifesting as psychopathology or in psychosomatic form, whether as a life threatening manic depressive disorder or as stuttering, were attributed to Oedipal conflicts. Was it any wonder that the psychosomatic conferences often resulted in heated arguments or that staff often left the meetings shaking their heads in disbelief at formulations that attributed libidinous functions to limbic structures? Psychiatry has become, if not wiser, at least far more precise since then. Although there were these theoretical extremes, let me cite some more balanced views. John Dewan and William Spaulding, director of the OPD at Toronto General Hospital (TGH), produced a balanced and useful clinical text for general medical use without the extremes;[12] and Jules Masserman produced a psychiatric text that was literate and neither mindless nor brainless.[13]

Group therapy in the OPD

The chance to be therapist or cotherapist in a series of psychotherapy groups organized by Tom Mallinson was greatly valued by residents in the OPD. In an era before video or even extensive use of audio taping in supervision, this was a chance to have one's behavior directly observed and critiqued by observers behind a one-way mirror. The therapy groups were assembled to run for six-month periods and varied widely in age, sex, pathology, personality. Though groups met at many times (including evenings), the best learning sessions were on Saturday mornings over a lot of coffee and lively criticism. Mallinson taught us to observe closely the interaction sequences in groups: the rise and fall of the group mood, the impact of absence or lateness of members. In other words, the emphasis was on detailed behavioral observations rather than verbal or symbolic content. In this way, it differed from the group psychotherapy offered in the forensic clinic and the daycare center, as well as from the training emphasis in individual psychotherapy. Mallinson's theoretical orientation owed much to Raymond Corsini and to George Bach,[14] but his teaching drew even more on his own experiences at the National Training Laboratory of Bethel, Maine, the original growth centre inspired by a mix of group dynamics, personal encounter experience, psychodrama, and field theory. Elsewhere, notably at McGill University, personal experience in a training or therapy group was becoming part of a psychiatric residency (as was personal analysis), but this came much later in Toronto.

The Journal Clubs

Many of my memories of the 1958 training program are associated with the biweekly Tuesday night journal club. Gathering the staff of all the psychiatry teaching programs, these were also social occasions frequently preceded by dinner at Little Denmark, a restaurant nearby on Bay Street, or followed by drinks at Maloney's, in the same block as TPH. The journal club was topic-focused and some of the best presentations were reports of ongoing research. I remember especially the visiting professors: Otto Jellinek, who spent a year with the Addiction Research Foundation and Rolv Gjessing, who reviewed the ongoing study of a small number of cases of periodic catatonia (a TPH specialty at the time, but long since abandoned in an age of neuroleptics), as well as John Lovett-Doust's studies on the microcirculation of schizophrenia and depression. The range of topics was also wide enough to include reports from the Crestwood Heights Project.[15] A major study of community mental health focused on families and children, it was conducted in Forest Hill Village and sponsored by the psychiatry department. The journal clubs were proudly conducted by Aldwyn Stokes and reflected his eclectic approach to psychiatry, to the "breakdowns in living," and his bullseye model—or chart with different factors in psychiatric illness drawn in concentric rings—which could accommodate a wide variety of viewpoints.

By 1958, Professor C.B. Farrar had long since abandoned his second floor office at TPH, becoming in our minds a legendary figure. So attendance of all residents was mandatory the night he returned to be honored and share some reminiscences. I remember his physical frailty and his vivid recall for detail. In one anecdote, he described an experience he had had while studying with the celebrated neuropathologist Franz Nissl. After spending some months working in Heidelberg with Nissl (whose staining techniques paved the way for mapping the layers of the human cortex), the two traveled together to Paris. After the long train journey from Germany, they made their way to the site of the Paris Exposition and just at sunset they climbed to the top of the Eiffel Tower. In the gathering dusk, they were each so overwhelmed by the grandeur that for a long while neither spoke a word. Finally, Nissl broke the silence by saying, "God must have a cortex that would stretch from here to Heidelberg."

OPD MEMORIES AS DIRECTOR: 1961–65

In 1961, I was attached to the Medical Research Council's social psychiatry research unit at the Maudsley Hospital in London, England. Out of the blue, I received a cable from Professor Stokes inviting me to return to Toronto as director of the OPD. A year earlier, John Dewan had become director of TPH and, because of his eight-year association with the OPD, there had been no rush to replace him. The offer was clearly linked to Stokes' dream, the opening of the Clarke Institute (then scheduled for 1964). Though I had worked in a variety of clinical contexts, I had no administrative experience and should have anticipated the trouble I would face dealing with "an eclectic group of professional colleagues," as Stokes put it. They were not only very senior and established psychiatrists, but also my former teachers; Bob Arthurs was my former therapist as well.[16] I accepted in blissful ignorance and so became involved with the OPD during one of its most productive periods, when it flowered as a center for teaching and exploring psychotherapy.

In describing the teaching program, I have already mentioned the conflict between two psychiatric schools, the organic-directive and the dynamic-psychotherapeutic. During my training, it became very clear another viewpoint was emerging—the social-community approach. Unlike the organic, biomedical perspective (which was clearly identified with Britain) and the dynamic (an offshoot of American psychoanalysis), the social school was not yet clearly formulated. Interest was rapidly growing in both countries at many levels: from detailed studies of the family to major epidemiological studies of whole countries. Community (as opposed to hospital) care was also strongly advocated, including preadmission and aftercare programs. In one regard the British were ahead, namely in the treatment of psychosis and major mental illness by brief hospital stays. With Stokes' sponsorship, I was lucky to be granted a McLaughlin Travelling Fellowship to study social psychiatry in Britain. I was one of the last to go to Britain; thereafter, the most prestigious training centers were in the U.S. But when I returned to the OPD, eager to teach and demonstrate the principles of social psychiatry, there was such overwhelming demand for psychotherapy training that few wanted to know even what I had learned in Britain.

I implemented a number of changes. Some reflect the atmosphere of the time. For example, the clinic maintained an anonymity (more appropriate to 1926 than 1961) which seemed to perpetuate the stigma associated with mental illness. Like all hospital mail, letters (even those offering appointments) were sent with a box number but with no other identification, in the approved Ontario Hospital manner. I sought permission and, after a while, was allowed to send letters bearing the address. Also, I recall my pleasure watching a sign painter write our name on the entrance door. The anachronism of an anonymous service just three or four years prior to the opening of the Clarke Institute should be apparent.

In the 1960s, bureaucratic rigidity was a constant irritant at TPH. Many Ontario Hospital practices and forms had been adopted. Although some of these were inevitable (for example, the rigid civil service classification and appointment rules for personnel), much professional time went into documenting the need for minor equipment or repairs. Additionally, there was tight financial control by Peter Thomson (a universal scapegoat for many clinical as well as administrative problems) and all prescriptions had to be endorsed by the bursar's office before being filled by the hospital pharmacy. While bureaucracy continued at the Clarke, it seemed less arbitrary and more amenable to discussion. The infusion of new staff allowed a break from TPH traditions and forms. Yet, examples of the pettiness of hospital organization still come to mind.

BLACK CHIFFON

The OPD coin had an obverse: It was a small enough place for rumours regarding staff members to spread unchecked. To illustrate, let me cite one dramatic example. Before I took over, the practice of assigning student nurses (from Ontario and general hospitals) to the OPD as part of their TPH rotation had lapsed, so it came as no surprise that the director of nursing, Marion Clark, reinstated this practice. It soon emerged that there was more to the appointment of a nursing instructor than I had suspected. For one thing, the nurse, Thelma Milsom, was exceptionally beautiful and very gentle with the students, patients, and staff. For another the nurse director kept after me for reports on her performance. Gradually over weeks I became aware that the two nurses had clashed violently while Milsom was working on the hospital wards. I never did learn the cause, though the difference in temperament was perhaps great enough to explain the clash. In any case, Clark took steps to have "our" nurse fired. Milsom grieved it as an Ontario civil servant and union member, and perhaps ten senior hospital staff were subpoenaed and required to testify under oath and cross-questioning by lawyers. The hearings were conveniently held in the Queen's Park Parliament Buildings, down the hall from the premier's office, which leant them a great deal of authority. Throughout the days of the trial the hospital was abuzz with gossip and rumour.

One of the strongest supporters of the nursing director was Mary Jackson, for years a token woman in this male domain. After the smoke cleared, "our" nurse (for by this time the whole OPD was her champion) had been vindicated and was able to continue her teaching. I found an occasion to ask Jackson what was behind the whole episode, and her response was "I can imagine that a nursing instructor, a role model for students, might under some circumstances abandon a uniform. But to wear black chiffon?" Some things clearly went too far.[17] The TPH was not a place to sanction impropriety. (I remain personally grateful, however, that black chiffon did not catch on with the student nurses.)

THE FORUM

As an offshoot of the Journal Club philosophy we ran a unique teaching conference: "The Forum." For a year, many clinic staff gave presentations, notably, resident Henry Fenigstein, who made us aware of the personal horror of the Holocaust and concentration camp experiences. We also invited guest speakers to share a wide range of interests, interests in fact so diverse that some colleagues thought the conference irrelevant and the residents were often clueless about its purpose. Among more memorable visitors was the sheriff of York County, who spoke on

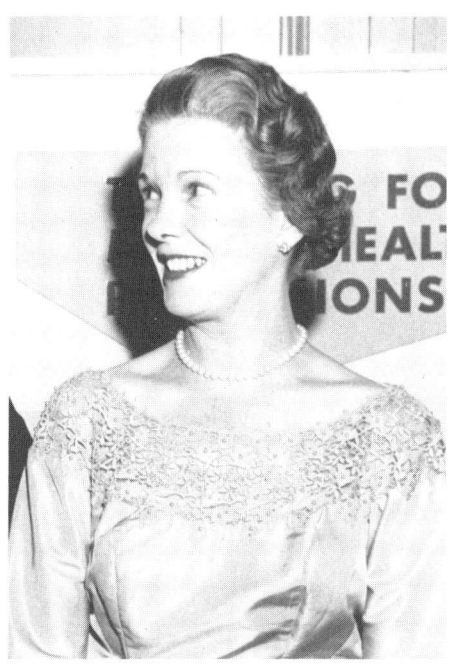

Mary Victoria Jackson (1905–1990), MD, University of Toronto, 1929; certificate in psychiatry, 1945; staff physician (women's services), TPH, 1934–1940; chief of staff, 1940–66; assistant director, 1960–66.

personnel selection. In his case, this entailed selecting an executioner (for the last official hanging at the Don Jail). Another speaker was Percy Saltzman, the television weather reporter, with whom we explored cyclical and lead-lag relationships. In his work, he predicted the weather from the day and week prior, and in ours, we anticipated behavior from foregoing events. Periodic catatonia was a particular specialty of TPH, and psychologist Bruce Quarrington was grappling with the analysis of complex data on women's mood and energy cycles. A number of people spoke to us of innovative community services. Especially memorable was a presentation by Peter Rowsell, an Oakville psychiatrist who, to our surprise, while giving an academic presentation on hypnosis had induced a trance state in the back row of the audience, even as others were protesting that the trance phenomenon was either imaginary or a voluntary collusion.

Closing the Waiting List

The nature of outpatient psychiatry had changed over time. In these years the public seemed to grow much more sensitive towards stress and neurotic suffering. Most people could differentiate between madness and neurosis, and seeking help for personal and self-defined problems was no longer stigmatized. It was the era of the sick joke and the whole society was sometimes called "sick, sick, sick." In Seeley's apt phrase, it was the time of the popularization or Americanization of the Unconscious.[18] Yet in the entire Toronto area there were few therapists in practice and only the most rudimentary adult community services were available. In the entire area, mental-health clinics existed only at Queen Street, New Toronto, and the TPH, with a few very small, municipally sponsored and child-oriented clinics operating in East York, North York, Weston, and Scarborough. The general hospitals provided follow-up to their own cases, but did not have the staff to take on many new cases. Thus, the demand for treatment far exceeded the resources available and, at times, even reached crisis proportions.

We had to meet this demand. The OPD, after an initial assessment interview, kept patients waiting up to a year for psychotherapy. In fact, one staff psychiatrist spent much of his time updating the waiting list. Being strongly influenced by crisis theory[19] and the advocates of early intervention from Boston, I found this an unconscionably long time and pressed hard to change the system. After a great deal of discussion within the clinic, we decided to specialize in teaching psychotherapy and to keep waiting only those who could be accommodated by residents within a six-month period. Initially, the idea of limiting the waiting list, or "closing the clinic" as it was widely interpreted, was opposed by both Drs. Dewan and Stokes, who later concurred.

The next step of advising the referral agencies went less well. The chief social worker in the OPD, Barry Katz, and I sent a letter to all the community agencies we could identify, saying that we would henceforth offer emergency appointments within a week, but that our waiting list for psychotherapy was temporarily closed until the next rotation of residents. In other words, we offered two responses, one of which was a crisis mode. Agencies did not understand our decisions and their reaction to this was immediate and severe.[20] Several agency heads protested that a badly needed resource could not be withdrawn; others cried that an essential service, particularly a public, provincial one, could not be abolished without more consultation. Then, reaction came from the tiny and precarious mental-health branch: Cyril Greenland and Bill Henderson were each sent to discipline me and to reestablish community goodwill. Throughout the entire incident, those in the clinic staff saw little change in the actual workload or caseload, and felt that we had simply made explicit that psychotherapy was a heavily time-consuming treatment.

The crisis provided opportunities for further innovation, such as going to other agencies to explain our role more fully and suggest ways they could manage cases. Most of all, our rapid response around crises markedly increased our contacts with outside agencies. We even made one or two token home visits. Inside the clinic, we organized into five effective multidisciplinary teams (one for each day's referrals and drop-ins), but staff resisted the erasure of professional boundaries.

More than anyone else, Barry Katz[21] recognized the learning opportunity that the crisis presented. He not only did much of the public relations work, he also studied the community response. One year later, he sent a questionnaire to the agencies originally notified and obtained a very supportive response. We interpreted this as the agency community looking for more psychiatric consultation in order to manage their own cases better. In a clinical presentation to the Toronto Medical Society, we gave a detailed accounting of the entire experience. Focusing on our experience, Tom Mallinson presented a timely interpretation of steady-state systems theory and chaos theory as proposed by Matthew Miles.

The crisis of the waiting list taught me a great deal about consulting and public relations, confirmed the considerable overlap in agency clientele, and identified similar management practices of psychiatric and social agencies. Morale within the clinic soared during this period of innovation and a number of papers were published, but, best of all, we were able to focus clearly on the teaching of psychotherapy.

STEPHEN NEIGER

One of the most memorable associates in the OPD was a Hungarian Jewish psychologist who was there both when I was a resident and when I became director. He and his wife, Trudy, equipped one of the larger offices with an espresso machine (a novelty in those days), and provided a gathering place for discussion in the clinic. Neiger might best be characterized as a mid-European intellectual, very well informed, witty and amusing, and, seen in retrospect, chronically depressed, often whining and desperate. His particular expertise was with the Rorschach ink blot test, far more accepted then than it is today. Throughout this period, he was constantly at work on the definitive dictionary of Rorschach responses, a project that entailed endlessly compiling the innumerable drafts typed and retyped by his wife Trudy, who was better organized and more stable than Stephen. I believe that the project was worthwhile, and that Neiger, having worked with Rorschach, was particularly appropriate to undertake it.

His comments on clinical case conferences were well-balanced and suited the burgeoning interest in psychodynamic formulations. Yet Neiger had a major problem: He had tired of his cataloguing and wanted to engage in more active (participant) research. Moreover, he had had some medical training in Hungary before the revolution and had a major interest in sexology. On my return, he looked to me for help to establish himself as a sexologist. I recall approaching both Stokes and Lovett-Doust, but their response implied that psychiatry was already a hard enough sell, particularly Freudian ideas, without identifying too closely with sexual behavior. They regarded the suggestion from a Jewish émigré as out of place. In fairness to them, their attitudes accurately reflected the prudery and conservatism of Toronto middle-class society. The senior staff of TPH were doubly sensitive as the funds for the Clarke Institute were only partially approved. Yet they failed to recognize that a social and sexual revolution was already well under way.

In addition to clinical duties, Neiger developed two research projects of merit: one on menstrual mood disorders, and the other on the prediction of suicidal risk. Both were refused funding, I maintain, because they were ahead of their time. Outside the OPD he was an endless source of ideas and projects. With his wife as manager, he started the first computerized dating service in Canada, using questionnaires as the basis for matching. He created enough interest among colleagues to start the Sexual Information and Education Council of Canada (SIECAN), following the pioneering efforts of Mary Calderone in the United States. A wonderfully curious and entertaining person, he was one of the first in Toronto to write about gay meeting places and rights, changing sexual morality, swingers clubs, and teenage sex.

Ernest (Van) Douglass

One of the more colourful characters in the OPD was Ernest ("Van") Douglass, an English speech therapist. Previously a travelling stage performer in Britain, he hid his quick wit behind talents for clowning, mind-reading, sleight-of-hand, and card-reading, which previously had been his livelihood. In particular, he had a gift for mime and his repertory of laughs ranged from a bark to an explosion to a slowly expanding, prolonged wheeze. All this stagecraft was put to work in his approach to stutterers, who made up the bulk of the cases treated by him and his two associates. At the earliest time of the clinic, speech therapy had been a strong specialty. By the early 1960s, this was bolstered by much experimental work, for example the clinical distinction between exteriorized (expressed) and interiorized (unevidenced) stuttering, the former being what one commonly thinks of as stuttering, that painful hesitancy for speech, the latter fluency gained at the expense of internal defenses and cover-up techniques. He helped non-stutterers understand the condition by using a tape loop for auditory delay (when wearing headphones one's own voice was heard so late that speech became disorganized and thought disrupted). This provided an experimental approach to stuttering behavior that related it theoretically to more general questions regarding neurotic behavior, anxiety; in short, to the mental mechanisms that were the main focus of the clinic. Moreover, the treatment largely consisted of deconditioning strategies not yet well developed in that era of "talking therapy." After due preparation, patients were taken into real social situations to practice their stutters in front of waiters, clerks, critical family, and strangers. Douglass thus described techniques of feedback, meaning both biofeedback and social responses to behavior in public—at the time a new field of theory—loosely grouping many specific mechanisms under the title "cybernetics." His interest in cybernetics was instrumental in bringing Warren McColluch, a distinguished scholar and leader in the field, to speak in Toronto. Later, Douglass founded a Canadian chapter of the American Cybernetic Society. Always adversarial, he sharpened thinking at our conferences, particularly the psychosomatic ones. It was a pity that, with failing health, he decided to retire rather than make the shift to the Clarke Institute.

Tom Mallinson

Tom Mallinson, a clinical psychologist and longstanding friend, figured in the well-developed group therapy program. He also helped reorganize the clinic when we concentrated on teaching psychotherapy. Originally from Vancouver, he took his master's degree under B.F. Skinner[22] and came to Toronto to continue similar studies of conditioning. Then he changed course dramatically after encountering John Seeley and William Line and joined the Crestwood Heights Project. His imagination was demonstrated by his work on non-directive human relations classes conducted in the Forest Hill grade schools ("talk sessions" in the eyes of more goal-directed critics). He and John Seeley were able to show a measurable impact on the personality of the children. Mallinson's interest in group dynamics led to his attending some of the earliest sessions of the National Training Labs in Bethel, Maine, in 1950, 1952, and 1953, and subsequently joining TPH inpatients where he and social worker Lon Lawson started a pre-discharge patients group.

At about this time, Burdett McNeel, director of the mental health branch, identified as a high priority the training of family doctors in rudimentary counselling and psychotherapy techniques. Mallinson, together with Ed Rosen of the children's service, developed a week-long training course which was given several times for up to 20 practitioners at a session. Concurrently, Mallinson had begun to conduct management seminars and workshops for a wide variety of organizations (including the CMHA and the YMCA). For Tom Mallinson I believe the OPD provided a more congenial professional home than for many other staff, where a high-energy setting of give-and-take resembled a high-level university seminar. Perhaps it is just nostalgia, but I share in his belief that in the late flowering of the OPD there was an openness to new ideas and experiments such as I have rarely experienced elsewhere.

Tom took full advantage of the OPD as a base from which to spread the lore of group dynamics and interpersonal relations. Within the clinic he was very active in running the group program, in organizing the teaching program, and in stimulating staff to publish their research. His own research ranged from the reports of the human relations classes,[23] to a study of treatment outcomes at Whitby Hospital with Cyril Greenland,[24] to a study of schizophrenics and their domestic relations[25] which we shared. A bright light not only in the OPD, but in TPH and the Department of Psychiatry, a major loss was felt when Mallinson left to start the communications department at Simon Fraser University.

AN END AND A BEGINNING

During the years prior to the closing of the OPD in 1965, a number of sociopolitical events occurred that had a considerable effect on outpatient practice everywhere. In Canada, the publication of *More For the Mind,*[26] which advocated a move away from mental hospitals and the establishment of psychiatric inpatient units in every general hospital above a certain size, shifted the locus of care to the community. It also shifted the locus in favour of inpatients. Similarly, the [Charles] Roberts Report of 1963 advocated the reattachment of freestanding mental health clinics to

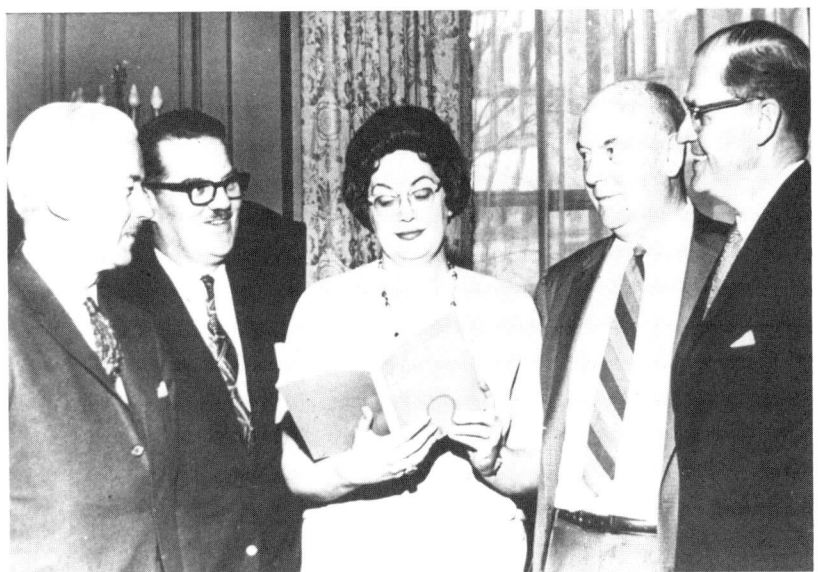

Canadian psychiatrists with Judy LaMarsh, federal minister of Health and Welfare, 1963-1965, celebrating the publication of *More for the Mind* in 1963. The book advocated shifting the locus of psychiatry to the general hospital. From left to right are Burdett McNeel, chief of the mental health branch of the Ontario government, Charles Roberts, F. S. Lawson, and John D. M. ("Jack") Griffin.

general or psychiatric hospitals. Part of a program to remedicalize psychiatry (and ensure its coverage under medicare), the report's effect was to lessen the commitment to social agencies and the "problems in living" model which had evolved throughout the life of the OPD. These major developments gave Canadian psychiatry (with its underpinning of medicare) a pattern uniquely different from the community mental health centres (CMHCs) which developed concurrently in the United States.

Though these developments provoked much interest and discussion amongst the OPD staff, they were overshadowed locally by the planning for the Clarke Institute. The reunion of the separate clinics under one roof was not as welcomed as one might have expected. In fact, for many, particularly longstanding civil servants, it was apprehensively viewed as a possible threat to benefits and a loss of freedom. Before my return, four staff[27] had planned for flexible, interdisciplinary research space for social psychiatry, as well as for a formal outpatient department. Ironically, by the time the research space was occupied, all four original planners had left. Clinical services in the Clarke Institute integrated programs for inpatients and outpatients in one space and with one team of therapists. Since so few of the OPD staff made the transition to the Clarke, very little of the practice pattern of the OPD was transferred. A new era had begun.

ENDNOTES

[1] Province of Ontario, Hospitals Division, Department of Health, *Toronto Psychiatric Hospital: Report Covering Period 1926-32.* (Toronto: Queens Printer, 1932).

[2] Ibid. Report does not indicate the psychiatrist's name.

[3] Ibid.

[4] Ibid. See Cyril Greenland, on eugenics and deportation.

[5] See Edward Shorter's chapter on Farrar (Chapter 3), which identified the involvement of Brock Chisholm, John Griffin, John Seeley, William Line, and others in World War II psychiatry.

[6] John R. Seeley, R. Alexander Sim, Elizabeth W. Loosley, *Crestwood Heights* (Toronto: University of Toronto Press, 1956).

[7] See Abraham Miller, *Lobotomy: A Clinical Study* [Toronto: Ontario Department of Health, 1954], for details on the lobotomy research study. Patients drawn from Ontario Hospitals were operated on by Harry Botterell at Toronto General Hospital.

[8] By 1952, the caseload had reached 1,400 cases a year. About 1,100 of these were new patients. In addition, as the focus shifted from diagnosis to treatment, visits increased in number, frequency and length. In 1958, the department reported 17,000 visits by about 1,400 patients (with a high of eighty visits and an average of eight visits per patient) that year. This high attendance pattern was maintained (with a few small shifts) until the department transferred to the Clarke in 1966.

[9] I protested this public display, only to find three or four years later that interviewing patients in front of a video or movie camera was even more controversial.

[10] W. Mayer-Gross, E.T.O. Slater, and Martin Roth, *Clinical Psychiatry* (London: Cassell, 1954).

[11] *American Handbook of Psychiatry*, 3 vols. edited by Silvio Arieti (New York: Basic Books, 1959).

[12] John Dewan and William Spaulding, *The Organic Psychoses* (Toronto: University of Toronto Press, 1952).

[13] Jules Masserman, *Practice of Dynamic Psychiatry* (Philadelphia: Saunders, 1961).

[14] Raymond J. Corsini, *Methods of Group Psychotherapy* (New York: McGraw-Hill, 1957). George Bach, *Intensive Group Therapy* (New York: Ronald Press, 1954).

[15] Seeley et al. Many investigations and reports of studies were subsequently published in technical journals.

[16] Efforts to get around TPH's rigid operating rules saw several special practices develop. Because of the sensitivity of certain university and civil service cases, the practice of keeping director's files had developed. These were filed separately with greater security. Curious to see what my file contained, I learned that all special files had been taken to John Dewan for safekeeping. My request to see it was unsuccessful.

[17] As a coda to this story, Milsom was married shortly after this incident (her fiancé had been a character witness during the trial). Several OPD staff were guests and I was surprised to be called on without warning to give a toast to the bride.

[18] John Seeley, *The Americanization of the Unconscious* (New York: International Science Press, 1967).

[19] See Gerald Caplan, *Principles of Preventive Psychiatry* (New York: Basic Books, 1964). Erich Lindeman demonstrated the benefits of early intervention after a crisis, but Caplan took crisis theory and developed it into a psychiatric theory.

[20] Barry Katz, "Community Reaction to Closure of Intake," *The Social Worker* 34 (1): 16-22 (February 1966).

[21] Barry Katz later edited *Canada's Mental Health*.

[22] Skinner was on loan to Harvard and Columbia universities from Indiana University. *Hamilton Alumni Review* 13 (1): 33 (October 1947).

[23] T.J. Mallinson, "Appplications of Group Processes to a Clinical (Psychiatric) Setting," *International Journal of Social Psychiatry*. Reprinted from 11 (1): (1965).

[24] A. Adams, C. Greenland, and T. Mallinson, "Measuring Remotivation," *Psychiatry, Journal for the Study of Interpersonal Processes* 25 (2): 135-45 (May 1962).

[25] D.B. Coates and T.J. Mallinson, "Family Interaction in Schizophrenia," *Canadian Psychiatric Association Journal*, 12: 387-401 (August 1967).

[26] Canadian Mental Health Association, *More for the Mind: The Study of Psychiatric Services in Canada* (Toronto: The Association, 1963).

[27] Tom Mallinson, John Seeley, Farrell Toombs, and Gordon Watson.

14

The Children's Service

Edward J. Rosen[*]

The term "child psychiatry" came into use with the publication of the text book *Child Psychiatry* by Leo Kanner in 1935. In the 1920s and 1930s, many children's clinics were established by the (U.S.) National Mental Hygiene Committee and the Commonwealth Fund. By 1950, there were 1,200 mental health clinics in the United States, of which about three-quarters were wholly or partly devoted to children. As part of that larger pattern we may view the history of child psychiatry in Toronto. In the outpatient department of the late 1920s, special days were reserved for particular groups of referrals (for example, child behaviour problems, juvenile delinquents, unmarried mothers, and inmates of industrial schools). The OPD clinicians would make diagnoses and give recommendations to the welfare and medical agencies from which the children came. It was not until psychiatrists, psychologists, and social workers returned at the end of World War II that child psychiatry began a period of expansion at TPH. After decades of being influenced by developments in the United States and Great Britain, Canadian child psychiatry was beginning to stand on its own.

In 1947, John Dewan became full-time director of the OPD with an expansion of full-time staff. After a slow start in the early 1930s, psychotherapy programs for children and parents began to replace the diagnostic and recommendation service to welfare agencies.[1] As the OPD grew, it moved out of the TPH building to larger quarters in an old house on College Street, where the Best Institute now stands. A few years later,

---

[*]Edward J. Rosen, M.D., McGill University, Dip. Psych., University of Toronto, 1947; F.R.C.P. (C), 1972, taught in the Department of Psychiatry of the University of Toronto from 1949-73 and at the University of British Columbia for 1974-75. A staff member of TPH and its successor, the Clarke Institute of Psychiatry, from 1947-71, he has been a consultant in custody assessment and mediation counselling since 1966.

the OPD moved into a section of the old Sick Children's Hospital building on Elizabeth Street.

In 1958, I became director of a separate child and adolescent service in a house on Grosvenor Street, with a full-time staff of social workers, psychologists, and psychiatrists. When the time came to move to the Clarke Institute in 1966, we designed our new space and moved into the first and second floors.

How did I come to child psychiatry? In 1944, Col. John D. ("Jack") Griffin of the psychiatry section of the Royal Canadian Army Medical Corps seconded me to TPH for a six-month course in psychiatry, taught by C.B. Farrar. Upon discharge from the army in 1946, I joined the Ontario Hospital Service and enrolled in the diploma course in psychiatry at the University of Toronto at TPH. The following year, on completion of this postgraduate course, I was appointed to the staff of the OPD at TPH. As director of the TPH during those years, Aldwyn Stokes initiated a steady expansion of the treatment and research facilities of the hospital. The growth of the OPD was part of that program.

The OPD moved out of TPH in 1947 and increased its permanent staff members in social work, psychology, psychiatry, and speech pathology. Pat Church (who left for Hamilton a year later) and I joined as senior staff psychiatrists. The teaching program included training for postgraduate psychiatrists, graduate students in the School of Social Work, psychology students, and clinics for medical students. The postgraduates were supervised by Caye Campbell (M.S.), Bruce Quarrington (Ph.D., psychology), and myself.

As senior psychiatrist, I was responsible for arranging case presentations at weekly conferences in general psychiatry, psychosomatic conditions, and child psychiatry. Although I was mainly involved in adult psychiatry in the army and at TPH, my interest in child psychiatry had begun when I was in medical school. In the summer of 1939, I had worked at a private children's treatment centre in Madison, Connecticut, and had become acquainted with the range of conditions and treatment of disturbed children.

In 1947, Aldwyn Stokes arranged a dual appointment for Morton Teicher, a psychiatric social worker, as head of the TPH social work department and professor of psychiatric social work at the University of Toronto School of Social Work. Teicher brought his experience in child and family therapy as practised in the Philadelphia Child Guidance Clinic and described in the book *Psychotherapy with Children* by Frederick Allen.

While the social worker saw the parents, Caye Campbell and I started the treatment of children's cases using play material play therapy or play technique). We then introduced this method to the clinic staff and students, after which the students were supervised in cases assigned to them. Prior to 1947, the service was essentially diagnostic assessment and recommendation to welfare agencies. It now became a community-based treatment service with referrals from physicians, schools, and the Children's Aid Society.

In 1957, Stokes asked me whether I would consider working on a full-time program for children. When I accepted this, he arranged for a one-year travelling fellowship in child psychiatry at the Harvard Medical School. On my return in 1958, Burdett McNeel, director of the mental hygiene division of the Ontario Health Department, offered to establish a child and adolescent clinic in a house on Grosvenor Street. This clinic was opened in 1958 with Al Slemon (psychologist), Catherine Campbell (social worker), and myself (as director). The staff quickly grew with the addition of psychologists, social workers, psychiatrists, and postgraduates in each of these disciplines.

In this new facility we soon added family therapy for parents, group therapy for children, special clinical assessment of children with learning disabilities, and the diagnosis of mental retardation. The Association for Children with Mental Retardation offered to support the appointment of a full-time specialist in mental retardation and a separate clinic was established in the building. The mental retardation unit consisted of visiting professors in mental retardation, clinic director John Fotheringham, social worker Mora Skelton, and a psychologist.

As for therapies, in 1947 the children's service initiated a child guidance treatment program, using play therapy with the child and case work with the parents. Twelve years later, we introduced group activity therapy with the children. In 1960, we began various new programs, including family therapy, special clinics for children with learning disabilities and mental retardation, and a special class for emotionally disturbed children in the Board of Education in Etobicoke, Ontario.[2]

In sum, the history of child psychiatry at TPH has been a mirror of larger changes. It reflects the increasing contribution of non-medical disciplines such as social work and psychology to disturbances that are, in the last analysis, disruptions of life situations and not just narrowly defined "diseases." It reflects the shift from diagnosis to therapy—from the resigned acceptance of "mental retardation" to active programs of group therapy and "normalization." And it reflects the growing acceptance within psychiatry of disturbances in children as being of equal gravity and legitimacy as those of adults.

Acknowledgements

Many thanks to the former children's unit staff members who gathered May 1, 1992, to share their memories of TPH. A transcript of the recording from that meeting was placed in the QSMHC Archives.

Endnotes

[1] Of the 775 new cases from November 1, 1931, to October 31, 1932, four were reportedly treated by psychotherapy. Province of Ontario, Hospitals Division, Department of Health. *Toronto Psychiatric Hospital: Report Covering Period 1926-1932* (Toronto: Queens Printer, 1932).

[2] I published several articles during that time. E. J. Rosen, *Mental Retardation* (Toronto: Ontario, Department of Health, Mental Health Services, 1960). E. J. Rosen, and C. Campbell, "A psychiatric, sociological and psychological study of illegitimate pregnancy in girls under the age of sixteen years," *Psychiat. Neurol. Basel* 142 (1): 44-60 (1961). E. J. Rosen, "Has Mental Health a Place in the School Curriculum?" *Journal of the Canadian Association for Health, Physical Education and Recreation* 27(1): 14-16 (October/November 1960). E. J. Rosen, "Current Attitudes as They Affect Neglected Children," *The Social Worker* 28 (4): 8-12 (October 1960). E. J. Rosen, John Bayles, C. Fine, et al. "A Research Project Using Activity Group Therapy in a Children's Outpatient Department," *The Social Worker* 29 (1): 24-30 (January 1961). E. J. Rosen, "Understanding the World of the Disturbed Child," *Child Study* 30 (2): 3-12 (Summer 1968). E. J. Rosen, "A Special Class Program for the Rehabilitation of Emotionally Disturbed Children," *International Psychiatry Clinics* 2 (1): 183-204 (January 1965).

15

The Mental Retardation Clinic

Mora Skelton

Opened in 1952, the mental retardation clinic was the fifth and last of the outpatient clinics of TPH. One of the moving forces was the Ontario Association for the Mentally Retarded (OAMR), a large and powerful group of parents and volunteers, with many local member associations. It should be noted that the term "mental retardation" could still be used in the 1960s to describe a condition which today is usually referred to by euphemisms such as "developmentally disabled" (DD). The association is still active under the name of the Ontario Association for Community Living.[1]

In 1961, representatives of the association met with Ted Rosen, head of the children's clinic, and Aldwyn Stokes, director of TPH, to request an outpatient clinic which would focus on the problem of mental retardation. By this time, the TPH children's clinic had specialized in a child guidance approach to helping children, using play therapy and group therapy. Many developmentally handicapped children were unable to make use of these forms of treatment, indicating the need for a separate clinic.

OAMR also offered TPH a considerable sum of money for a one-shot project focusing on mental retardation. In 1962 Stokes and John Lovett-Doust, professor of psychiatry, recruited John Fotheringham, a recent graduate of the course in psychiatry, to head up a new mental retardation clinic. At the beginning, the team staffing the clinic included John Fotheringham, child psychiatrist; Mary Morrison, nurse; a psychologist; and Helen Coleman and myself, social workers.

The third floor of the old Victorian house used by the children's clinic was made available to the new clinic. As time went by, other full- and part-time staff, social work and other students, research assistants, clients, and visitors climbed the three flights of stairs to the clinic at 34 Grosvenor Street. We accepted referrals from doctors, nurses, schools, social agencies, OAMR and families themselves.

Helen Coleman remembered the story of a little boy, "Marvin," who arrived at school for the first time at approximately age six and was found to be unintelligible when he spoke. The school referred him to us. When Helen drove the family to the clinic, she noticed that the mother did not speak to any of her children (two little boys ages six and five, and a baby), nor did they speak to her. Helen heard the "unintelligible" language when the little boys talked to each other. Later, when she met the father, it was obvious that he had a marked speech defect. In the home, there were very few toys and the children seemed to play only with each other. On intelligence tests Marvin scored badly, but Dr. Fotheringham detected some hopeful signs.

Helen suggested that the mother talk to the children, read to them at bedtime, buy some yard toys, and let neighbour children join in the fun. To the school, she suggested that the two boys be permitted to attend, with very little pressure on formal learning but praise for even modest achievements in talking or socialization. When last seen, the boys had been admitted to a regular grade one class.

Usually, the service given by our clinic achieved less spectacular results, but very often handicapped and sheltered children could be stimulated and helped to reach their potential more fully. The days when some parents felt so ashamed and guilty about having a handicapped child that they hid such children away in the attic or basement were not quite over, and we saw one or two such terrible cases. Most of the parents we saw were suffering the "chronic sorrow" described by social workers writing at that time. Sometimes differing parental attitudes toward the child or resentment felt by the siblings was tearing the family apart. Other parents were cooperative, highly motivated people, who were willing to do almost anything to help their handicapped child. For them, the group efforts and mutual support of OAMR and its local associations offered a perfect vehicle to make their own efforts effective.

Service at the clinic was a matter of carefully assessing the child's abilities and discussing the implications of this condition for other family members (since the causes of some forms of developmental disabilities are genetic). We also counselled parents with regard to stimulating and teaching their child and managing related tensions within the home.

Sometimes we saw the siblings only, other times the whole family together.

VISITING PROFESSORS

One of the most interesting features of the mental retardation clinic was the sojourn, one at a time, of four outstanding authorities on this type of handicap. These four experts were brought from England and the United States to lecture at the Department of Psychiatry of the University of Toronto, at TPH, and in the community. They were also to visit the large, government-supported Ontario Hospital Schools (institutions for developmentally handicapped young people) on a consultative basis. They would inhabit an office in our tiny establishment and be resource people to the staff.

This was the special project decided upon to make use of the funds offered to TPH by OAMR. The money was raised by the association in January 1961 during an eighteen-hour telethon, the first such effort by OAMR. The proceeds from the telethon were carefully invested, the income used to pay the costs of the telethon, and the sum raised spent on four or five projects of which the plan for the visiting professors was one. A description of these visiting professors is given in Betty Anglin and Jane Braaten's *Twenty-five Years of Growing Together: A History of the Ontario Association for the Mentally Retarded.*[2]

First to arrive, in 1961, was Leslie T. Hilliard, superintendent of the Fountain Hospital in London, England (which taught basic skills to developmentally disabled children for many years), who was an expert on large institutions for developmentally disabled persons, as they were understood at that time. John Fotheringham and I accompanied him on some of his visits to Ontario Hospital Schools. He was seldom completely satisfied with what he saw and prefaced many of his remarks with the phrase: "I should have thought..." (finishing up with some vigorously worded suggestions).

Joseph M. Berg followed in 1962. He came from the Galton Centre in England where he worked with Lionel Penrose, a world authority on Down's Syndrome (which is a major cause of developmental disability). We accompanied him to numerous meetings with groups sponsored by the OAMR, where he explained over and over again, with perfect courtesy, the nature of this condition, and answered parents' questions. Berg was invited to stay in Canada at the end of his official visit and still serves as a consultant to the Hospital for Sick Children, Surrey Place Centre, and others.

Barry W. Richards came to TPH in 1963 on loan from St. Lawrence's Hospital (formerly Caterham [Mental] Hospital) in Caterham, England.[3] For many years, he edited the *British Journal of Mental Deficiency Research*. A quiet scholarly type, he was occupied chiefly in writing and lecturing at the university and at TPH during his stay with us.

The final visitor arrived in 1965 and contrasted with those who had come before him. Carl Haywood was an American, a psychology professor interested in special education. He demonstrated teaching methods which integrated children who were developmentally disabled into regular classes. He worked at the John F. Kennedy Center for Research in Education and Human Development at Vanderbilt University of Nashville, Tennessee. Later, he became editor of the *Journal of the American Association for Mental Deficiency* (AAMD). After returning to the US, Haywood continued his contact with Fotheringham. In the following years, he repeatedly invited Fotheringham (and sometimes other members of our staff) to present papers at AAMD conferences in the United States.

These four men were most helpful and accommodating and they greatly enlarged the knowledge and experience of the staff.

Research and publications

A major study by clinic staff resulted in a monograph titled *The Retarded Child and His Family*, written by Fotheringham, Skelton, and Bernard Hoddinott (a psychologist).[4] All the material was gathered prior to 1966, while the clinic was still part of TPH, but was not fully worked up until later. The study was published by the Ontario Institute for Studies in Education in 1971.

The project was a longitudinal study of the effects of home and institutional care on mentally retarded children and their families. To investigate these two options for care (the only alternatives available to many families at that time), a group of children who were institutionalized and their families were compared with a similar group residing in the community. The two groups were seen twice: just prior to institutionalization of the children in the first group and again one year later. The findings stressed the importance of the provision of a range of supports for retarded persons (schools, nursery schools, sheltered workshops, group homes), a suggestion vigorously acted upon by the OAMR. It should be noted that the day of integration in the community, rather than segregation, had not yet dawned.

An ongoing project of the clinic social worker was the production of a booklet titled *Directory of Services for the Mentally Retarded in Ontario*, which was updated occasionally and given free on request.[5] The final directory in the series was published in 1970 by the Ontario Department of Health. A chapter on "Social Work and Mental Retardation," written much later for a text on mental retardation, was based on my learning and experience at the mental retardation clinic and the Surrey Place Centre.[6]

John Fotheringham, head of the clinic, published a number of articles on aspects of mental retardation while at the clinic. Some reflected his increasing interest in prevention of this condition, where this is possible. Later, he (with others) wrote two books on the subject, the last of which, *Prevention of Intellectual Handicaps*, is a recognized text.[7] While still at the clinic, Fotheringham became very active with the OAMR by leading discussions and presenting papers at conferences. His interest continued and he was for many years the chairman of the professional advisory committee of the OAMR, which honored him with a life membership in the association.

THE LARGER PICTURE

Fotheringham points out that the mental retardation clinic at TPH played its part in an era of tremendous change in attitude toward people with developmental disabilities and in planning for their school, work, and housing. When the clinic began, the institutionalization (often for life) of persons thought to have a developmental disability was generally felt to be the best disposition for them, for their own and their families' sake.

"Orillia Hospital School in those days had about 2,700 residents; today it has about 700," Fotheringham recalls.

> Admissions came heavily from Metro Toronto. About one third of all admissions from Toronto were Children's Aid Society wards, admitted before they turned 16, when CAS wardship ended. Many were mildly retarded young women, and the major

concern was that they were "interested in boys" and might become pregnant.

Residents in Orillia were rigidly segregated by gender to prevent any sexual activity with the opposite sex. All residents were certified as incompetent and if they escaped they were brought back. Once, when I was in the Orillia Hospital, they brought back a woman who had escaped three years previously. She was discovered working in a restaurant as a waitress and supporting herself.[8]

When a child was born with Down's Syndrome in the 1960s, the parents were frequently asked to decide whether they were going to take the child home, or send it to an institution. Children born with Down's Syndrome frequently have a serious congenital heart disorder or pyloric stenosis of the stomach. The tendency was not to operate on such babies, but to let them die. On occasion, our clinic heard of such cases in time to call the Children's Aid Society, who could make such children wards and so save their lives. "Today, virtually no children with developmental disabilities are admitted to large institutions," noted Fotheringham.

In Rideau Regional Hospital, for instance, there are now approximately 800 residents, all adults, who tend to be severely handicapped intellectually, with serious physical or behavioral problems. At the time our clinic was operating, Rideau housed some 3,500 persons.[9]

During the four-year life of the clinic, the mindset of treatment personnel, government, parents, (and particularly the powerful OAMR) began to swing away from care in institutions toward community living for people with developmental disabilities. Looking back, one can see that the move to community living was made in two stages and is still under way.

During the first stage, parents' councils and the OAMR with its local associations made tremendous efforts to provide special schooling, nursery schools, sheltered workshops, residences, and group homes for persons with developmental handicaps. The first "experimental class" for retarded children was opened in 1947 in Kirkland Lake. The Department of Education made a grant of $2,000 per year, with the remaining costs to be covered by local groups. During the next decades, members of the associations raised great amounts of money, and spent some of the best years of their lives trying to provide special services for those who seemed to need them. Those years of effort were just getting under way when our clinic opened.

Then, in 1971, the Declaration on the Rights of the Retarded Persons of the United Nations General Assembly stated: "The mentally retarded person has, to the maximum degree of feasibility, the same rights as other human beings."

The second stage in the move toward community living represented normalization: the view that, rather than segregate persons with a developmental disability in special services in the community, every effort should be made to include them in the range of options open to everyone, with special supports where needed. The philosophy of service of OAMR changed during the 1970s and in 1978 was stated as follows: "OAMR and its member local associations want to ensure that retarded people are able to live in a state of dignity, share in all elements of living in the community and have the opportunity to participate effectively."[10] As we have seen, the institutions have greatly reduced their populations with this goal in mind (sometimes before the community was ready). The struggle to realize the goal continues.

Looking back over the years since 1962, and taking into account the difficulties change brought, Fotheringham says, "It's all been ninety percent good."

The Move to Surrey Place

In 1966, when most of the staff of TPH moved to the new Clarke Institute, the mental retardation clinic took over the former TPH building at 2 Surrey Place. The new service was first called the Mental Retardation Centre; then, in deference to our clients' wishes, simply Surrey Place Centre. With an enlarged staff and mandate, the centre has continued to serve its community till the present day. It should not be forgotten that the centre might not have come into being without the planning and encouragement of TPH and the foresight of the OAMR back in 1961.

Endnotes

Many thanks go to John Fotheringham for his many contributions to the content of this chapter. His kind assistance has been greatly appreciated.

[1] For an excellent history of the association see Betty Anglin and Jane Braaten, *Twenty-five Years of Growing Together: A History of the Ontario Association for the Mentally Retarded* (Toronto: Canadian Association for the Mentally Retarded, 1978).
[2] Ibid.

[3] For more on British institutions see Gwendoline M. Ayers, *England's First State Hospitals and the Metropolitan Asylums Board* (Berkeley, Los Angeles: University of California Press, 1971).

[4] John B. Fotheringham, Mora Skelton, Bernard A. Hoddinott, *The Retarded Child and his Family* (Toronto: Ontario Institute for Studies in Education, Monograph Series/11, 1971).

[5] Mora Skelton and Richard Wong, *Directory of Services for the Mentally Retarded in Ontario* (Toronto: Ontario Department of Health, 1970).

[6] Mora Skelton and Cyril Greenland, "Social Work and Mental Retardation," in Michael Craft, ed., *Treadgold's Mental Retardation* 12th ed. (London: Balliere Tindall, 1979).

[7] John B. Fotheringham, Walter D. Hambley, Harriet W. Haddad-Curran, *Prevention of Intellectual Handicaps* (Toronto: The Martin Group, 1983).

[8] Personal communication with John Fotheringham, summer 1992.

[9] Ibid.

[10] Ontario Association for the Mentally Retarded, *Positions on Social Issues Affecting People Who Are Mentally Retarded* (Toronto: The Association, 1978).

16

THE FORENSIC CLINIC

R.E. TURNER AND ERIKA STEFFER*

When the clinic was founded in 1956, there was no precedent to guide its planning. No one knew to what extent the courts would use it. No one knew what types of offenders would be referred, how many would be suitable for treatment or how many would benefit from attendance at the clinic.

The courts had been referring cases to the in-patient clinic since the Toronto Psychiatric Hospital began in 1925 and it was likely they would make some use of the new service. It was known that many people were in need of treatment which was not available. By coincidence the probation service was advocating the establishment of a clinical service for probationers.

...Magistrates and probation officers are making extensive use of the clinic. It is gratifying to see that the clinic has reached the stage where it can conduct a scientific appraisal of its successes and failures in the treatment of deviant behaviour...

Thus, lawyer-psychiatrist Ken Gray summarized in his foreword to the 1960 annual report the value of the forensic clinic in the context of forensic psychiatry at Toronto Psychiatric Hospital.[1] In fact, forensic psychiatry at TPH during the postwar period was dominated by Gray. A 1928 graduate in medicine of the University of Toronto, Kenneth George

---

*R. Edward ("Ed") Turner, born 1926, graduated M.D. from the University of Toronto in 1952. He trained at psychiatric hospitals in Canada and England and joined the Forensic Clinic of TPH in 1955, becoming director in 1958. Erika Steffer, M.L.I.S., University of Western Ontario. Erika Steffer is a Toronto-based information specialist, an associate of Clear Language and Design consulting service, and an active volunteer with East End Literacy. She is currently a researcher with the Bank of Montreal and has worked as a freelance researcher, writer, and editor since 1991.

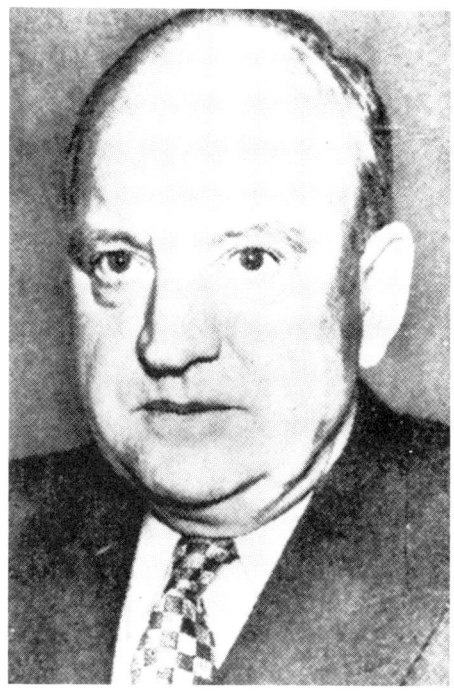

Kenneth G. Gray (1905-1970), the first forensic psychiatrist in Toronto, graduated MD from the University of Toronto in 1928 and joined the Law Society of Upper Canada in 1935. He began lecturing on medical jurisprudence in 1937 and established a formal clinic in 1956.

Gray studied psychiatry at the Ontario Hospital, New Toronto, in 1931, and, after working for the Ontario Hospital, Mimico, began at the Toronto Psychiatric Hospital in 1933.

Shortly afterward, he graduated from Osgoode Hall Law School and was retained by the Attorney General of Ontario to assist with the drafting of a new mental hospitals act. Passed in 1935, this act, which introduced advanced procedures for the caring of the mentally ill and included entirely new terminology, remained in force essentially unchanged until 1967. Gray was next appointed lecturer in medical jurisprudence in 1937, and gave a course of lectures to senior law students on psychiatric problems in law, sharing the podium with pathologist William Robinson.

Throughout his career, Gray built the bridge between law and psychiatry over which all subsequent forensic staff have passed. After serving as a lieutenant colonel in the Royal Canadian Army Medical Corps during World War II, Gray became "special lecturer" in forensic psychiatry while working for the Prime Minister's Office. During this period, he delivered a paper entitled "What is Forensic Psychiatry" to the Ontario Neuropsychiatric Association, a paper that Turner used for many years in introductory lectures to Forensic Psychiatry.

Gray joined the University of Toronto Department of Psychiatry in 1949 and was instrumental in the development of the forensic psychiatry program. Department chair A.B. Stokes, in his letter to Claude Bissell, university president, promoted the appointment, noting that Gray had "already made a contribution to the development of those legal aspects of social psychiatry which are bound to have important repercussions in any Health programme."[2] He was later appointed professor of forensic psychiatry (the first such chair in Canada) in 1960.

During these early years after World War II, Gray authored two books[3] and joined the executive of numerous provincial, national, and international associations and committees. He was president of the Ontario Psychiatric Association and the Medico-Legal Society of Toronto. Legal counsel at the founding of the Canadian Psychiatric Association in 1951, Gray remained honorary counsel until his death in 1970.

While his contemporaries Bruno Cormier at McGill and George Scott at Kingston seemed motivated on "humanistic grounds with the wish to ensure adequate care to mentally ill prisoners in the correctional system," Gray emphasized the "fitness to stand trial, competency and remand assessment with a later emphasis on the sexual offender."[4] In his approach to forensic psychiatry, Gray:

> not only developed the servicing end of it, but the research side as well... [He] directed a lot of attention to the question of homosexuality, for example, and all the sexual deviations, trying to find out more about what it is all about, and how to categorize them, what's the best treatment, what's the best approach from the law, and from society's point of view.[5]

Alex Finlayson (a resident assigned to the forensic service in 1954) relates some of his experiences:

> Dr. Ken Gray was a very kind, quiet, supporting person who was well respected both in the Forensic Service and in the Judiciary. On my return to Orillia, I was still called upon to do forensic cases in some of which I was supported by Gray. There are two instances which I recall with pleasure when I valued his support. On the one occasion I was called to give testimony in Parry Sound before Justice J.D. Stewart in the case of a manslaughter charge against a male in the death of his teenage daughter. As a somewhat inexperienced forensic psychiatrist I was trying to explain to the judge the nature of the accused's mental state in that he was both mentally retarded and suffering from a paranoid schizophrenia. I was describing to the judge that some patients,

although regarded as being insane, still had their lucid moments. My explanation seemed to upset the judge. He replied I was describing "an alarm clock" insanity which could be turned on and off according to the psychiatrist. Dr. Gray, however, was able to smooth things over by first of all explaining in depth the nature of paranoid schizophrenia, and in the recess in the judge's chambers was able to convince Justice Stewart that the father was not guilty by reason of insanity...

The second occasion occurred when Dr. Gray and I were involved in giving evidence in the historic case of Marvin McKay, who was found guilty as charged and was the last man to be hanged in Canada for a capital crime...

I always admired Dr. Gray's approach to the bench and [how] in his quiet, deliberate way, [he] could not be ruffled in his testimony despite hours of vigorous cross examination. I mourned his untimely passing but always associate him with the implementation of Forensic Psychiatry at the Toronto Psychiatric Hospital and its development through the years by his former students both at the Clarke Institute of Psychiatry and METFORS.[6]

In addition to Gray, TPH staff working in forensics included Alex Finlayson, John Atcheson (director of the juvenile and family court clinic), and Gordon Watson. In 1954 and 1955, Gray and Watson followed up on persons admitted to the forensic unit five years prior, while Finlayson and his tutor, Alan Parkin (who had recently completed analysis under Mildred Creak in London, England), set up two or three group programs at the old outpatient department at Elizabeth Street. Yet while forensic psychiatry had been a concern for TPH since its inception, it was the much publicized murder of three children in 1956 and the residual mayhem that led to legislative changes affecting forensic psychiatry at TPH.

FOUNDING A FORENSIC CLINIC

In 1956, public outcry over sexual deviation (prompted by the murders of these three children) precipitated the development of a forensic clinic. Alarm in the press led to a public forum (sponsored by the Toronto Star) at Massey Hall in January 1956. Edson L. Haines, Q.C., (past vice-president of the Canadian Bar Association and later Ontario Supreme Court judge) chaired a panel of four experts discussing the problem of the sexual offender.[7] A provincial committee was subsequently formed which recommended that a forensic clinic be established.[8] Parkin encouraged using group psychotherapy to treat patients in the new forensic service, so several sexually dysfunctional males were referred to the group and with Parkin's help they experienced the therapeutic process.

The clinic was set up in May 1956 in the former Nurses Building at 7 Queen's Park Crescent, and Peter Thomson (a graduate of the Toronto program) moved from the Queen Street Mental Health Centre to become the first director of this town, crown, gown arrangement. The staff included Lorraine Williams as chief social worker, Daniel Paitich as psychologist, Elsie Russell as secretary, and Margaret McKeen as receptionist. Harry Hutchison was chief psychologist of the forensic service throughout TPH. In 1956, Thomson was also secretary of the Toronto Psychoanalytical Study Circle during its first year and continued his studies at the Canadian Psychoanalytic Society in Montreal on alternate weekends (the first Toronto student to do so).

In July 1956, after completing his residency, Finlayson also joined the forensic service. Because of a shortage of senior consultants, he divided his time between TPH's male service with Abe Miller and the forensic service with Gray and Atcheson. Under Gray's direction, they proceeded to establish the individual forensic service and Finlayson led the sexually dysfunctional group as part of the outpatient structure. Due to a severe hearing loss, he asked Ken Gray and Aldwyn B. Stokes, head of TPH, to transfer him to the clinical administration post at the Ontario Hospital School in Orillia, a position he took up in September 1956.

Turner recalls: "I had the good fortune to be assigned to the clinic as a third-year resident, the first such appointment, starting July 1, 1956. By the time I became director in May 1958, Val Hartman had become the chief social worker; Peter Thomson, Sam Jedwab, and Elliot Markson were psychiatric consultants; one resident had been on staff in 1957, and four residents had been assigned for 1958."[9] The clinic provided diagnosis and assessment, treatment, research, and teaching services.

McRuer Commission

In 1959, the Royal Commission on the Criminal Law related to Criminal Sexual Psychopaths published its report.[10] Chaired by J.C. McRuer, then Chief Justice of Ontario, the commission noted the need for research:

We believe that there is great necessity for concentration on ways and means of clinical study and experiment to arrest the development of sexual deviation. The responsibility for this extends far beyond the jurisdiction of the courts, and even of the legislative bodies.

The commission said of the forensic clinic,

We think the proper authorities should embark on a program of education of parents, teachers and all those in charge of young persons, to co-operate with clinics established on the principle of the Forensic Clinic of Toronto, so that all known effective measures may be taken to arrest the development in young persons of tendencies toward sexual deviation... In addition, diagnostic centres equipped with proper medical facilities should be established in conjunction with special institutional treatment under the direction and auspices of universities. These diagnostic centres should operate in close relationship with the courts. When these centres have been set up and have functioned for a sufficient period of time to appraise their success, the legislation we recommend ought to be reviewed in the light of known results.[11]

The commission concluded that (a) "The courts should be given power to refer any prisoner convicted of any indictable offense for psychiatric examination before sentence" and (b) "There is urgent need in Canada for research in all aspects of sexual deviation , with a view to development of means of correction and prevention."[12] The report recommended that "special clinics be set up in co-operation with the courts and penal institutions, to which a person found guilty of any sexual offense may be required to report for study and treatment."[13]

This was the climate in which forensic psychiatry entered a new stage at TPH—with an elevated status, in a setting where research and teaching were closely allied to service.

Diagnosis and assessment

The clinic brought systematic diagnosis and assessment to Ontario's courts. The 1958 annual report notes that the clinic studied and appraised cases that were

selected and referred by Magistrates and Judges under section 92(d) of the Ontario Mental Hospitals Act, which states "...a Mental Health clinic shall have authority to conduct an examination of the physical and mental condition of...any person on the Order of a Magistrate."[14]

The clinic had four to six weeks to conduct an investigation and report the results to the magistrate under provision section 96(c). "The Officer in charge of a Mental Health Clinic may report the results of examination under section 92...(c)...to any person or organization upon whose order and request the examination was undertaken..."[15]

The clinic also offered diagnostic and assessment services to probation officers, private physicians, outpatient clinics, hospitals, and community agencies. (Probation officers were terribly overworked and were pleased to have the clinic lessen their caseload.) Other cases were voluntary; some were suggested by the Metropolitan Toronto Police. The 1958 annual report also states that,

> In addition to the psychological and social service contributions to the clinic, several ancillary tests, such as electroencephalogram and X-ray can be carried out at the Toronto Psychiatric Hospital. The Medical and Neurological Consultant Staff of the hospital are also available.[16]

Ron Stokes, who gave evidence at 210 murder trials and was in court more than once a week while on staff, experienced the excitement of trial work as an expert witness preparing a thorough work-up for important cases. Medical and hospital information about the patient would be gathered and a team approach used to perform psychological tests and social work studies.[17] A psychiatric examination was intended to provide a complete picture of the patient. Stokes noted, "I learned more general psychiatry in forensic than in any of the locations I was at." He stressed the importance of being credible as an unbiased professional and noted there was "none of this battle of the experts" since there were times when clinic staff were on the same case—on opposing sides. A psychiatrist would check with counsel and ask what they wanted the psychiatrist to do since (1) cases might be difficult, not just clinically, but also in how one might choose to present them, and (2) it "often turned out it wasn't a subject for psychiatry at all."[18]

TREATMENT

According to social worker Lorraine Williams, the team approach used for court cases to provide a well-researched investigation also served for clinic cases in general. A social worker would complete a social history form used as the basis for research, a psychologist would do psychometric testing, and the psychiatrist would see the patient. At a weekly conference, staff would decide who would treat individual cases: A few were treated by a psychologist, those with disturbed functioning were seen by a social worker, and those who were quite disturbed were seen by the psychiatrist. In general, there was a lack of damaging hierarchy and in lieu of inter-office rivalry, there was good *esprit de corps*.

Forensic staff treated offenders on an outpatient basis, which was unique at the time. The offenders were

> able to remain in the community, having been discharged from the Court and/or placed on probation. If treatment in the form of psychotherapy is recommended in the pre-sentence report, the Forensic Clinic can carry out such a form of treatment. Several types of therapy are available, including long-term intensive treatment, re-educative, and supportive psychotherapy. The majority of cases are dealt with on a once-weekly basis. Specially selected cases of homosexuality, exhibitionism, and pedophilia are studied on an intensive basis over a long period of time. Particular efforts are being made in the use of group psychotherapy.[19]

Although data from their programs were collected for future analysis, the demands of the service limited the amount of research performed at the clinic in the early years. Particular areas of interest were the psychodynamics of sexual deviation and the efficacy of group therapy.

Research

Yet over the years clinic staff were very active in research. Ron Stokes, assistant director from 1963–65 describes the work environment at the clinic.

> Research and writing of papers [were] just a part of the job. It was something that automatically came and there was a lot of inspiration. I think one of the things that played a big role in that was that Ed [Turner] and Ken Gray always gave credit to the person who did the work (contrary to many other departments where the head of the department would take the credit). So they inspired people to work. There was a mutual respect for achievements and they were always encouraged in younger professionals.[20]

Responding to courts and magistrates looking for information on sexual offenses, forensic staff researched and wrote *Pedophilia and Exhibitionism: A Handbook* by J.W. Hans Mohr, R. Edward Turner, and Marion B. Jerry, a work the University of Toronto Press published in September 1964. In June 1992 Mohr recalled that there was "reliance in knowledge" and a feeling that "research was important."[21] But in a pre-computer era, data sorting took a long time. The book, which provided a full sample of voluntary and referred cases, was first reviewed by Bruno Cormier, in the *Canadian Psychiatric Association Journal* of December 1964.[22] The book was selected by the Behavioural Science Book Club to appear on their list in spring 1964.

Another notable study was *Mental Illness and Homicide* by Ken McKnight. McKnight analyzed the 122 cases of homicide admitted to the Oak Ridge division of the Ontario Hospital, Penetanguishene, over a 30-year period. In 100 of these 122 cases, the question of mental illness was raised at the time of trial. The other 22 cases either represented homicides in other mental hospitals or patients who became mentally ill after being sentenced to penitentiary. The analysis included: the offender-victim relationship; social and family background; personal background; diagnosis; age at time of murder; place, time, and method of offense; behavior after offense; etc.[23]

TEACHING

Because of its association with TPH, the clinic was closely linked with the University of Toronto's Department of Psychiatry.

> Teaching has been involved at both undergraduate and postgraduate levels. Two postgraduate physicians in psychiatry are assigned to the clinic for training for periods of six months. They participate in the Seminar programme, receive teaching and experience in group psychotherapy, and have a number of tutorial sessions individually in psychodynamics and psychotherapy. The clinical staff participate in the medical undergraduate teaching programme. Teaching is offered also to other groups and disciplines, such as psychologists, nurses, social workers and Probation Officers, particularly through case conferences.[24]

Senior members of the staff participated in the teaching programs in many areas. Thomson, Markson, and Turner were clinical teachers in the Department of Psychiatry in the Faculty of Medicine. The postgraduate physicians in psychiatry had individual tutorial sessions from each of these clinical teachers. Jedwab, a "marvellous teacher" Ron Stokes noted, assisted these postgraduate physicians in the preparation of their seminar papers. Hutchison was a superb teaching fellow in psychology, and several summer internships were provided for postgraduate psychology students on a rotation basis. Joe Rubin was a lecturer in the University of Toronto Extension Department. Val Hartman, who counted as resident wine connoisseur and LCBO consultant, supervised students from the School of Social Work assigned to the clinic for the year. Ken McKnight participated in the teaching of fourth-year medical students. Said Turner, "I was appointed also as a psychiatric teacher in the university's new diploma course in speech pathology and audiology. Along with Markson, I lectured to the ministers and pastors in the Toronto Institute for Pastoral Training."

Informally, staff members extended teaching in practical ways (1) to several officers of the probation service in the form of clinical case conferences and (2) through a weekly seminar convened Tuesday mornings from September to the end of June. For two hours each week staff would present formal papers, which were followed by spirited discussion. Approximately once a month a special guest was invited from outside the immediate staff to speak on common problems and related subjects, thus keeping our orientation broad and practical. Ron Stokes noted that people worked together and the teaching was "inspirational." He added,

> When you were being corrected, it was done in a manner that provoked thought, further study and reading to get on with it...the learning process kept going on and on. There was a fine flow of information while at the same time you were carrying a pretty hectic patient load.[25]

He compared the atmosphere to MASH, saying that with "rats frolick[ing] in the basement...under adverse conditions the job was done well and with humour."

In the foreword to the clinic's eighth (and final) annual report in 1965, Charles Roberts, executive director of TPH, stated:

> The clinic has provided considerable leadership in forensic psychiatry. The development of similar clinics in Glasgow, Rochester and Philadelphia, and the planning of those for Vancouver and Winnipeg, has been largely influenced by the experience of this clinic.

As we look forward to further contributions from the Forensic Clinic we can hope for a better understanding of and more effective treatment for such patients.[26]

Prior to being included in the Clarke Institute of Psychiatry, the small clinic had created a feeling of being part of the group, a group that worked on all fronts to understand its cases and to improve treatments. Because it was small and had fostered that MASH-like intensity and creativity, it succeeded, a success it would take time to re-establish at the Clarke.

Endnotes

[1] Province of Ontario, Department of Health, Hospitals Division, *Toronto Psychiatric Hospital: Report Covering Period 1926-1932* (Toronto: Queens Printer, 1932), p. 5. [C.B. Farrar authored the report.] The vision of TPH founders was that it provide a "Centre for the observation of persons coming before the courts and requiring investigation as to their mental status." Their approach established forensic psychiatry as one of the two major functions of TPH (the other being to "provide a receiving centre for mental patients in the earliest stages of their illness with a service as closely similar as possible to that of a general hospital") and carried out a provision of the Ontario Statutes of 1914 whereby "persons suffering or believed to be suffering from mental disabilities may not be confined in gaols or other similar places of detention." Warrant cases were important in the life of TPH, comprising 40% of its cases in its initial seven years. "[A]ll cases appearing in court in which a mental disability is present or suspected are remanded for observation" (p. 7). After observation, cases were either transferred to provincial hospitals or referred back to the courts with recommendations based on personality and social group studies of the patients. The court was cooperative and routinely considered these recommendations about particular cases.

[2] A.B. Stokes, letter to C.T. Bissell dated July 25, 1949.

[3] K.G. Gray, *Law in the Practice of Medicine*, rev. and enlarged ed. (Toronto: Ryerson, 1955); K.G. Gray and N. Fidler, *Law in the Practice of Nursing* (Toronto: Ryerson, 1947).

[4] C.A. Roberts, "More for the Mind: Thirty Years Later," presented at the conference on the "Organization and Delivery of Services to the Chronic Mentally Ill" at the Health Science Centre, University of Calgary, May 11-12, 1992.

[5] J. Dewan, "Psychiatry in Ontario 1930-1970" presented at the Clarke Institute of Psychiatry Historical Seminar, March 11, 1978.

[6] METFORS is the acronym for the Metropolitan Toronto Forensic Service, established in 1977, which provides psychiatric assessment to the courts in York Region and elsewhere in the province based on bed availability and need for the service from outside of York.

[7] Participants were (1) Ralph Brancale, Director of the State of New Jersey's Diagnostic Center for Sex Offenders; (2) Kenneth George Gray; (3) Manfred Guttmacher, Chief Medical Officer of the Supreme Bench, Baltimore, Maryland; (4) Frederick Van Nostrand, Chief of Treatment Services, Department of Reform Institutions of Ontario.

[8] This committee consisted of the (1) Attorney General, A. Kelso Roberts; (2) Minister of Reform Institutions, J.W. Foote, V.C.; (3) Minister of Health, W. MacKinnon Phillips; (4) William J. Stewart, M.P.P. for Parkdale and (5) representatives of the Parents Action League, who had been a vocal part of the cry for change.

THE FORENSIC CLINIC 315

[9] The residents were G. Cormack, H. Freedman, D. Squire, K. McKnight, and J. O'Shaughnessy.

[10] J.C. McRuer, *Report of the Royal Commission on the Criminal Law Relating to Criminal Sexual Psychopaths* (Ottawa: Queens Printer, 1958).

[11] "Research," ibid., pp. 117-19, quote p. 117.

[12] "Summary of Conclusions," ibid., pp. 123-25, quote p. 124.

[13] "Recommendations," ibid., pp. 127-30, quote p. 130.

[14] Forensic Clinic, *Annual Report 1958*. R.E. Turner files.

[15] Ibid.

[16] Ibid.

[17] Interview with Lorraine Williams, June 22, 1992. She noted that social work studies could be simple or very complex. The patient was interviewed to detail the social history for the case. Afterwards, staff would determine whether to involve other family members. Lastly, the social work study was put in the record.

[18] Interview with Ron Stokes, June 25, 1992.

[19] Ibid.

[20] Ibid.

[21] Interview with J.W. Hans Mohr, June 29, 1992.

[22] B.M. Cormier et al., "The Persistent Offender and his Sentences: A Problem for Law and Psychiatry," *Canadian Psychiatric Association Journal* 9 (6): 462-480 (December 1964).

[23] C.K. McKnight and J.W. Mohr, "Oak Ridge Study: Report of the Preliminary Survey." Unpublished. Clarke Institute of Psychiatry archives.

[24] Forensic Clinic, *Annual Report 1965*. R.E. Turner files.

[25] Interview with Ron Stokes, June 25, 1992.

[26] Forensic Clinic, *Annual Report*, 1965. R.E. Turner files.

17

Farewell to TPH

Charles Roberts[*]

I served as the fourth superintendent of the Toronto Psychiatric Hospital from January 1, 1965 to June 1966.

During the fall of 1964 I had a phone call from a Mr. Ian Davidson, who introduced himself as Chairman of the Board of the Clarke Institute of Psychiatry, then under construction in Toronto. He wished to visit me in Montreal to discuss hospital organization and management.

A year of so before I had prepared a report on mental health services in Ontario for the then Minister of Health, Dr. Matthew Dymond. While studying the Ontario services and preparing my report, I became convinced that a new facility to replace the old Toronto Psychiatric Hospital might not be in the best interests of psychiatry. I would have preferred to see those services integrated with the general medical and mental health services already in place.

In a letter to Dr. Dymond, I recommended that the institute not be built. I suggested that the money instead be divided among the main teaching hospitals in Toronto—the Toronto General Hospital, the Toronto Western Hospital, Wellesley Hospital, Women's College Hospital, and the Sick Children's Hospital—and perhaps "999," the Queen Street Mental Health Centre. Dr. Dymond, I was told, gave very serious consideration to my views, but indicated that the situation had already developed too far for the government to reverse its position.

---

[*]Charles Roberts, born in 1918 in St. John's, Newfoundland, graduated M.D. in 1942 from Dalhousie University. After training in psychiatry in Nova Scotia and Toronto, he was superintendent from 1945 to 1950 at the Hospital for Nervous and Mental Diseases in St. John's. He served in the early 1950s in the Department of National Health and Welfare in Ottawa, and in 1957 became superintendent of the Verdun Protestant Hospital in Montreal. In 1965 he came to Toronto as the last director, or superintendent, of TPH.

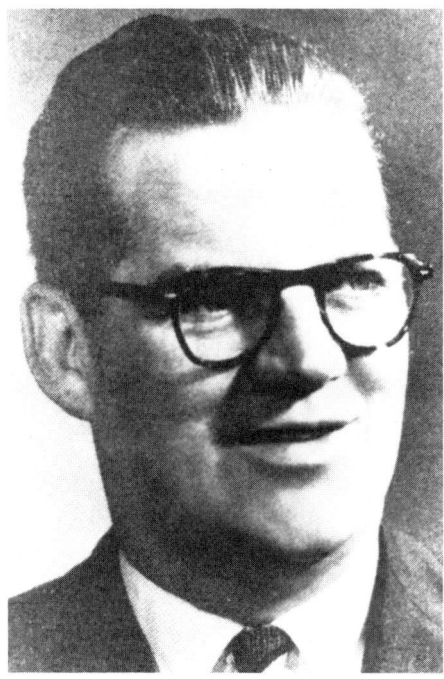

Charles A. Roberts (b. 1918), the final director of TPH, 1965-1966.

After Mr. Davidson's visit, I received the first of a series of calls from him, ironically leading me to become executive director of the very institution I had suggested should not exist.

While I was in Ottawa with the Department of National Health and Welfare, I had come to know most of the senior psychiatrists in Ontario very well. Burdett McNeel, by then a very good friend, became director of mental health in the Ontario Department of Health; shortly thereafter Dr. W.H. Henderson became director of community psychiatric services. Dr. McNeel and I had developed an effective working relationship while I was in Ottawa.

By the time I moved to Toronto, Dr. McNeel had retired as director of mental health and had been succeeded by Dr. Henderson, whom I had known when he was director of the mental health clinic at the Ottawa Civic Hospital. Without his support it would have been much more difficult to close a public service hospital, the Toronto Psychiatric Hospital, and open a board-operated, university affiliated hospital, the Clarke Institute.

The long-time assistant medical superintendent of the Toronto Psychiatric Hospital was Dr. Mary Jackson. It soon became apparent to me that she had been responsible for the day-to-day operation of the hospital for many years. She was one of a small number of outstanding women in psychiatry in Ontario at that time. Dr. Jackson was quietly effective in her role, which continued at the Clarke Institute after we closed the TPH.

I cannot think of the Toronto Psychiatric Hospital without recalling Doris Leggett and the part she played both there and at the Clarke. She was very knowledgeable about the organization and administration of the hospital and the University of Toronto, and was unfailingly kind and considerate to all who encountered her. Like so many of the senior secretaries I have known across the country, she played a major part in the operation of the hospital and the Department of Psychiatry. She moved to the Clarke with Dr. Stokes and continued as his secretary until the time of his death.

When I arrived in Toronto in 1965, my mandate was as follows:

1. To close the Toronto Psychiatric Hospital

2. To open the Clarke Institute of Psychiatry

3. To develop teaching programs in mental health and psychiatry for students in health administration and public health at the School of Hygiene, University of Toronto.

I held concurrent appointments as executive director of the Clarke and medical superintendent of the Toronto Psychiatric Hospital. My responsibility with respect to the latter was to oversee its smooth operation and, in due time, to transfer all of its functions to the new institute and close the old one down.

My association with Dr. Aldwyn Stokes was most gratifying. He was an outstanding influence upon my work as a psychiatrist, and as a former medical superintendent of the facility, I was appointed to wind down. I first met him in the late forties when I represented Newfoundland on the Advisory Committee on Mental Health to the Minister of National Health and Welfare in Ottawa.

The next major contact I had with Dr. Stokes was during the Hall Commission study on medical care insurance for Canada. The board of directors of the Canadian Psychiatric Association appointed Dr. Stokes and myself to prepare a submission to the Hall Commission. I still remember the weekend we spent in Ottawa from late Friday afternoon through to Sunday evening preparing that draft report. We essentially completed our task that weekend.

Although I knew that Dr. Stokes was heavily involved in the development of the Clarke Institute, and was aware of the suggestion that I become director, I did not discuss this matter with him. However, I greatly appreciated the warm welcome he gave me when I arrived to assume my duties in Toronto.

Dr. Stokes and his wife, Margaret, made an effective team. Early in his career, Dr. Stokes became aware of a neurological deficit that made it very difficult for him to drive a car. He gave up driving and relied on Mrs. Stokes as his chauffeur, a duty she carried out without complaint or bitterness throughout their life together. Although Dr. Stokes was willing to use taxis much of the time, he would certainly have found it difficult to function as effectively without Margaret's support.

Aldwyn Stokes has, I believe, been given insufficient credit for his contributions to Canadian psychiatry. Like Dr. Ewen Cameron at the Allan Memorial Institute in Montreal, he took full advantage of the National Health Grants Program when it was introduced. He spearheaded the rapid post-war expansion of postgraduate training programs in psychiatry at the University of Toronto, as well as the training of clinical psychologists, social workers, occupational therapists, liaison psychologists, and teacher psychologists. He sponsored valuable research and brought a number of eminent psychiatrists to Canada from the United Kingdom. One of the most outstanding pieces of research done during the TPH years was the Crestwood Heights Study, also known as the Forest Hill Village Project, which dealt with the mental health of children in the local school system. The study catalyzed a number of efforts to minimize psychiatric symptoms in that community and promote better mental health.

Credit is due to the work done at the Toronto Psychiatric Hospital during its forty years of operation. Its highly successful two-year diploma course in psychiatry was the first and the largest in Canada until the Allen Memorial Institute came into its own in the 1940s. The TPH improved the staffing of Ontario psychiatric hospitals by providing formal education for staff recruited from across the province. The hospital also served as a resource for other provinces in the areas of education and program development, and enjoyed an international reputation. Its accomplishments in research were significant, particularly after the National Health Grants Program became available in 1948.

The actual closing of the Toronto Psychiatric Hospital took place with relatively little fanfare. There were no protests or objections from the

Ontario Civil Service Association, the union of the day. A few clinical staff elected to stay in government service and appropriate positions were found for them. A number of administrative support personnel chose to remain with the Toronto Psychiatric Hospital as it was converted into a mental retardation centre. As I recollect only one staff member—a social worker from the United State—resigned because he did not agree with the plans for the Clarke: He wanted us to develop a mental health centre such as those arising in the United States at that time.

Clinical and research records were transferred to the Clarke Institute of Psychiatry; all other records remained with the Ontario Ministry of Health.

After appropriate decisions had been made regarding the organization and administration of the Clarke, including such matters as salary scales, pension plans, vacations, and other benefits, the time came to involve the existing staff at TPH. A decision was made to send a letter to all individuals working at that hospital—regardless of their area—offering them an appointment on the staff of the Clarke Institute. As we had decided to participate in all of the Ontario Hospital Association's programs, our employees' working conditions and benefits would be similar to those prevailing in Ontario's general hospitals.

While planning the Clarke, we learned much from the numerous operating difficulties at the Toronto Psychiatric Hospital in the days when it was administered by the provincial Ministry of Health. For example, while many employees of the hospital were provincial public servants, others were hired by the university or taken on independently by the hospital for research projects. There were thus at least three sets of personnel policies, and it was not uncommon for some departments to be open on particular days while others had a statutory holiday.

During the years at TPH an organization of volunteers, the "White Cross Guild," had been established. The Guild was one of the hospital's strengths and continued at the Clarke Institute.

I remember being given a very big send-off when I left Toronto in 1969. On the one hand, this was quite touching, as I had only been there about four and a half years. However, I could not help but feel that the enthusiasm at my farewell was fostered in part by a sense of relief as I, with my heightened sense of administrative order, cheerfully took my leave, and new hands, perhaps more flexible than mine, took over the helm.

INDEX

A

Abbey, Susan, 12
Academy of Medicine, Toronto, 35
Addiction Research Foundation, 279
Advisory Committee on Mental Health, 125, 136, 318
Aikens, H. Wilberforce, 79
Ainsworth, Mary (Salter), 230
Alexander, Franz, 88
Allan Memorial Institute, Montreal, 319
Allemang, Margaret, 204
Allen, Frederick, 294
Alvirez, Ann (Adams), 245
Alzheimer, Alois, 14, 28, 54, 65, 72, 162
American Association of Psychiatric Social Workers, 243
American Cybernetic Society, 287
American Handbook of Psychiatry (1957), 278
American Journal of Insanity (later *American Journal of Psychiatry*), 77
 history of, 156-158
American Journal of Psychiatry (*AJP*), 80, 89, 107, 155-168
 Canadian involvement in, 155
 centennial issue, 167
 growth of, 166
American Medico-Psychological Association, 157
American Psychiatric Association, 158-159, 206
 and tributes to Farrar, 167
 annual meetings, 166
 centenary, 166-167
 growth of, 166
 Toronto meeting (1931), 158
Anglin, Betty, 298
Angus, Leslie, R., 122-123
anorexia nervosa, 7-8, 275
antidepressants, 3, 135
antipsychotic drugs, 135, 174
 impact on occupational therapy, 267
aptitude testing, 219-220
Argue, John, 78

Armstrong, S.A., 22
Arnold, Magda, 230
art therapy, 275
Arthurs, Bob, 276, 280
Aschaffenburg, Gustav, 85
Association for Children with Mental Retardation, 294
Association of Medical Superintendents of American Institutions for the Insane, 155-157
Atcheson, John, 307
autointoxication theory, 72-75, 83

B

Bach, George, 279
Banting Foundation, 120
Banting Institute, 115
Banting, Sir Frederick, 113-115, 119
Barnes, Edward, 79
Barrett, Albert Moore, 185
Bäumler, Professor Christian, 65
Beech Grove Infirmary, Kingston, 22
Beers, Clifford, 164
Belyea, Ed, 230
Benedict, Nathan D., 157
Bennett, Hilda, 203
Berg, Joseph, M., 298
Berger, Hans, 119
Berrios, German, 1, 9
Best, Charles H., 119
Bethe, Albrecht, 65
biological psychiatry, vii, 3, 14, 63-68, 89, 99, 104, 111, 120
 established in Ontario, 28
 Farrar's emphasis on, 14, 83-84
 preserved at TPH, 138
 resurgence of, 3
 See also neuropsychiatry— organicism
Biringer, Barbro, 227
Bissell, Claude, 306
Blain, Emile, 160
Blatz, William, 231
Bleuler, Eugen, 83, 184

Blumer, G. Alder, 157
Board of Psychiatric Examiners, 107
Bonkalo, Alec, 226
Boothroyd, Eric, 136
Borden Committee, 104, 125, 139-140
Bott, Edward, 230
Braaten, Jane, 298
Braceland, Francis J., 167
"breakdowns in living," 275, 279, 289, 295
Bregg, Elizabeth ("Betty"), theory of nursing, 208-209
brief psychotic disorder, 177
Brigham, Amariah, 156-158
Brockville Reception Hospital, 22, 38, 134
Brown, Jean, 100, 218-224, 233, 272
Bruce, Herbert A., 261
Brush, Edward, 63, 65, 71, 77, 155, 158
Bucke, Richard M., 78, 260
Burgess, T.J.W., 21
Burns, Margaret ("Marg"), 242
Bynum, William F., 10-11

C

Calderone, Mary, 286
Cameron, D. Ewen, 319
Campbell Meyers, Donald, 30, 33-36, 50, 97, 184
Campbell, Catherine ("Caye"), 242, 293-294
Campbell, Charles Macfie, 157
Canadian and Ontario Occupational Therapy Associations, 261
Canadian Army Medical Corps, 120
Canadian Association of Occupational Therapists, 261, 264
Canadian Mental Health Association (formerly CNCMH), 273
Canadian National Committee for Mental Hygiene (CNCMH) (later Canadian Mental Health Association), 42-43, 50-51, 100, 106, 118
Canadian Psychiatric Association, 318
Canadian Psychoanalytic Society, 308
Cappon, Daniel, 227-228, 277
Cassidy, Harry, 241
Castellano, Vincent, 245
Catell, Raymond, 226
Cerletti, Ugo, 117
Chant, Sperrin, 230
child guidance, 242, 273, 294, 296
child psychiatry, 292
Children's Aid Society, 218, 223, 274, 300-301
children's services, 272-274, 294-295

Chisholm, Brock, 87-89
attack on Farrar, 87
Chisholm, D., 49-50
chlorpromazine, 135, 179
Christian Brothers, 218
Chronic Fatigue Syndrome, 2, 10
Church, Pat, 293
City of Toronto, 52
and Reception Hospital obligations, 37-38, 41, 44, 48-51
Civil Service Commission, 205
Clare, Harvey, 35, 38, 40, 51, 53
Clark, Daniel, 23
Clark, Marion, 282
Clarke Institute of Psychiatry, 19, 142, 212, 232, 271, 280-281, 286, 289, 293, 302, 314, 316-320
construction delays, 142
Clarke, C.K., 19, 21-38, 42-43, 46, 48-49, 51-54, 56, 77-81, 97, 99, 107, 121-122, 132, 155, 195, 260, 263, 265
and C.B. Farrar, 77-78, 80-81
and Canadian National Committee for Mental Hygiene, 42
and conflict with Campbell Meyers, 33-34
and Department of Psychiatry (proposed), 28-29
and Ernest Jones, 27-29
and hospital reforms, 22
and support for occupational therapy, 260, 263, 265
and Symposium on Mental Hygiene, 35-36
and Willoughby Commission, 25-27
appointment to University of Toronto, 24
proposes psychiatric clinic, 24-25
Clarke, Emma, 82
Clarke, Eric Kent, 52-53, 132
Clarke, Lieutenant Colonel Charles, 21
Clarke, Marion, 209, 212
Cody, Henry J., 55, 107
colectomy, 73, 75
Coleman, Helen, 296-297
Collins, Mary, 224
Commonwealth Fund, 292
community psychiatry, 129, 142, 267, 281
"community psychology," 228, 231
Conolly, John, 162
continuous baths, 31, 111, 135, 173, 176, 189, 199, 206, 242
Cormier, Bruno, 306, 312
Corsini, Raymond, 279
Cotton, Henry, 72-75
court cases, 102-103, 185, 304, 309-310
Crawford, Clarence, 183

Creak, Mildred, 307
Crestwood Heights Project, 136, 273, 279, 287, 319
crisis theory, 284
curare, 117
Currie, Bill, 233
Cushing, Harvey, 131
cybernetics, 287

D

Davidson, Ian, 316
Davies, Austin M., 159
Dejerine, Jules, 86
dementia praecox, 64, 67, 83, 113
  See also schizophrenia
Department of Health (Ontario), 97, 100, 104, 109-111, 116, 120, 130, 218, 222, 262, 294, 300, 317
  leucotomy program, 132-134
  mental health branch, 243-244
  See also Ministry of Health (Ontario)
Department of Health and Welfare (Federal), 97
Department of Pathological Chemistry, 138
Department of Public Health, 219
  Mental Hygiene Division, *See* Mental Hygiene Division, Toronto Department of Health
Department of Soldiers' Civil Re-establishment, 42, 76, 78, 163
Department of Veteran's Affairs (DVA), (Federal), 230
depression, 2-3, 9, 111, 117
  neurochemistry of, 275
Devaux, Albert, 67
developmental disabilities, 128, 138, 212, 271, 273, 294, 296-302
  and integration in the community, 299-302
Dewan, John, 82, 111, 120, 124, 128, 137-138, 140, 239, 272, 276, 278, 280, 284, 292
  and interviewing skills, 276
Dewey, Richard S., 157
Dick, Edith, 203
Digby, Anne, 10
Ditchburn, Eileen, 109, 194, 203
Don Jail, Toronto, 223
Dörner, Klaus, 4
Douglass, Ernest ("Van"), 136, 286-287
Down's Syndrome, 298, 301
Draper, John W., 75
Drever, James, 224
Drury, E.C., 43
Dubois, Paul, 70, 86

Dunbar, Flanders, 161
Dunlop, W.W., 40, 44-48, 50-51, 54
Dymond, Matthew, 142, 316

E

Earhart, Amelia, 263
Earle, Pliny, 156
Easton, Norman L., 112, 115-118
Edinger, Ludwig, 65
electroconvulsive therapy (ECT), 3, 98, 117-118, 173, 179-180, 189, 207, 275
  injured patient, 177
  in Ontario Hospitals, 118-119
electroencephalogram (EEG), 119, 176
electrotherapy, 31
Ellenberger, Henri, 13
Elliot, G., 128
Ellis, Havelock, 164
Ellis, Louise (McDonald), 246
English, O. Spurgeon, 88
Etobicoke Board of Education, 294
eugenics, 273
Exner, Sigmund, 66
Eysenck, H.J., 234

F

Falconer, Sir Robert, 29, 44, 52, 54, 81, 99, 106
family therapy, 293-294
Farquharson, Ray F., 123, 126
Farrar, Clarence B., 13-15, 25, 42, 48, 53, 55, 59-96, 99, 102-103, 106, 117, 119, 121-122, 130, 155, 183-186, 198-200, 202, 224, 227, 260-262, 280, 293
  and American Journal of Psychiatry 155-168
  and Clifford Beers, 164
  and "menstrual psychosis," 71, 83
  and Osler's influence, 161
  and research, 113-120
  and "rest cure," 69-72
  and *AJP* editorial philosophy, 160, 165
  and biological psychiatry, 83-84, 104
  and C.K. Clarke, 76, 78, 80-81
  and Canadian army, 75-76
  and changes in psychiatry, 59, 68, 86-89
  and hereditary influences, 71, 83-84
  and history of psychiatry, 156
  and insulin coma therapy, 112-115
  and Ontario licence, 79-80
  and Osler's influence, 62-63, 85
  and political interference, 107-111

Farrar, Clarence B. *(continued)*
   and psychiatric nursing education, 196-197
   and psychosomatic illness, 85, 89
   and psychotherapy, 70, 85-86, 89
   and social psychiatry, 84
   and training of psychiatrists, 82-83, 89, 104, 184
   appointments to university and TPH, 54-55
   as neo-Kraepelinian, 184
   at Homewood Sanitarium, Guelph, 78-81
   at Johns Hopkins, 61-63
   attitudes to nurses, 200-201
   Carnegie Institute research grant, 68
   compared to Adolf Meyer, 184-185
   denigration by psychoanalysts, 86-89
   European trip, 63-67, 162
   historical significance of, 59
   honours, 167-168
   in Baltimore, 68-72
   in Cattaraugus, New York, 59-60
   in Toronto, 80-89
   in Trenton, NJ, 72-75
   opposition to pseudo-scientific sects, 163
   opposition to psychoanalysis, 86, 122-123, 163
   publications, 167
   reminiscences about, 183-186, 280
   support for occupational therapy, 260, 264
Farrar, Evelyn Linwood (Lewis), 74, 108
Farrar, Joan, 76-77, 86
Farrar, Thomas Jefferson, 59
Faulkner, James A., 107
Federal grants-in-aid program
   See National Health Grants
"female insanity," cultural artifact, 12, 179
Fenigstein, Henry, 282
Ferguson, Howard, 43
Fidler, Nettie, 105, 109, 194, 197, 214
   and nursing education, 201-203
Fine, Reuben, 4
Finlayson, Alex, 307
Fischer, Martin, 134
Fisher, Martin, 275
FitzGerald, John G., 28, 35, 107
Flavelle, Sir Joseph, 30, 35
Fletcher, D.R., 116
Foley, Ken, 160
Foley, Myrtle, 109, 195, 203, 206
forensic clinic, 307-314
   research, 311-312
   teaching program, 312-314
   treatment, 310-311

forensic psychiatry, 55, 164, 306-307
Forest Hill Project
   See Crestwood Heights Project
Forster, J.M., 35
Foster, D.J., 205
Foster, Mayor, 55
Fotheringham, John, 80, 294, 296-302
"Foucauldian" theory, 4-5, 15
Foucault, Michel, 4-5
Franks, Ruth MacLachlan, 82-83, 105
Freeman, Walter, 130
French, David, 243
Freud, Sigmund, vii, 4, 13, 15, 27-29, 86, 163, 184, 245
Fromm-Reichmann, Frieda, 3

G

Garfinkel, Paul, 12
Geary, George R., 49
Gerstein, Reva Appleby, 229
Gibney, Doris, 207-209
Gilman, Sander, 180
Gjessing, Rolv, 137, 227, 279
Goderich Hospital, 245
Goldie, Lincoln, 47, 53-55, 101, 108
Gornall, Allan, 138
Gosling, F.G., 12
Govan, James, 51
Graduate Nurses' Association of Ontario, 196
Graham, Duncan, 52, 120-122
Grant, James, 275
Grant, Robert, 51
Gray, John P., 157
Gray, Kenneth, 128, 139, 155, 304-308 311
Greenland, Cyril, 244-245, 284, 288
Gregg, Alan, 113-115, 119-120, 122
Griesinger, Wilhelm, 84
Griffin, John D. ("Jack"), 11, 82, 293
Grob, Gerald, 10
group dynamics, 136, 279, 288
group therapy, 136, 287, 294, 296, 308, 311
Grune and Stratton Publishing Co., 160
Gunn, Jean, 50

H

Hackney, Mary, 229
Haines, Edson L., 307
Hall Commission, 318
Halsted, William, 61
Hamilton Hospital, 133
Hanna, Charles, 132, 134
Hanna, William J., 23-27, 29

Hannah, Jason A., 110
Hanover Press, 160
Hare, Edward, 9
Hargreaves, Ronald, 88
Hartman, Val, 308, 313
Hastings, Charles, 35, 50
Haultain, Herbert, 261
Hawkins, Marie, 59
Haywood, Carl, 299
Health Survey Committee Report (1951), 139
Heidelberg school, 11, 14-15, 65
Heldt, Thomas, 185
Henderson, Bill, 284
Henry, Rev. Edwin, 53
Hepburn, Mitchell, 109
Hilliard, Leslie T., 298
Hincks, Clarence, 42-43, 106, 114, 122, 159, 261
Hippocrates, 168
history of psychiatry, vii, 1-15, 245
   changing theories, 3, 12
   growth of interest in, 1-2, 5-13
   institutional histories, 10
   lack of diagnostic detail, 10-11
   trends in historiography, 7, 13
Hobbs, Alfred T., 78-79, 108
Hoch, Marjorie, 262
Hoche, Alfred, 65
Hoddinott, Bernard, 299
Hodgins Commission (1919), 49
Hodgins, Justice, 49
Homewood Sanitarium, Guelph, 15, 54, 78-81, 108
Hone, William, 168
Hospital for Sick Children, 299
Howland, Goldwin W., 46-47, 261
Huerkamp, Claudia, 7
Huestis, Mrs. Archibald, 50
Hueston, Doris (Franks), 198-199, 203
Huntington's chorea, 190
Hurd, Henry M., 71, 158, 167
Hutchison, Alan, 233
Hutchison, Harry, 233, 308, 313
hydrotherapy
   See continuous baths
Hyland, Herbert, 275
hypnosis, 283
hysteria, 8, 12

I

illegitimacy, 223
insulin coma therapy, 98, 111-113, 116, 119, 207-208, 267, 275
   Toronto studies, 113-116
intelligence testing, 100

Inter-Hospital Psychiatric Society seminars, 104
Irvine, Sheila (Dunn), 264, 267-268

J

Jackson, Mary, 131, 140, 282, 317
   support for occupational therapy, 264
Jackson, Robert, 230
Jackson, Stanley, 9
James, William, 61, 161-164
Janet, Pierre, 164
Janzarik, Werner, 11
Jarvis, Frederick C., 79
Jedwab, Sam, 308, 313
Jellinek, Otto, 279
Jerry, Marion B., 312
Johns Hopkins Faculty of Medicine, 68
Johns Hopkins Hospital, Henry Phipps Clinic, 194
Johns Hopkins Medical School, 61-63
Jones, Arthur, 233
Jones, Ernest, 27-29, 36, 245
Jones, Maxwell, 212
Jonys, Birute (Petrulis), 234
Jung, Carl G., 28, 164
Jungian therapy, 277

K

Kanner, Leo, 292
Karrick, Joan, 199, 208
Katz, Barry, 284-285
Kelly, Arthur, 141
Kelly, Howard, 61
Kilgour, Archibald ("Archie"), 82, 198
Kingston Hospital (formerly Rockwood), 263
Kohs' Block Test, 221
Kraepelin, Emil, 11, 14, 28-29, 54, 65, 72, 85, 122, 162, 164
   clinic in Heidelberg, 63, 70
   clinic in Munich, 24, 26-28, 65, 97
   lack of biography, 15
Kraepelinian classification, 28, 31
Kraepelinian school
   See Heidelberg school
Krasnick Warsh, Cheryl, 10
Kubie, Lawrence, 87-88

L

Lambert, Robert A., 114
Lane, William Arbuthnot ("Willy"), 72
Langley, Peg (Lewis), 262, 264
Lawrence, Bill, 234

Lawson, Lon, 288
learning disabilities, 294
Leggett, Doris, 318
Lett, Stephen, 78
leucotomy, 130-135, 208, 242
  patients, 177, 189, 190, 208, 267
LeVesconte, Helen Primrose, 110, 262-265
Levine, Helen, 241
Levinson, Toby, 223-225
Lewis, C.H., 205
Lewis, Edmund P., 100, 219, 221-223, 272
Lewis, Sir Aubrey, 88, 160
Lindenfield, Rita, 246
Line, William, 82, 228, 230-231, 287
lobotomy
  See leucotomy
London Asylum (Ontario), 78, 260
London Hospital (Ontario), 38
Lord Baltimore Press, 159
Lovett-Doust, John, 136, 138, 278-279, 286, 296
Lucas, C.C., 115
Lucas, Isaac, 49

M

Macdonald, Michael, 11
MacFarlane, John A., 122-124, 141
MacFie Campbell, Charles, 47, 54, 67
Mackey, Myrtle (MacArthur), 264, 266
Maclay, L.S., 124
MacPhee, Earle, 218, 222-223
Magnan, Valentin, 67
Maguire, Mayor, 52
Mallinson, Tom, 234, 245, 279, 285, 287-288
Maloney, Patrick, 21
manic-depressive illness, 9, 64, 83, 190
Markson, Elliot, 308, 312-313
Martin, Charles, 42
Marxist theory, 3-4, 6-7, 15
Masserman, Jules, 278
Mathers, Alvin, 155
McColluch, Warren, 287
McCullough, John, 35
McDairmid, Finlay, 49
McGhie, Bernard T., 108, 112-114, 131, 183, 198, 205-206
McKay, Marvin, 307
McKeen, Margaret, 308
McKenzie, Kenneth, 130, 132-133, 135
McKnight, Ken, 312-313
McLaughlin Travelling Fellowship, 281
McLean, William, 38-40
McLeod, Hugh, 226, 228, 232-233

McNeel, Burdett, 115, 134, 140, 288, 294, 317
McPherson, William, 48-50
McRuer Commission, 308-309
McRuer, J.C., 308
medicare, 289, 318
Meduna Joseph Ladislas von, 116
Melville, Phillip, 211, 130, 225-226
Menninger, William, 88, 160
"menstrual psychosis," 71, 83
Mental Health Grants
  See National Health Grants
mental health professions, 100, 240-242, 294
  gender issues, 190
  interaction among, 15, 231, 241-242, 267-268, 294, 311
Mental Hygiene Division, Ontario Department of Health
  See Department of Health (Ontario)
Mental Hygiene Division, Toronto, 100, 219
mental retardation
  See developmental disabilities
mental retardation clinic, 296-302
  and visiting professors, 298-299
  move to Surrey Place, 302
  research, 299-300
  services, 297-300
  See also Surrey Place Centre
Merskey, Harold, 10
Metcalf, William, 21
metrazol, 116-118
metrazol shock therapy, 116-117
Meyer, Adolf, 72, 74, 79-81, 181, 184-185, 197
  support for occupational therapy, 260, 265
Meynert, Theodor, 4
Micale, Mark, 12
Miles, Matthew, 285
milieu therapy, 129, 211-213, 267
Mill, John Stuart, 168
Miller, Abraham ("Abe"), 124, 127, 134-135, 275, 308
Milsom, Thelma, 282
Ministry of Health (Ontario), 139, 320
  Mental Health Branch, 140-142
  See also Department of Health (Ontario)
Mitchell, Eileen, 208, 210
Mitchell, Silas Weir, 69-70, 227
Mitchell, William, 173-174, 176, 180, 209
Möbius, Paul Julius, 9
Mohr, J.W. Hans, 312
Moniz, Egas, 130
Montgomery, Richard, 116, 126, 132

INDEX 327

More for the Mind, 288
Morin, Elizabeth (Locke), 242
Morrison, Mary, 296
Mott, Dr. (English pathologist), 27
Mott, Frederick, 65
Muller, Claire, 135
Multiple Chemical Sensitivities, 2
multiple-personality disorder, 10
Munns, Evangeline (Scraba), 234
Myers, Roger, 229-230

N

Napier, Sir Richard, 11
National Committee for Mental Hygiene (US), 106, 292
National Health Grants, 98, 126, 136, 241, 244, 319
National Society for the Promotion of Occupational Therapy, 260
National Training Laboratory, Bethel, Maine, 279, 288
Neiger, Stephen, 233-234, 285-286
Neiger, Trudy, 285-286
Nesbitt, Russell, 103
neurasthenia, 12
neurobiology, 14
neurohistology, 14, 63
neuroleptics, 2-3, 98, 275, 279
neuropathology, 14, 28, 64, 66
neuropsychiatry, 84, 275, 278
neuroses, 130, 191, 275, 284
neurosyphilis, 9, 63, 190
New Jersey state asylum, Trenton, 72, 74-75
New Toronto Hospital, 112-113, 133-134
Nightingale, Florence, 195
999 Queen Street West
  See Toronto Hospital—Queen Street Hospital
Nissl, Franz, 14, 65, 67, 162, 280
Nixon, Harry, 43, 51
Noble, Robert, 159
Northway, Mary Louise, 229
Noyes, Alfred P., 156-157
nurses, graduate, 196, 200
nursing at TPH, 197-214
  and closing of hospital, 212
  and nurse/patient relationship, 197, 208, 213
  directors of, 109, 194-195, 201, 203, 206, 209
  varying qualifications, 109, 201
nursing education, 193
  at TPH, 105, 187-188, 201-204, 206, 210, 213-214
  in general hospitals, 187, 196, 201
  in Ontario asylums, 31, 195

nursing qualifications, 194-195
nursing, psychiatric, 197-198
  history of, 195
  impact of new treatments, 207-208, 212
  lack of standardized regulations, 195-196
  qualifications, 193

O

obsessive-compulsive disorders, 275
occupational therapy at TPH, 198-199, 262-269
  activities, 264-267
  community outings, 266
  directors, 110, 262, 264
Occupational Therapy Society, 261
occupational therapy, psychiatric ("Psych OT"), 259-262
Ontario Association for the Mentally Retarded (OAMR), later Ontario Association for Community Living, 296-298, 300-302
Ontario asylums
  See Ontario Hospitals
Ontario Board of Examiners in Psychology, 228
Ontario Civil Service Association, 320
Ontario College of Physicians and Surgeons, 79
Ontario Department of Health
  See Department of Health (Ontario)
Ontario Health Survey (1952), 98
Ontario Hospital Association, 320
Ontario Hospital Schools, 298
Ontario Hospital Service, 122, 129, 139-141, 293
  and married nurses, 205
  low salaries, 107, 125, 199-200
  political interference, 107-111
  postgraduate course at TPH, 105, 107
Ontario Hospital, Toronto, 206
Ontario Hospitals, 28, 30-31, 97-100, 111, 115, 202, 239, 260, 262, 272, 319
  and occupational therapy, 262
  and shock therapies, 116-119
  and social work, 245
  expansion of, 125
  leucotomy program, 133-134
  name change from "asylums," 22-23, 37
Orillia, 272
outpatient services, 125
overcrowding in, 20, 38, 125, 132-134
psychology in, 218
shortage of personnel, 125, 204-206

Ontario Institute for Studies in Education (OISE), 229
Ontario Medical Association (OMA), 55
Ontario Medical Council, 78
Ontario Mental Health Survey (1937), 100
Ontario Mental Hospitals Act (1935), 305, 309
Ontario Nurses' Registration Act (1922), 196
Ontario Psychological Association, 228
organic psychoses, 138
organicism, 66, 83, 85, 138, 278
Orillia Hospital School, 300-301
Osler, Sir William, 27, 61, 64, 85, 161, 164
    and informal psychotherapy, 62-63
Otto, Bill, 234
outpatient department (OPD), 128, 271-290
    and waiting list crisis, 283, 285
    directors of, 272, 280, 292
    expansion of, 272, 274, 293
    group therapy, 278-279
    programs, 272
    psychiatric training programs, 127, 274, 277-280, 293
    referrals, 271, 273-274, 292, 294
    reminiscences, 276-280
    speech therapy, 286-287
    weekly psychosomatic conferences, 278
Owen, Trevor, 123
Ozarin, Lucy D., 168

P

packs, 199, 206, 242
Paitich, Daniel, 234, 308
paraldehyde, 242
Parkin, Alan, 136, 307-308
Parry-Jones, William, 10
Parsons, Sara May, 197
Paskauskas, Richard, 27, 29-30
patients
    anecdotes about, 188, 191-192, 266, 297
    subjective account of hospital experience, 171-177
patients' records
    at TPH, 178
    Farrar's at Sheppard, 69-72
    Farrar's at TPH, 118-119
Paton, Stewart, 63-64, 67-68, 74-75
Penetanguishene Hospital, Oak Ridge Division, 312
Penfield, Wilder, 261, 275
Penrose, Lionel, 131, 298

Pepleau, Hildegarde, 209
periodic catatonia, 137, 279, 283
Perretz, Edgar, 243-244
Phair, J. T., 123
Philadelphia Child Guidance Clinic, 293
Phipps, Henry, 36
physical therapies, vii, 14, 111-119, 130, 135, 206, 213
Pinel, Philippe, 5
Piotrowski, Zygmunt, 224
Pivnick, C., 128
play therapy, 294, 296
political interference, 19-21, 23, 36, 54, 107-111, 183
Pollock, Jack, 267
Ponoka Hospital for the Insane, Alberta, 203
Porter, Roy, 6, 10-11
Pos, Robert, 34, 89, 140
post-traumatic stress disorder, 177, 180
postgraduate medical students
    See psychiatric residents "PG"s
Pound, Ezra, 186
Price, Colonel, 54
Price, G.F.W., 51
Primrose, Alexander, 50, 53, 261
Proctor, Lorne, 118, 155
projective testing, 224, 228, 230
Provincial Lunatic Asylum (later Toronto Hospital), 20
psychiatric care in Canada
    changes in, 288, 290
psychiatric care in Ontario, 20-56, 97-98
    and new psychiatric institute (proposal), 138-142, 316
    changes in, 120-122, 128, 136, 142
    expansion, 125, 274
    federal funding, 126
Psychiatric Hospitals Act (1926), 101, 103
psychiatric illness, 273
    as "breakdown in living", 129
    changes in diagnosis and treatment, 190
    description and diagnosis, 14
    historical studies, 9-13
    influence of culture on, 8
    misdiagnosis, 174, 177, 179-181
    stigmatization of, 2, 12, 33, 243, 281
psychiatric residents ("PGS"), 241, 274-275, 293
    reminiscences of, 276-280
psychiatry
    changes in, 2-3, vi-vii, 283
    conflicting theories in, 70, 278, 280
    in general hospitals, 33-34, 97-98, 122, 127, 129, 140, 273-274, 288, 316

psychiatry *(continued)*
  military, 42, 76, 87, 120, 261, 264, 273, 293, 305
  relationship with social forces, vii-ix, 11-13
psychoactive drugs, 208
psychoanalysis, 82, 86, 89, 120, 127, 129, 136
  decline of, 3, 13
  historiography, 4, 13
  rise of, 86-89
  psychoanalytic theory, 278
psychodrama, 279
psychological testing, 178, 225, 219-230
  of hearing-impaired, 218, 224
psychological therapies, 129, 135, 188, 190
  "breakdowns in living," 130
psychology, 127, 129, 210
  professionalization of, 232
psychology, applied (later known as clinical psychology), 218-219, 222
  denigrated by academic psychologists, 224
  evolution into clinical psychology, 224, 228
  low status of, 220, 222, 224
psychology at TPH, 218-234
  and professional chauvinism, 219, 221-222, 232
  and training in psychology, 228
  eclecticism, 226-227, 233
  expansion, 224-225, 227
psychology, academic, 229
  impact of Second World War, 230
psychology, clinical, 218, 224
  education for, 229, 231
psychology, professionalization of, 228
psychometrics, 136, 218-219, 311
  applications, 220
  limitations of, 220-221, 223
psychoneuroses, 2, 10-13, 180
psychopharmacology, 135-136
  early resistance to, 2-3
psychoses, 129-130, 178, 190, 271, 281
psychosomatic illness, 85
psychosurgery, 130, 207
psychotherapy, 86, 127, 129, 136, 232, 276-277
  demand for training, 281
  group, 278-279
  increased demand for, 274, 283, 285
  training for family doctors, 288
Pyne, Robert A., 53

Q

Quarrington, Bruce, 225-227, 229, 231-234, 245, 293
Queen Street Hospital, Toronto (later Queen Street Mental Health Centre), 104, 121-122, 133, 135, 175, 212, 273, 275, 308, 316
Quirk, Douglas, 234

R

Ray, Mary, (Clark), 264
Read, Kathleen (Robb)
  See Robb, Kathleen
Reception Hospital Act (1914), 37-38, 41, 100, 101
reception hospitals, 22, 30
  introduced by Clarke, 31, 38
  legislative foundation, 37-38
reflex theory, 8, 71-72, 74, 78, 83
Richards, Barry W., 299
Richardson, Agnes, 76
Richardson, J. Clifford, 82, 275
Richardson, John C., 136
Riddell, Dorothy, 202
Rideau Regional Hospital, 301
Roazen, Paul, 13
Robb, Kathleen ("Kay") (Read), 110, 262, 266
Robbins, H.M., 101-103
Roberts Report (1963), 288-316
Roberts, Charles, 140, 232, 288, 313
Robinson, William, 305
Rockefeller Foundation grants, 43, 48, 106-107, 113-115, 119-120, 131, 136
Rockefeller, John D., 106
Rockwood (Asylum) Hospital, Kingston (later Kingston Hospital), 21, 23, 31-32, 38, 260, 263
Rogers, Joy, 212
Rooney, Thomas, 102-103
Rorschach test, 228, 285
Rorschach, Hermann, 286
Rosen, Edward ("Ted"), 128, 239, 242, 288, 296
Ross, T.A., 184
Rowsell, Peter, 283
Royal Canadian Army Medical Corps, 293, 305
Royal College of Physicians and Surgeons, 122
Royal Commission on Health Services (1966), 98
Rubin, Joseph, 233, 313
Rubinstein, Frank, 225-226
Russell, Elsie, 308

Russell, Kathleen, 202
Ryan, Edward, 23, 25-27, 34, 46, 51, 97, 104
　attack on Clarke, 31-32, 35

S

Sagert, Grace, 209
St. Michael's Hospital, 135
Sakel, Manfred Joshua, 111-112
Saltzman, Percy, 283
Santayana, George, 61
Sargant, William, 163
Schär, Markus, 9
schizophrenia, 2-3, 9, 64, 66, 83, 112, 115-116, 118, 120, 137-138, 179, 190
Schofield Gwynneth (Thompson), 262
Scott, Clifford, 34, 54
Scott, George, 306
Scott, John, 20
Scull, Andrew, 5, 9, 177
Scull-Hare debate, 9, 11
Seeley, John, 128, 284, 287
Senn, John, 133
sexual abuse, 179
sexual disorders, 164, 309
Sexual Information and Education Council of Canada (SIECAN), 286
sexual offenders, 306-307, 309, 311
shellshock, 13, 76
Shepherd, Michael, 10
Sheppard and Enoch Pratt Hospital, Baltimore, 63, 68-71, 74, 159
shock therapies, 111-119, 129, 135, 207
　erroneous theoretic basis, 116
Shortt, S.E.D., 10
Showalter, Elaine, 8, 179
Sicherman, Barbara, 12
Sidle, Nancy (Cornish), 268
Silverman, Harry, 228
Simmons, Harvey, 11
Skelton, Mora, 294, 299
Skinner, B.F., 287
Slemon, Al, 233-234, 294
Smith Kline and French, 3
Smith, Bruce, 35-36
Smith, Sidney, 87-88, 123
Smith-Rosenberg, Carroll, 12
social psychiatry
　See community psychiatry
social service exchange, 243
social work, 210, 239-244
　directors, 240, 243-244
Social Work Journal, 243
social work, psychiatric, 240
　education, 241-243
sociology, 127
sodium amytal, 179, 189

Southard, Elmer, 75
Spaulding, Harrison, 106
Spaulding, William, 138, 278
special education, 299
specialization, impact on nursing, 210-211
speech pathology, 136
"speech training," 272
Spielmeyer, Walter, 82
Spree, Reinhard, 7
Stanford-Binet Intelligence Test (IQ test), 220-221, 223
Stevenson, George H., 133
Stewart, Justice J.D., 306-307
Stewart, Marion E., 100
Stokes, Aldwyn, 14, 82, 88, 126-127, 129, 132-133, 136-138, 140-141, 224, 232-233, 245-246, 264, 275, 280, 284, 286, 293, 296, 306, 308, 318-319
　and biological research, 137-138
　and eclecticism, 14, 124, 127, 279
　and leucotomy, 132-133
　and mental-health education, 319
　and psychiatry in general hospitals, 127
　and research, 136-138
　and social work education, 241, 293
　interest in psychology, 136, 225-227
　support for occupational therapy, 264
Stokes, Margaret, 319
Stokes, Ron, 310-311, 313
straitjackets, 176
Stringer, Robert Melbourne, 108
Sullivan, Harry Stack, 157, 209
Sulloway, Frank, 13
Sunnybrook Veterans Hospital,
　psychiatric unit, 191, 276
Surrey Place Centre, 212, 299-300, 302, 320
Symposium on Mental Hygiene (1915), 35-36

T

Taylor, Euphemia ("Effie"), 193, 197
Teicher, Morton I. ("Mort"), 128, 136, 240-243, 293
Thematic Appercetion Test (TAT), 228
therapeutic community
　See milieu therapy
therapeutic milieu
　See milieu therapy
Thompson, Edward, 6
Thomson, Peter, 281, 308, 312
Tischler, G., 1
Tomes, Nancy, 10

Toronto asylum
    See Toronto Hospital—Queen Street
    Hospital
Toronto Board of Education Child
    Adjustment Service, 274
Toronto General Hospital (TGH), 28, 30,
    120, 126, 141
    and Committee on Psychological
        Medicine, 140
    and psychoneurology, 122
    connections with University of
        Toronto, 41, 121
    nervous diseases ward, 30, 33-34,
        50, 97
    psychiatric outpatient clinic, 43, 172
Toronto Hospital (later Queen Street
    Hospital/Mental Health Centre), 20-21,
    23, 31, 37-38, 41, 48, 260
    overcrowding in, 41, 51
    See also Queen Street Hospital,
        Toronto
Toronto Institute for Pastoral Training,
    313
Toronto Jail, 51
Toronto Medical Society, 285
Toronto Mental Health Clinic, 274
Toronto psychiatric clinic (proposed),
    24-25, 43
    delays, 29-30, 35
    objections to, 30, 32
    See also Toronto Psychiatric
        Hospital
Toronto Psychiatric Hospital (TPH),
    97-142
    accomplishments of, 319
    administration, 99-103, 122,
        140-142, 281, 320
    admissions, 101-103
    and community psychiatry, 129-130,
        211-212, 225-226
    and integration of psychiatry into
        medicine, 99, 126-127, 142
    and mental health education, 105
    and move to Clarke Institute, 232,
        289, 293, 314, 317-320
    and public pressure, 132
    annexed buildings, 226, 239, 265,
        273, 276, 292, 296
    as psychometric resource centre, 223
    as reception hospital, 99-103
    as research centre, 99, 105, 115-
        120, 131, 134-137, 319
    biological research, 137-138
    child psychiatry, 128, 239, 292-295
    children's clinic, 128, 225, 232, 272,
        293-297
    clinical psychology, 128

Toronto Psychiatric Hospital (TPH)
    (continued),
    community outreach, 128-129, 223,
        284-285
    day hospital, 267, 272
    directors, 59, 80, 82, 87-88,
        122-124, 140, 224, 232, 272, 293,
        313, 316, 318-319
    expansion, 100, 128-129, 293
    forensic clinic, 225, 232, 272,
        304-314
    forensic psychiatry, 128, 305, 307
    journal clubs, 279-280, 282
    leucotomy program, 130-134, 208,
        276
    limited facilities, 45, 111, 124-126,
        139
    mental retardation clinic, 296-302
    metabolic clinic and laboratory, 137
    name change from Psychopathic,
        183
    occupational therapy, 100, 188,
        259-269
    opening, 55
    origins of, 19, 24-55
    outpatient department (OPD), 100,
        128, 223, 225, 232, 239, 242,
        271-294, 307
    patient care, 188-189, 197-199
    PhD program, 105
    postgraduate courses, 105-107, 293
    psychiatric residents ("PGs"),
        129-239
    psychology services at, 100, 136
    psychology group, 225-228, 232-233
    reminiscences of patients, 172-177
    resemblance to Kraepelin's clinic, 51
    social work, 100, 128, 228, 239,
        276, 293
    social work, inpatient, 242
    sociology, 128
    speech pathology, 228
    speech therapy, 276
    staff disputes, 281-282
    staffing problems, 109-110
    student nurses' recollections,
        187-192, 203-204
    teaching forum, 282-283
    training programs, 82, 104-107,
        126-127, 319
    treatment, 129-130, 189, 199
    See also Toronto psychiatric clinic
        (proposed)
Toronto Psychoanalytical Study Circle,
    308

Toronto Reception Hospital, 38-41, 44-45, 48-53
and appointment of director, 46-48
and cornerstone laying ceremony, 52-53
and delegations meeting, 49
and planning committee, 51-52
See also Toronto Psychiatric Hospital
Torrey, Fuller, 9
Total Push project, Whitby Hospital, 245
Tuke, William, 5
"turf struggles," 30, 210-211, 222, 229
Turner, R. Edward, 305, 308, 311-313

U

uniforms, 211-212, 268
University of Toronto, 13, 24, 28-29, 41, 52, 80, 87, 121, 261
and establishment of TPH, 41, 43-48
and psychiatric residency program, 275-276
and new psychiatric institute (proposed), 140-142
and Reception Hospital, 44-45
and Rockefeller Foundation grants, 43, 115
Department of Medical Research, 113, 115
Department of Psychiatry, 28, 104-107, 124-125, 129, 139, 141, 241, 312, 318
and social work, 241
expanded training program, 126-127, 288, 298, 319
forensic psychiatry program, 306
Department of Psychology
and antipathy to clinical psychology, 229-230, 231
postwar programs, 230, 231
Extension Department, 313
Faculty of Medicine, 43, 54, 312
health service, 276
occupational therapy course, 262-264
psychology programs, 218, 224-225, 228-231
School of Hygiene, 318
School of Nursing, 202, 206, 209-210
School of Social Work, 241, 243, 293, 313
speech pathology course, 313
war aides program, 262
University-Provincial Drug Research Committee, 135

Utica State Hospital, 156-158

V

Van Wagenen, Dr., 130
Veith, Ilza, 4
Vincent, George E., 106
volunteers, 320

W

Walters, Allan, 275
Watson, Gordon, 307
Watts, James, 130
Wayne State Hospital, compared to TPH, 226-227
Welch, William, 61, 64
Wellesley Hospital, 127,
psychiatric unit, 126, 275
Wernicke, Carl, 65
Wessely, Simon, 12
Whitby Hospital, 20, 24, 37, 41, 48, 116, 135, 174, 177, 202, 214, 244, 288
Pavilion 2B, 245
White Cross Guild, 320
White, Owen, 226, 234
White, William Allanson, 69
Whitney, J.P., 23
Wideman, Harley, 225-227, 229, 232
Williams, Lorraine, 308, 310
Willoughby Commission, 25-27, 32, 35
Willoughby, W.A., 26, 32, 97
Wilshire, Bernice ("Bunnie"), 223, 272
Wilson, Jean, 209
Women's College Hospital, 187
Workman, Joseph, 21, 260
Wortis, Joseph, 117
Wright, Mary, 222
Wundt, Wilhelm, 14

Y

Yale University, School of Nursing, 194
York, Lydia (Senyshyn), 233
Young, George, 80

Z

Zilboorg, Gregory, 4